Management of Head and Neck Vascular Lesions

Sanjiv C. Nair • Srinivasa R. Chandra
Editors

Management of Head and Neck Vascular Lesions

A Guide for Surgeons

Springer

Editors
Sanjiv C. Nair
Department of Maxillofacial Surgery
B.M. Jain Hospital
Bangalore Institute of Dental Science
Bangalore, Karnataka, India

Srinivasa R. Chandra
Oral & Maxillofacial- Head & Neck
Oncology Reconstructive Surgery
Oregon Health & Science
University Portland
Portland, OR, USA

ISBN 978-981-15-2320-5 ISBN 978-981-15-2321-2 (eBook)
https://doi.org/10.1007/978-981-15-2321-2

This Springer imprint is published by the registered company Springer Nature Singapore Pte Ltd.
The registered company address is: 152 Beach Road, #21-01/04 Gateway East, Singapore 189721, Singapore

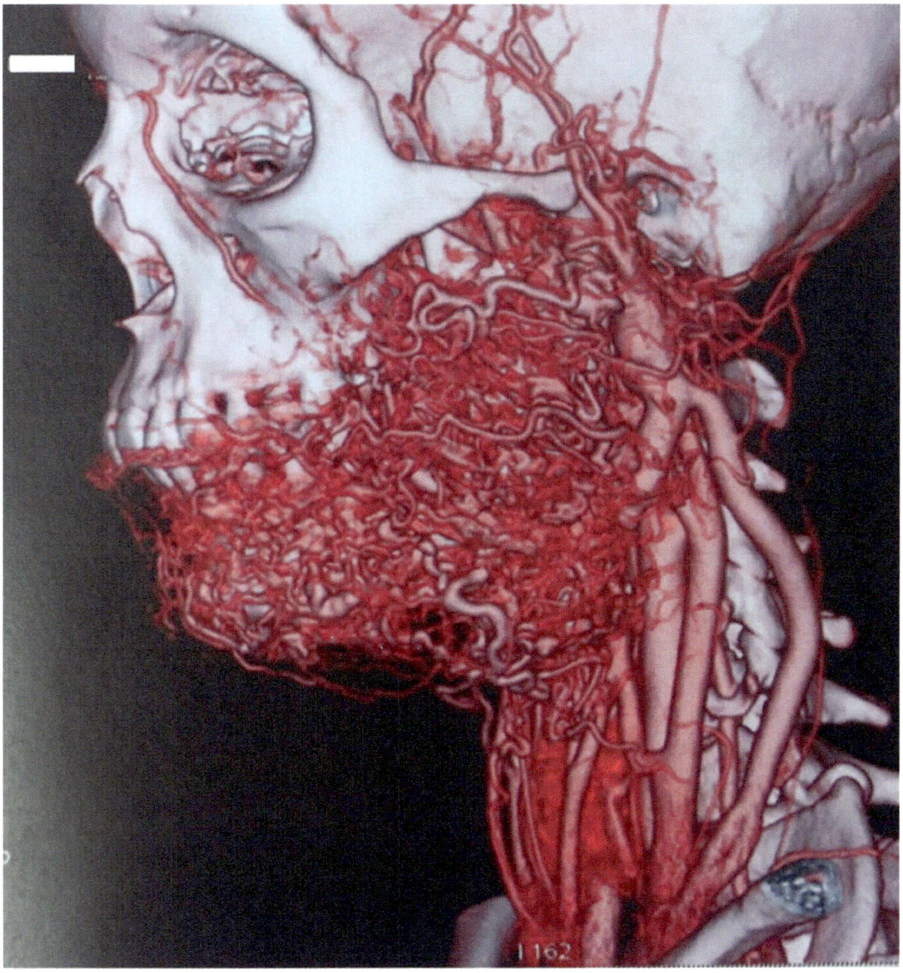
I 162

Patient's Testimony

If you're reading this, chances are good that you're knowledgeable on vascular lesions and their different forms. Maybe this is because you're a surgeon, or studying to be a surgeon, or maybe just because you're highly interested in or invested in the subject. Whatever the reason is, I'm going to assume that your knowledge on the subject is already superior to mine, so I'm not going to attempt to use medical jargon or to pretend that my understanding of vascular lesions is greater than it actually is. Instead, I'm going to give you something that I'm more familiar with, the perspective of a patient.

Let me introduce myself. My name is Marissa, I'm 23 years old, and I've been a patient of the vascular lesions medical field more times than I can count on my two hands. I was diagnosed with microcystic lymphangioma of the tongue when I was about 2 years old. Since then I've undergone sclerotherapy, multiple reduction surgeries, laser ablations, and bleomycin injections. These procedures have taken place in the United States spanning from West Coast to East Coast, providing me the good fortune to meet and be helped by a collection of surgeons and their staff. I was asked to write this foreword to help elucidate the thoughts of a patient by taking into account my myriad interactions with doctors. As a patient, I've had good doctors and I've had great doctors, the following discussion outlines some actions that I believe sets the two apart.

Be Personable It's a common stereotype that doctors are too impersonal, too clinical. With the sheer number of patients a doctor sees in a day it seems like this would be an easy persona to adopt, but for a patient that one interaction with the doctor is likely all that they have. An introduction, asking the patient their name, and offering a handshake all go a long way in the initial establishment of the doctor–patient relationship. Because, as patients we want to be helped by our doctor, but on a more basic human level we also want a relationship with our doctor. We want to trust our doctor, to feel that they care about us not only as a patient but also as a regular person. The initial meeting between doctor and patient is important, but the continuation and development of that relationship is what really builds the connection. Some key elements of this include remembering the patient's preferred name, asking about their life outside the medical sphere, and checking-in at the patient's bedside after a procedure.

Engage with the Patient This is a clear derivative of being personable, but I believe it is important enough to warrant its own explanation. Doctors interact with patients every day, providing vital input and information to their patients. Just like any human interaction, there are more effective and less effective ways of interacting and communicating with patients. The more effective methods serve to strengthen the doctor–patient relationship through increased trust and sense of connection on the patient's side, which can be gained multiple ways.

Provide the Patient with Undivided Attention No interruptions from phones, no typing on the computer, just listening to the patient's questions, concerns, and thoughts on their medical situation. Facing the patient, making eye contact, and giving non-verbal listening cues, like a nod of the head, are great indicators to a patient that they're being listened to and that is what they're saying matters.

Have a Clear, Open Dialogue Rather than talking at a patient, talk with them. Give them explanations and answers that are as easy as possible to understand, pose questions to them and ask for questions in return. As a former patient, I know that the easiest, most comfortable interactions with doctors are the ones that feel like a conversation, not a lecture or an interrogation.

Dont Rush Out of The door As patients, we realize that doctors are incredibly busy, but it feels quite impersonal to have a few hurried minutes of a doctor's time before they rush off to the next patient. It will most often have the effect of making a patient feel frustrated and insignificant. So, please, let the conversation and questions take place at a reasonable pace before exiting stage left.

Although these actions I discussed may seem basic, I know from personal experience that they make a world of difference in the dynamics of the doctor–patient relationship. All the doctors that have helped me were respectable and skilled in their own right, but not all of them displayed these actions. The one doctor who displayed these actions, who remembered my name, who asked about my daily life and family, who made themselves unfailingly available and open for questions and concerns, that doctor is the one who stands head and shoulders above the rest. From a doctor's perspective, it must be easy to recognize that patients need medical counsel, they need prescriptions, and they need procedures, but I believe that it's the great doctors who also recognize that patients want to be cared for by someone who cares.

—C. Marissa Shields

Acknowledgments

As the science of vascular anomalies evolves, it is for us, clinicians to propose management with the understanding that no science is perfect. We have seen the dilemma that exists between the two, it needs a good clinician and a compliant patient to go ahead with treatment of an anomaly that one has no control over. It is not life-threatening, not cancer but is disfiguring. So, we try to present an effort at some unique surgical techniques and the science for better therapies for vascular lesions.

Our efforts are to ameliorate the suffering.

We would acknowledge the contribution of our colleagues in this effort

Dr Praveen Kumar Pampapati Choudri, MBBS, MDRD, DNBRD

Dr. Advaith Nair MBBS

Dr. Robert Woodwards MD FDS FRCS

Dr. Kishore Nayak FDSRCS FDSRCI

Dr. Basavaraj Ghodke MD

Dr. Rui Fernandes MD DMD FRCS

Contents

List of Contributors

Jack Burt Department of Radiology, University of Nebraska Medical Center, Omaha, NE, USA

Srinivasa R. Chandra Oral & Maxillofacial- Head & Neck Oncology Reconstructive Surgery, Oregon Health & Science University Portland, Portland, OR, USA

Amelia Christabel Rajasekaran UIH Chicago, Chicago, IL, USA

Steven Curry Department of Otolaryngology, University of Nebraska Medical Center, Omaha, NE, USA

Madanagopalan Ethunandan Department of Oral and Maxillofacial Surgery, University Hospital Southampton, Southampton, UK

Basavaraj Ghodke Department of Neuroradiology and Neurosurgery, University of Washington, Seattle, WA, USA

Subramania Iyer Department of Plastic and Reconstructive Surgery, Head and Neck Surgery, Amrita School of Medicine, Kochi, India

Balasubramanya Kumar Department of Maxillofacial Surgery, B.M. Jain Hospital, Bangalore Institute of Dental Science, Bangalore, Karnataka, India

Jagadeesh Kumar Elkton Dermatology, Elkton, MD, USA

Victoria A. Manon Katz Department of Oral & Maxillofacial Surgery, The University of Texas at Houston, University of Texas Health Science Center at Houston, Houston, TX, USA

James C. Melville Katz Department of Oral & Maxillofacial Surgery, The University of Texas at Houston, University of Texas Health Science Center at Houston, Houston, TX, USA

Oral, Head, and Neck Oncologic and Microvascular Reconstructive Surgery, Katz Department of Oral & Maxillofacial Surgery, The University of Texas at Houston, University of Texas Health Science Center at Houston, Houston, TX, USA

Sanjiv C. Nair Department of Maxillofacial Surgery, B.M. Jain Hospital, Bangalore Institute of Dental Science, Bangalore, Karnataka, India

Janarthanan Ramu Department of Plastic and Reconstructive Surgery, Amrita School of Medicine, Kochi, India

Jose Rodriguez-Vasquez Department of Radiology, University of Nebraska Medical Center, Omaha, NE, USA

Sunil Shroff Department of Oral and Maxillofacial Surgery, Bhagwan Mahaveer Jain Hospital, Bengaluru, India

Huy Q. Tran Katz Department of Oral & Maxillofacial Surgery, The University of Texas at Houston, University of Texas Health Science Center at Houston, Houston, TX, USA

Simon Young Katz Department of Oral & Maxillofacial Surgery, The University of Texas at Houston, University of Texas Health Science Center at Houston, Houston, TX, USA

Lei Yu Radiology, University of Nebraska Medical Center, Omaha, NE, USA

History, Terminology, and Classifications of Vascular Anomalies

1

Srinivasa R. Chandra and Sanjiv C. Nair

1.1 Introduction

The objective of this chapter is to present a ready reckoner for the understanding of the history, incidence and a review of all noted classifications. This may provide a comprehensive understanding of this group of vascular-related entities.

Majority of the vascular anomalies are seen in the head and neck region. Even though the incidence of this anomaly could be construed as a rare disease entity, with only 5% of overall affliction, the lack of knowledgeable management has disfigured many. A comprehensive understanding of this benign yet complex life-changing entity is essential. A historical perspective, pathophysiological evolution, and the current knowledge of management modalities are essential for rendering clinical care in this subspecialty care.

The core points to consider in vascular lesions management -

1. Majority are benign entities and not "cancers." The high-flow vascular malformations can be treated effectively too.
2. Lesion eradication should not be a piecemeal methodology.
3. There is no one treatment modality that would fit every vascular anomaly.
4. Biopsy of the lesions may not be necessary; malformations are more common. Biopsy only if you understand the malignant behavior.
5. Vascular anomalies have a" dynamic lifecycle."
6. Between vascular tumors and malformations- tumors are more common, but you may encounter "malformation" more often as they persist and need varied care.
7. Vascular anomalies are a "group" of different entities of varied etiopathological which may not share the same treatment approaches. The grouping is for logistical convenience.
8. Airway has to be a consideration in managing head and neck anomalies, especially with syndromes and segmental presentations.
9. No single susceptible population group has been identified.
10. Patients usually present with multiple earlier investigations and interventions.
11. That is a great potential for molecular and genetic research in this field-so consented patients could save tissue samples for laboratories discovering targeted therapies.

S. R. Chandra (✉)
Oral & Maxillofacial- Head & Neck Oncology Reconstructive Surgery, Oregon Health & Science University Portland, Portland, OR, USA
e-mail: chandrsr@ohsu.edu

S. C. Nair
Department of Maxillofacial Surgery, B.M. Jain Hospital, Bangalore Institute of Dental Science, Bangalore, Karnataka, India

S. C. Nair, S. R. Chandra (eds.), *Management of Head and Neck Vascular Lesions*,
https://doi.org/10.1007/978-981-15-2321-2_1

1.2 History

The first scientifically documented "surgery under an ether anesthetic agent" by Morton in 1846 done in Boston, Massachusetts USA, was for excision of a "low flow" vascular malformation. Rudolph Virchow, in 1863 first categorized vascular anomalies by microscopic architectural patterns. From earlier use words "Port wine stain," "Angiomas," etc. Virchow's attempted an acceptable Cellular classification as angioma simplex, angioma cavernosum and angioma racemosum. His trainee Wagner further studied lymphatic malformations and contributed to the understanding of their challenging clinical management. The further biological classification was proposed in 1982 by Mulliken and Glowacki [1]. The international collaborative group ISSVA-International Society for the Study of Vascular Anomalies is a way forward to advance constant review of the current and updated science in this field. In this rapidly changing understanding of the molecular basis of disease, we may need a constant redefinition of our comprehension and learning.

Classifications for vascular lesions are complex. It serves as a means of communication between the clinicians. Today, the ISSVA is an umbrella association for the classification of vascular lesions. At the broadest level, the ISSVA classifies vascular lesions as Vascular Tumors and Vascular Malformations (Table 1.1) [2]. Vascular malformations are structural abnormality that is always present at birth but may not become apparent until later in life [3]. They include capillary (arteriole and venule), venous, arteriovenous, lymphatic, and a combination of these vessels. Vascular tumors have increased mitotic activity and will appear soon after birth, with approximately 30% already apparent at the time of birth [1, 3]. Vascular tumors are divided by the ISSVA as benign, locally aggressive or borderline, and malignant. Benign tumors include hemangiomas. Locally aggressive or borderline tumors include Kaposi Sarcoma and hemangioendothelioma. Malignant tumors include angiosarcomas and epithelioid hemangioendothelioma. Intraosseous vascular lesions have not been classified by the ISSVA. Table 1.1 is a summary of individual authors who proposed vascular anomaly

Table 1.1 Various classifications of vascular anomalies

Year	Author	Basis of classification
1863	Virchow RLK	Microscopic channel architecture
1877	Wegener	Histomorphic subclassification of Virchow's classification
1973	Degni and coworkers	Site of origin of the detect
1974	Malan	Embryologic site of origin of the defect
1982	Mulliken JB and Glowacki J	Endothelial characters
1983	Burrows and colleagues	Angiographic flow patterns
1988	International Society for the Study of Vascular Anomalies (ISSVA), Hamburg	Anatomopathologic classification of vascular defects (Hamburg classification)
1989	Belov	Etiologic and pathophysiologic classification system
1992	ISSVA, Colorado	Cellular features, vascular flow characteristics, and clinical behavior
1993	Jackson and associates	Flow rate
1996	ISSVA, Rome	Modified ISSVA classification
2011	S C Nair	Anatomical presentation
2014	ISSVA, Melbourne	Modified ISSVA classification

classification and the basis of their effort to differentiate various presentations.

Head and Neck Vascular anomalies can cause significant morbidity. There are various misguided attempts to treat with the "one size fits all" approaches. Chemotherapy, Interferons, chemical agents with no long-term outcome reviews have disfigured many an individual seeking care.

We have attempted to give you a list of classifications more for a perspective and the efforts which have gone to well-intentioned methods to care in Table 1.1 above.

The international Society proposed its fast classification in 1988 in Hamburg. In multiple meetings have happened in Hamburg, Germany, Colorado, USA, and Rome, Italy etc. an ongoing. Occasionally the names of the meetings have been associated with the classifications (Hamburg classification). Multiple societies like the oculoplastic association have its own classification of vascular anomalies of the orbit.

1.3 Incidence

The overall incidence of vascular lesions is around 5% [4]. Among tumors, infantile hemangiomas have the same percentage of incidence. Among vascular lesions, venous malformations are commonly similar to lymphatic malformations with an incidence of 1: 5000 to 1:10000. More than 50% of them are present in the head and neck anatomical area.

1.4 Terminology and Classifications

Terminology of Vascular lesions evolved from descriptive to the more scientific basis for nomenclature, the former possibly arising from maternal explanations of the lesions. It posted 1982 after Mulliken and Glowacki et al. [1] attributed biologic differences within the lesion that they were described as separate entities. A neoplastic Hemangioma was found to be distinctly different from the developmental VM.

1.4.1 Historical Terminology on Appearances

Descriptive terms and historical nosology of vascular anomalies offers an array of overlapping descriptive and histopathologic terms (Figs. 1.1, 1.2, and 1.3)

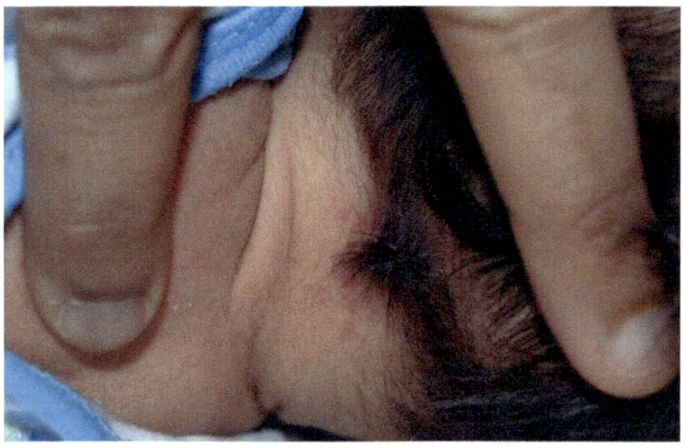

Fig. 1.1 Superficial vascular lesion was seen on the neck of infant. Historically was also referred to as "stork bite"

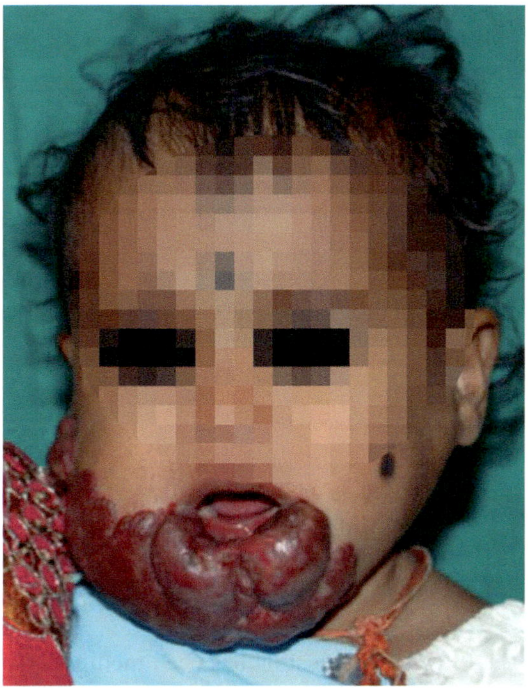

Fig. 1.2 Capillary malformation of lower lip, chin, and right cheek

- Port wine, as illustrated below it can be used for "capillary hemangiomas" historically. It can be as small and superficial.

1.4.2 Histopathologic Terms Used Historically

- Capillary
- Cavernous
- Arterial
- Mixed

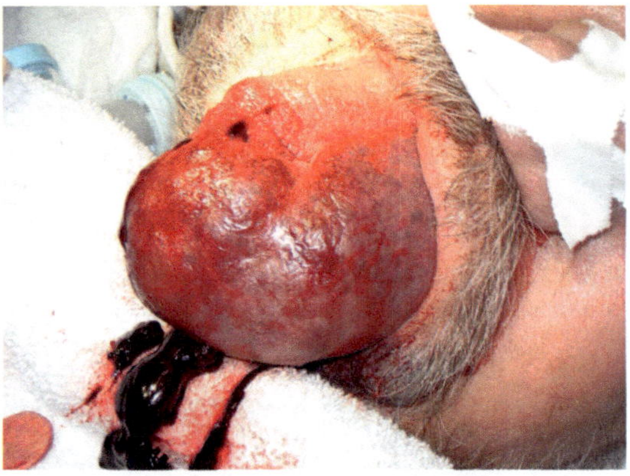

Fig. 1.3 Strawberry lesion or a "capillary-cavernous hemangioma" was commonly used for lesions like present on the tongue as illustrated in Fig. 1.3. Such terminology added to the confusion as shown in the tongue vascular lesion, which is a low flow vascular lesion, with sequela of trauma

Biologic behaviour-based terminology [1]—This is the current ISSVA terminology simplified and widely accepted. The classification is elaborated below.
Vascular Tumors
Vascular malformations

1.5 Mulliken and Glowacki's Biological Classification (1982)

The ISSVA classification has been modified and based on the biologic classification by Mulliken and Glowacki [1] and further with the mutational knowledge.

Hemangiomas

- Proliferating phase.
- Involuting phase.

Malformations

- Capillary
- Venous
- Arterial
- Lymphatic
- Fistulas

- Hemangioma (Fig. 1.4)

1.6 Vascular Malformations (Figs. 1.5 and 1.6)

1.6.1 Classifications

Here we have listed all relevant classifications espoused by various groups. Each has their merits. The current International Society for the study of Vascular Anomalies classification system. There have been various editions over the years.

Here is a link to the entire extensive classification

- https://www.issva.org/classification
- https://www.issva.org/UserFiles/file/ISSVA-Classification-2018.pdf

International Society for the study of Vascular Anomalies classification system (ISSVA, last revision May 2018)
Vascular tumors
Benign
Locally aggressive or borderline
Malignant
Vascular malformations
Simple
Capillary malformations
Lymphatic malformations
Venous malformations
Arteriovenous malformations
Arteriovenous fistula
Combined (2 or more VMs in one lesion)
CVM, CLM, LVM, CLVM, CAVM, CLAVM, others

(C-capillary, V-venous, L-lymphatic, AV-arteriovenous)
Anomalies of major named vessels
Vascular malformations associated with other anomalies

Based on the anatomic location, Hemangiomas were described by Waner and Suen [3] **as:**

Classification by Waner and Suen:
• Superficial hemangioma
• Deep hemangioma
• Combined hemangioma

M.Ethunandan et al., [5] **bjoms 44(2006) described a flow chart that correlated the various clinical signs, which helped differentiate a Vascular malformation from a Hemangioma.**

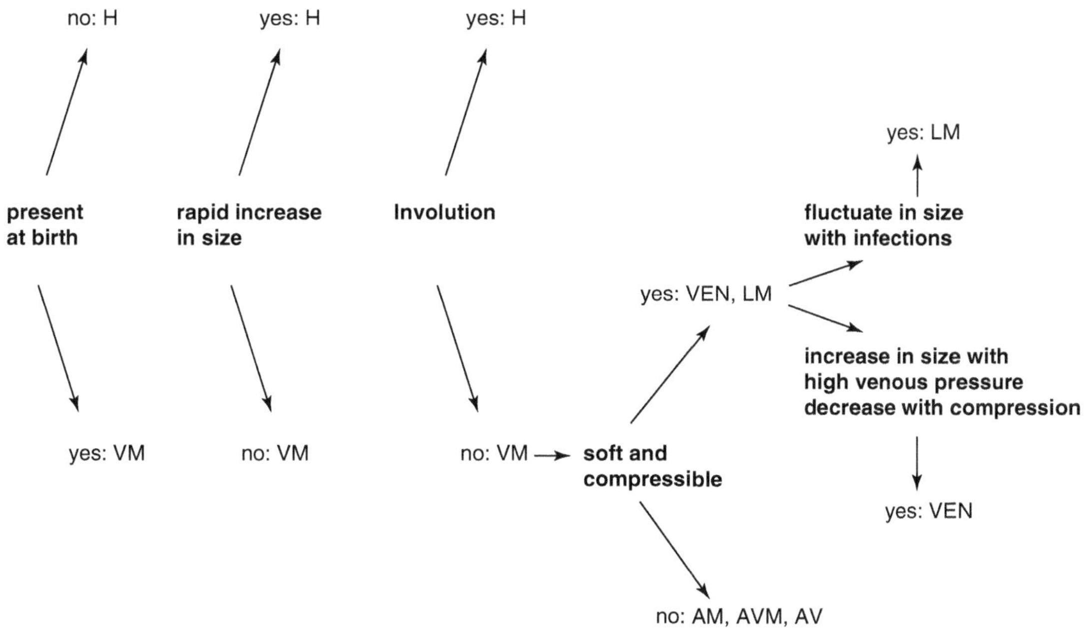

H **hemangioma;** ***VM*** **vascular malformation;** ***VEN*** **venous malformation;** ***LM*** **lymphatic malformation;** ***AM*** **arterial malformation;** ***AVM*** **arteriovenous malformation;** ***AV*** **AV-fistula.**

Further advances in the understanding of the vascular dynamics allowed changes in the classification, and this was first proposed by Ian Jackson et al., allowing major breakthroughs in treatment planning and management of vascular lesions.

Box 1 Classification of vascular anomalies by vascular dynamics according to Jackson

I.	Hemangiomas
II.	Vascular malformations
	(a) Low-flow (VM)
	(b) High-flow (AVM)
III.	LMs

From Jackson IT, Carreno R, Potparic Z, et al. Hemangiomas, vascular malformations, and lympho-venous malformations: classification and methods of treatment. Plast Reconstr Surg 1993;91:1217

1.7 CNS and Non-CNS List of Vascular Lesions

Central nervous system vascular malformations are rare abnormalities of blood vessels in your brain or spinal cord and their membranes. They distinctly differ in their appearance and management. A classification differentiating the CNS VM from its non-CNS variant is presented.

Table I Classification of CNS vascular malformations

Arteriovenous shunts
Classical AV Malformations
Pial AV fistulas
Dural AV shunts
Galenic shunts
Cavernous malformations
Capillary telangiectasias
Venous malformations
Developmental venous
Anomalies
Mixed malformations

Table II Classification of non-CNS vascular malformations

Haemangiomas (proliferative lesions or tumours)
Vascular malformations (non-proliferative)
High flow
• Arteriovenous malformations
Low flow:
• Capillary malformations
• Venous malformations
• Lymphatic malformations
• Mixed malformations

The severity of Artery venous malformation was scored by Schobinger into four stages based on their clinical appearance and behavior. From lesions exhibiting minimal symptoms to the severe malformations that resulted in hi-output cardiac failure consequent to the decompensatory phenomenon. Priority in therapeutic management decisions evolved.

1.8 Schobinger Classification

Schobinger clinical staging system of arteriovenous malformations

Stage I	Quiescence	Cutaneous blush, skin warmth, arteriovenous shunt on Doppler ultrasound
Stage II	Expansion	Darkening blush, lesion shows pulsation, thrill and bruit
Stage III	Destruction	Steal, distal ischemia, pain, dystrophic skin changes, ulceration, necrosis, soft tissue and bony changes
Stage IV	Decompensation	High-output cardiac failure

Based on Eighth Meeting of the International Workshop on Vascular Malformations. Amsterdam, Netherlands, 1990

Adapted from Kohout MP, Hansen M, Pribaz JJ, et al. Arteriovenous malformations of the head and neck: natural history and management. Plast Reconstr Surg 1998;102:643–54

1.8.1 Jackson's Classification

IAN JACKSON IN 1992 further expanded on the earlier classification. Based on this, Hemangiomas were described on their location and VM on the dynamics of blood flow.

Hemangiomas
Superficial (capillary hemangioma) (Fig. 1.2)
Deep (cavernous hemangioma)
Compound (capillary-cavernous hemangioma)
Vascular malformations
Simple lesions
Low flow lesions
Capillary malformations (capillary hemangioma, port wine stain)
Venous malformation (cavernous hemangioma)
Lymphatic malformation (lymphangioma, cystic hygroma)
High-flow lesions
Arterial malformation
Combined lesions
Arteriovenous malformations
Lymph venous malformations (Fig. 1.6)
Other combinations

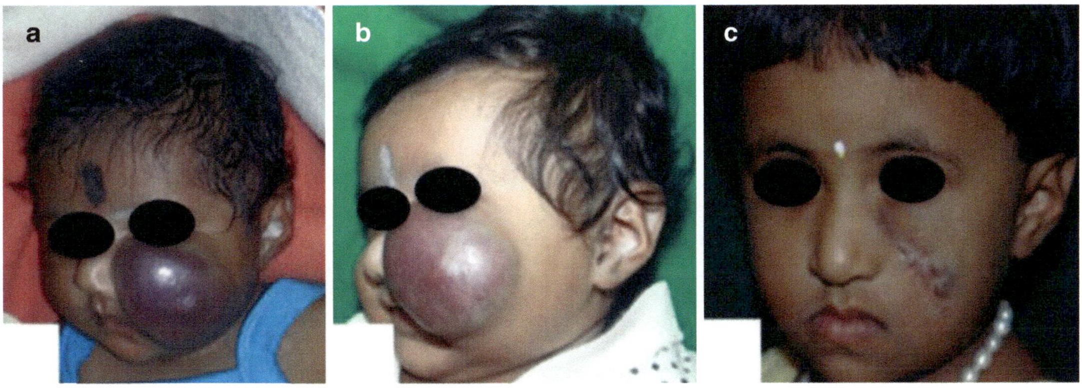

Fig. 1.4 Non-involuting congenital Hemangioma (NICH) of the left cheek ((**a**) initial therapy with propranolol 10 days post-birth, (**b**) 6 months following propranolol therapy, (**c**) excision of lesion at 2 years age)

1.8.2 Surgical Management Based Classification for Head and Neck Lesions

More recently Sanjiv Nair et al. [4] classified both Hemangiomas and VM based on their anatomic location. This helped understand the depth of the lesion and allowed a surgical treatment plan .The classification has been effectively used in the surgical ablation of the lesions, as will be described in Chap. 7.

Type I	Mucosal/cutaneous
Type II	Subcutaneous/juxta muscular
Type III	Glandular
Type IV	Skeletal (intra bony)
Type V	Deep visceral (temporal, infra temporal, parapharyngeal)

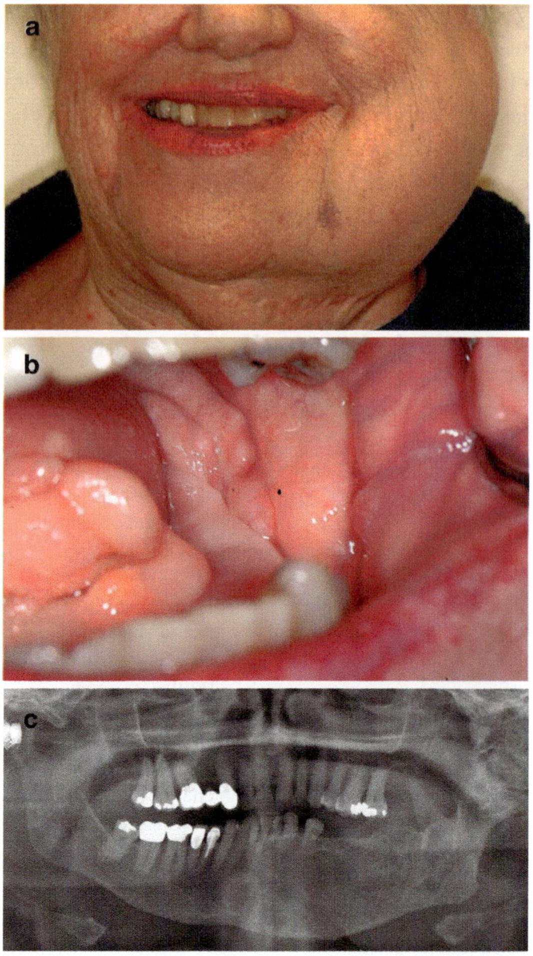

Fig. 1.5 Left facial low flow lymphovenous malformation of an intraosseous type of the left lower facial skeleton. (**a**) Noted left lower facial asymmetry with no superficial vessels. (**b**) Mucosal area of the intraoral picture with tissue expansion and no surface ulceration or superficial vessels. (**c**) Left mandibular and condylar hypertrophy of the skeleton involved. Courtesy: O Ross Bernie DDS PhD

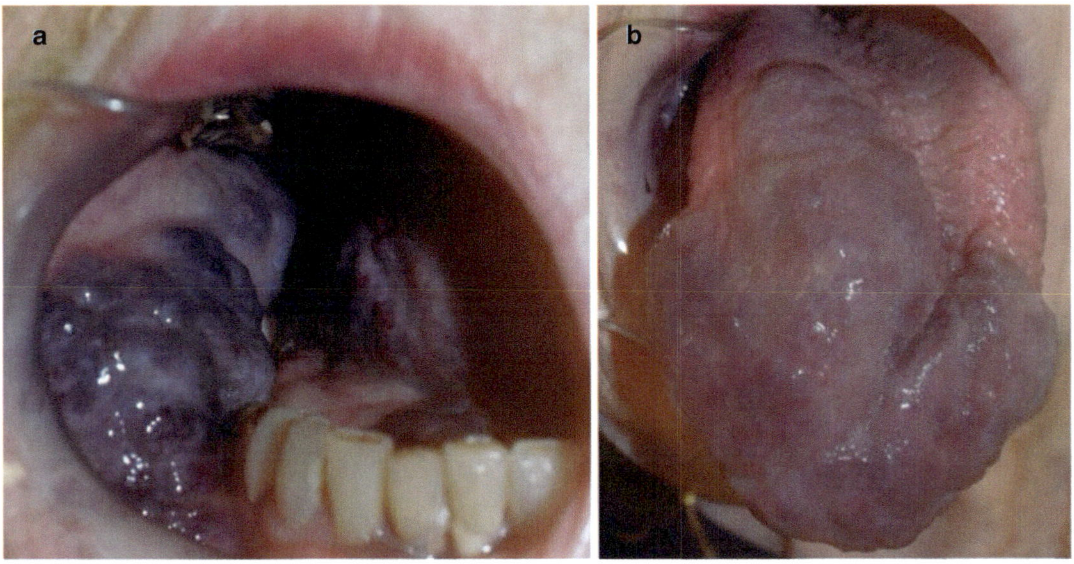

Fig. 1.6 The appearance is easy to be remarked as "berry" or "purple" which caused the historic confusion in nomenclature (**a**) Notice extensive dark purple lesions of right buccal mucosa extending to tongue and floor of the mouth. (**b**) Shows extensive growth and discoloration of anterior ventral tongue

1.9 Conclusion

The evolution of various classification has been based on the increased understanding of both clinical and biologic behavior of VA. Earlier confusion in terminology has been largely dispelled with a better understanding of the clinical features aided by advances in imaging techniques.

Vascular lesions have a varied clinical and radiographical presentations. A surgical plan and approach based on Nair's Clinical Classifications and imaging data can minimize complications. The radiologist, pathologist, and surgeon must consider clinical, radiographic, and histological data. A classification system for intraosseous vascular lesions needs to be established and is a work in progress.

References

1. Mulliken JB, Glowacki J. Hemangiomas and vascular malformations in infants and children: a classification based on endothelial characteristics. P Reconstr Surg. 1982;69(3):412–22.
2. Wassef M, Borsik M, Cerceau P, Faucon B, Laurian C, Le Clerc N, Lemarchand-Venencie F, Massoni C, Salvan D, Bisdorff-Bresson A. Classification des tumeurs et malformations vasculaires. Apport de la classification ISSVA 2014/2018 [Classification of vascular tumours and vascular malformations. Contribution of the ISSVA 2014/2018 classification]. Ann Pathol. 2021;41(1):58–70. French. https://doi.org/10.1016/j.annpat.2020.11.004. Epub 2020 Dec 10. PMID: 33309330.
3. Waner M, Suen JY. Hemangiomas and vascular malformations of the head and neck. New York: Wiley-Liss; 1999.
4. Nair SC. Vascular anomalies of the head and neck region. J Maxillofac Oral Surg. 2018;17:1–12. https://doi.org/10.1007/s12663-017-1063-2.
5. Ethunandan M, Mellor TK. Hemangiomas and vascular malformations of the maxillofacial region – review. Br J Maxillofac Surg. 2006;44:263–72.

Pathogenesis, Genetics, and Molecular Developments in Vascular Lesion Therapy and Diagnosis

2

Srinivasa R. Chandra, Balasubramanya Kumar, Sunil Shroff, and Sanjiv C. Nair

Key Points

- Genomic research, Next-generation sequencing, and disease-specific therapeutic options to treat vascular lesions are the future due to genetic testing. Exploring genetic mutations of inherited or somatic types has opened up an understanding of the underlying molecular mechanisms.
- RAS/MAPK/ERK altered signaling due to mutations in GNAQ and GNA11 in congenital hemangiomas and capillary malformation (CM), in GNAQ, KRAS and BRAF in pyogenic granuloma (PG), in RASA1 in CM-AVM1, in EPHB4 in CM-AVM2, in KRIT1 in HCCVM, and MAP3K3 in verrucous venous malformations have established for the therapeutics.
- PI3K/AKT/mTOR pathway regulation alterations in hereditary hemorrhagic telangiectasia (HHT) are noted with mutations in BMP9/10, ALK1, and endoglin, in sporadic venous malformations (VM and MVM). Blue rubber bleb nevus syndrome (BRBN), inherited cutaneous-mucosal venous malformations (VMCM), all with mutations in TIE2, and in sporadic VM and lymphatic malformations (LM) with mutations in PIK3CA.
- Glomuvenous malformations (GVM)-have mutations in glomulin with a hyperactive hepatocyte growth factor/c-Met and TGF-ß is signaling.
- Infantile hemangioma (IH)- VEGFR1 expression is downregulated; VEGF-A/VEGFR2 signaling is upregulated, with mutations in TEM8 and VEGFR2.
- Acquired vascular lesions—paraganglioma of neural crest origin—APUD—DNES cells—cells—located in extra-adrenal locations like the carotid, vagus, orbit, tympanic, larynx, jugular, thyroid, nasal cavity, aortic arch, intracranial, etc. that are mostly benign.

S. R. Chandra (✉)
Oral & Maxillofacial- Head & Neck Oncology Reconstructive Surgery, Oregon Health & Science University Portland, Portland, OR, USA
e-mail: chandrsr@ohsu.edu

B. Kumar · S. C. Nair
Department of Maxillofacial Surgery, B.M. Jain Hospital, Bangalore Institute of Dental Science, Bangalore, Karnataka, India

S. Shroff
Department of Oral and Maxillofacial Surgery, Bhagwan Mahaveer Jain Hospital, Bengaluru, India

S. C. Nair, S. R. Chandra (eds.), *Management of Head and Neck Vascular Lesions*,
https://doi.org/10.1007/978-981-15-2321-2_2

2.1 Introduction

Vascular lesions have been better understood recently with pathogenesis, mutational, and immune-expression with advances in immunohistology-chemical staining as well as genetics and mutational defects.

2.2 Pathogenesis

Blood vessels form consolidated aberrations in limited anatomic sites of the human body. They result in sporadic anomalies or hereditary occurrences. The classification helps differentiate the anomalies based on their morphology, histology, and dynamics of blood flow. The primary differentiating features divide these lesions into Vascular neoplasms and vascular malformations.

Histologically the vascular lumen is lined with young endothelial cells (Fig. 2.1). These are underlined by smooth muscle cells and pericytes that are more seen in a vascular network than lymphatic channels [1].

The formation of the blood vessel network begins with vasculogenesis. Hemangioblasts are the precursor cells forming an island of endothelial cells. The peripheral cells in the island differentiate into primordial endothelium and core cells as precursors of blood cells [2].

The primary capillaries are formed from tubular structures made of differentiated endothelial cells.

Arteries, veins, and capillaries are developed from the maturation and remodeling of the primary capillary plexus. This phenomenon is referred to as Angiogenesis. This represents the sprouting of newer capillaries, formation of transcapillary connections, and maturation of the vascular network [4].

Non-perfused blood vessels disappear, and the rest further modify and strengthen to form the mature vascular network.

Lymphangiogenesis follows angiogenesis and arises from endothelial cells. Theory that lymph vessels derive from lymphangioblasts and not vascular endothelial cells do exist. Various angiogenic and anti-angiogenic factors influence the formation of both vascular and lymphatic networks. Therefore, the occurrence of vascular anomalies may be consequent to their disharmonious behavior.

Hemangiomas are vascular neoplasms that have different phases of development. They go

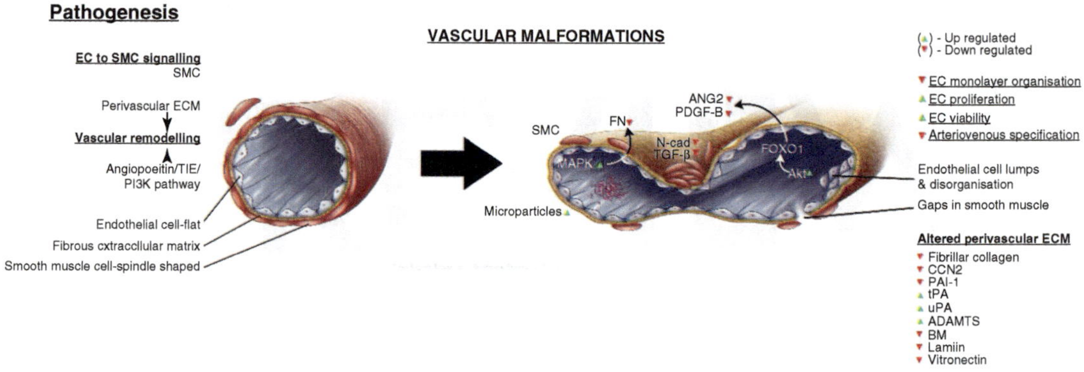

Fig. 2.1 Normal vascular lumen lined with endothelial cells with normal radiation, surrounding fibrosis extracellular matrix, and spindle-shaped smooth muscle cell layer. *SMC* Smooth muscle cell, *EC* Endothelial cell, *ECM* Extracellular matrix; Somatic mutations causing 'gain of function' in the tyrosine kinase receptor of -ANG (Angiopoietin) type, TIE and PIK3CA encoding genes activated cell signaling pathway leading to vascular malformations. In experimental mouse models of angiogenesis ANG/TIE/PIK3CA cause cell signaling and perivascular extracellular matrix remodeling, degradation, etc. Adapted from Kangas J, Nätynki M, Eklund L. Development of Molecular Therapies for Venous Malformations. Basic Clin Pharmacol Toxicol. 2018 Sep;123 Suppl 5:6–19. https://doi.org/10.1111/bcpt.13027. Epub 2018 May 29. PMID: 29668117

through the proliferative phase, quiescent phase, and finally involutory phase. Histologically they are characterized by the proliferation of plump endothelial cells with mast cell infiltration [5, 6]. The latter phases show flattened endothelial cells. Infantile hemangiomas show increased expression of glucose transporter-1 (GLUT-1).

Typically, most hemangiomas may not be visible at birth but present with telltale signs such as a pigmentation, a macule, or papular eruption. They attain prominence in the first month or two. Proliferation then occurs with a rapid enhancement of its clinical appearance. The phases to follow are quiescence and involution. The cellular activity during involution shows the reduction in angiogenesis with apoptosis of endothelial cells. The vascular channels now are replaced with fibrofatty tissue. Congenital hemangiomas in contrast are fully mature at birth and do not show a proliferative phase.

Pathogenesis is a complex interaction of genetic and environmental factors. The role of HPV-8 infection, chronic villus sampling, and hormonal, especially estrogen disturbances with possible hypoxia causing endothelial cell proliferation is another theory [4–6]. Multiple angiogenic factors play a role in proliferating hemangiomas in contrast with VEGFR1 being down regulated [8]. The role and efficacy of beta 2 blockers in the management of proliferating hemangiomas are documented [9–11]. Its effect on the VEGF, fibroblast growth factor, and matrix metalloproteinase are thought to be the method of action. Vasoconstriction and apoptosis of the capillary endothelial cells occur consequently.

Vascular Malformations are the result of errors in angiogenesis. The commonest among them is venous malformation. Depending on the involved vascular subunit, they may be capillary, arterial, venous, lymphatic, or a combination of these resulting in artery venous malformation or lympho-venous malformation. The differentiation can be picked up with an ultrasound doppler augmented with an MRA.

Venous malformations are thin-walled, and dilated channels with normal endothelial cell lining occurring on the skin or subcutaneous (Type 1/Type 2) (refer authors classification [11]). The VM vary in their clinical presentation. From small blush discolored, soft compressible swellings in the head and neck region to large vascular spaces invading deeper anatomic spaces in the head and neck region. They gradually expand over a period with enhancement associated with hormonal changes or trauma. Mostly isolated in appearance and rarely multiple manifestations occur. The lesions enhance with dependent positions like lying down or Valsalva maneuver. The increasingly static nature of flow causes the formation of phleboliths which are easily palpable as hard masses and result in pain. The plane radiographs or an US easily demonstrate the phlebolith. Local intravascular coagulation (LIC) shows a rise in D-dimer level in the presence of normal fibrinogen. The VM is often present unilateral and result in pressure on the surrounding structures. Skeletal deformity or hypo-plastic muscular tissue may be seen. Those within the orbital cavity cause exophthalmos globe as well as orbital dystopia. Intraorally large VMs of the tongue and floor of the mouth deform mandible or maxilla resulting in malocclusion of the teeth (see clinical figures in Chaps. 1, 3 & 5). Speech impairment and impairment of functions such as swallowing, respiration may be compromised. Histologically the venous channels are dilated with a lack of smooth muscle cells around the endothelial cells which can be demonstrated with IHC markers (Fig. 2.1). Thus, defective recruitment of SMC with lack of proliferation of EC probably result in dilation of the venous spaces. The molecular basis of the development of the anomaly is discussed later in this chapter.

Capillary Malformations because of their appearance are referred to as port-wine stains. They occur in 0.3 of newborns as flat, reddish, or deep red patches in the head and neck [1–9]. The histological picture is that of a dilated capillary network which is more in number. The primitive capillary plexus fails to mature or modify resulting in normally appearing endothelial cells on the vessel wall.

The significant reduction in innervation may be the cause of capillary vessel wall dilatation and resultant abnormal blood flow pattern. VEGF secreted by the cutaneous nerves reduces, leading to an abnormality in the capillary network. CM occurs on the face distributed along the Trigeminal nerve dermatomes [12–14]. The presence of Sturge Weber syndrome must be ruled out. The maxilla, or mandible and the skin or gingiva may overgrow and appear deep red or purple in appearance as age advances.

Arterial Malformations and Arteriovenous Malformations are anomalies with absent or imperfect capillary intermediaries between arteries and veins. The presence of a 'nidus' which is a dilated vascular sac replaces the capillary network of vessels. This dilated sac acts as a pressure break between the arterial and venous systems and is comparable to a cardiac chamber. Transmitted pulsations from the arterial system is palpable over the nidus. Local warmth and increased coloration over the swelling are other features. Large AVMs show the phenomenon of vascular steal resulting in high output cardiac failure. Schobinnger [18] in 1990 has staged the AVMs clinically into [Ref. 18]:

Stage I (quiescence): Discolored skin with arteriovenous shunting demonstrated with an US doppler.
Stage II (expansion): Like stage I with pulsatile enlargement.
Stage III: Stage II with ulceration, necrosis, bleeding, and pain of overlying skin.
Stage IV: Presence of cardiac failure.

Histologically the endothelial cells are proliferated in the absence of sensitivity to inhibitory cytokines (IL-1 B, TNF- alpha, TGF- Beta, and interferon- Gama [4, 5, 7]. Their sporadic appearance, therefore, contradicts any genetic influence.

Lymphatic malformations are also common in the head and neck and extremities. Their development is unknown. Clinically they appear as venous malformations without the discolouration [19]. The spaces within the lesion differentiate them into macrocystic, microcystic, or combined. Preoperative imaging help differentiate the types of lymphatic lesions [7, 9, 11]. Cystic Hygroma is a variant of a macro cystic LM. The surface lesions appear as minute blisters that appear dark red because of intra-vesicular bleeding.

Like VM the LM shows pressure effects on the skeletal structure causing deformity [20]. Large lesions in the tongue and floor of the mouth result in the anterior open bite as well as macroglossia. Functional impairment and airway distress may necessitate even tracheostomy.

2.3 Genetic Basis of Vascular Lesions with Mutation and Inheritance

2.3.1 Mutations (Table 2.1, See Also Fig. 2.6 Consolidated Review)

The majority of Vascular anomalies are of a ***sporadic type***. There are a few rare reported types of familial inheritance (germline type) [15–17].

2.3.2 Cancer and Vascular Lesions

Mutations causing Malignancies and vascular lesions share similar pathways (Figs. 2.2, 2.3, 2.4, 2.6). However, surprisingly causation and phenotype are poorly understood between oncogenesis and vasculogenesis [18–23, 34]. The Growth and differentiation of vascular lesion and endothelium are driven by two major pathways- RAS/RAF and PIK3CA (Fig. 2.1 of RAF/RAS).

Table 2.1 Germline versus Somatic Mutation differences [24–31]

Germline mutation in vascular lesions	Somatic mutation in vascular lesions
Inherited	Nonheritable
Syndromes & malignancy association	Sporadic
Mutations present in egg/sperm	Non-germline tissue
All the offspring affected	Most vascular lesions

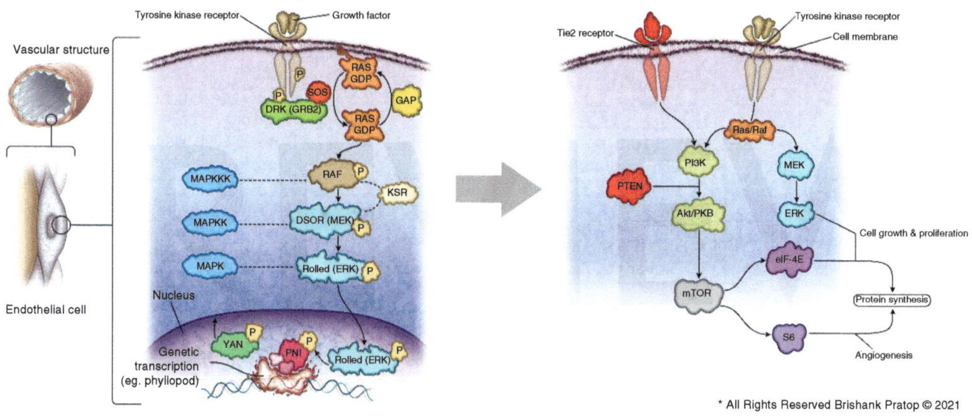

Fig. 2.2 Transmembrane tyrosine kinase receptors like ANG (angiopoietin) homologs TIE1 & TIE 2 (tyrosine kinase with immunoglobulin and epithelial growth factor (EGF) homology domain) are present on vascular endothelial cells. The activation of the Ras-Raf-MEK-ERK pathway leads to angiogenesis and cell growth and proliferation. Various growth factor receptor mutations in downstream have been identified in vascular and lymphatic endothelial cells leading to vascular malformation

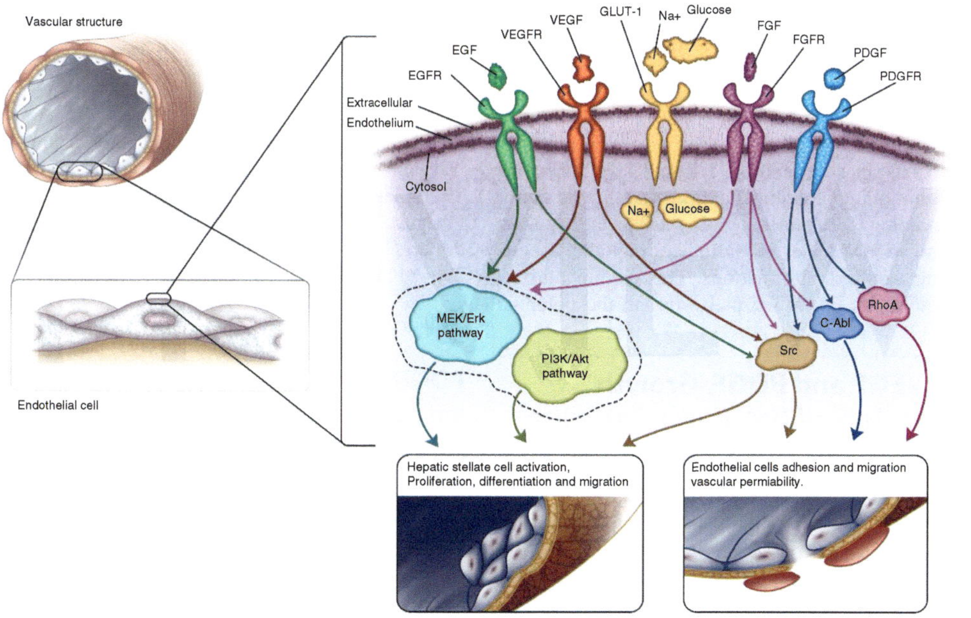

Fig. 2.3 Tyrosine kinase receptors picture. Receptor Tyrosine Kinases (R TKs): Cell surface expresses two peptide amino acid tyrosine class receptors of growth factors like EGFR: Endothelial growth factor receptor family (Receptor, TK class I), PDGFR: Platelet-derived growth factor receptor (receptor tyrosine kinase class III), VEGFR: Vascular endothelial growth factor receptor (Receptor, TK class IV), FGFR: Fibroblast growth factor receptor (Receptor tyrosine kinase class V). These polypeptide, cell surface, transmembrane, high-affinity receptors for cytokine, growth factors and hormones are responsible for angiogenesis and growth. This growth, proliferation, DNA synthesis by Ras–Raf–MEK–ERK pathway downstream is similar in vascular lesions as well as oncogenesis. The vascular endothelial cells proliferate once the surface RKTs get activated and can cause hepatic cell proliferation or endothelial cell migration and adhesion. In vascular lesions, the adhesion is defective leading to dilated and tortuous pools. The defect can extend to the smooth muscle cell layer. *EGF* Endothelial growth factor, *VEGF* Vascular growth factor, *GLUT-1* Glucose transporter 1, *FGF* Fibroblast growth factor, *PDGF* Platelet-derived growth factor

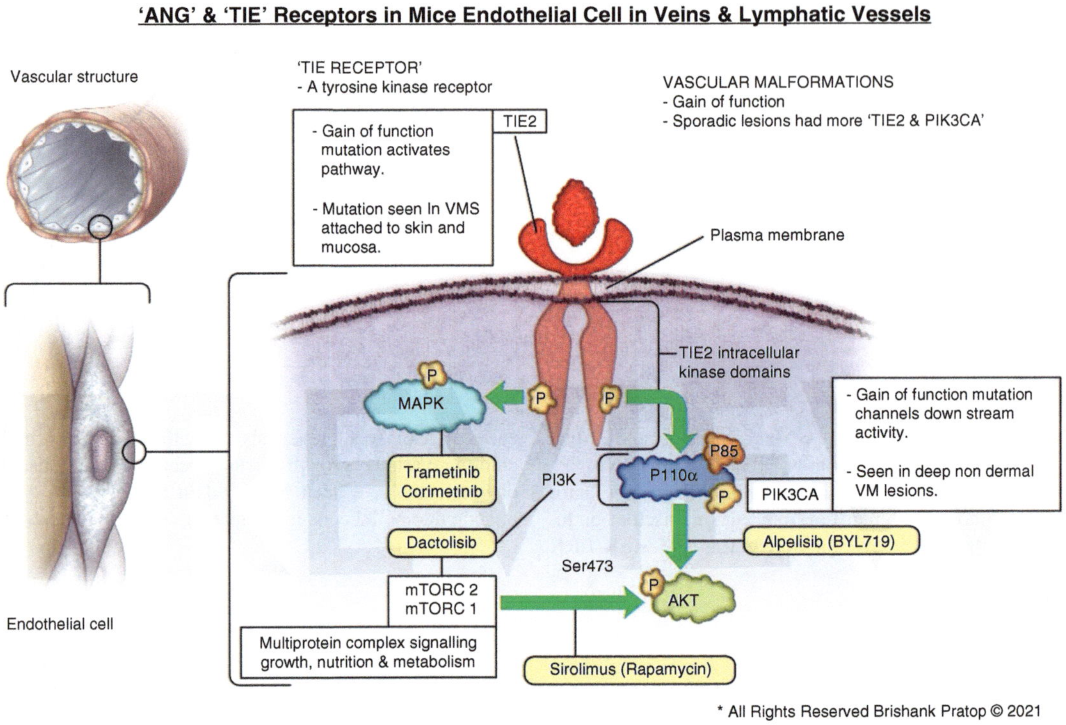

Fig. 2.4 Angiopoietin (ANG) based on two transmembrane tyrosine kinase receptors-TIE1 and TIE 2 (tyrosine kinase with immunoglobulin and epithelial growth factor (EGF) homology domain) homologous receptors have been identified in vascular and lymphatic endothelial cells leading to vascular malformations. This picture illustration represents the identified pathway and the potential therapeutic molecular therapies. Adapted from Kangas J, Nätynki M, Eklund L. Development of Molecular Therapies for Venous Malformations. Basic Clin Pharmacol Toxicol. 2018 Sep;123 Suppl 5:6–19. https://doi.org/10.1111/bcpt.13027. Epub 2018 May 29. PMID: 29668117

2.4 VEGF and PDGF, Growth factors of Raf, Ras in Tyrosine class receptors

Ras and Raf are downstream from the two-peptide amino acid class tyrosine kinase, which is the first step receptor in cancer and vascular cell upregulation.

Upregulation of the receptor or function of the tyrosine kinase (TIE or TK) group of receptors is known to cause cell division and proliferation. Cascade activation of TK to the cell nucleus leads to Growth, virus-directed replication, sepsis, inflammation, oncogenesis, etc.

Vascular endothelial growth factor (VEGF), Platelet-derived endothelial growth factor (PDGF), Epidermal growth factor (EGF), EGFR, PDGF, V EGF, etc. are all tyrosine kinase receptors. There is an extracellular receptor binding site. This sequential protein to protein communication of a phosphorylated cascade is known as RAS–RAF–MEK–ERK/or MAPK/ERK (mitogen-activated protein kinase/extracellular signaled regulated kinase).

RAS is activated by the phosphorylation of the tyrosine kinase class receptor in the cell wall. Activated Ras then activates Raf kinase (both GTPases). Activated Raf downstream phosphorylates MEK the next step of the chain (MEK 1 and 2). Phosphorylated MEK activates the ERK pathway. ERK and MAPK (mitogen-activated protein kinase), well known as RAS–RAF–MEK–ERK cell signaling cascade from the cell surface to the nucleus for growth and proliferation.

2.5 G Protein-related Spectrum

There are multiple G protein receptors related mutations on genes of GNA Q/GNA 11/GNA 14 [30, 31]. This G protein-related spectrum is GNA-vascular anomaly (GNAVA). A few instances of this GNA VA spectrum anomalies are congenital hemangioma, capillary hemangioma, kaposiform hemangioendothelioma. So evidently, these G protein-related receptor mutations can manifest in both tumors and malformations [30].

2.6 PIK3CA-related Overgrowth Spectrum (PROS) [31–36]

Vascular anomalies caused by PIK3CA related mutations are known as PIK3CA-related overgrowth spectrum (PROS). As previously classified independently currently grouped as PROS spectrum. There is a potential targeted therapy for these receptor-related malignant tumors—many PROS-related anomalies present as malformations of a similar kind.

Multiple mutations can give rise to various manifestations in different stages of cell proliferation. Some mutations can give rise to both tumors and malformations. Mutations of a single gene can manifest varying phenotypic characteristics clinically. The mutated gene can express varied manifestations depending on the up-regulation or down-regulation of proliferating, differentiation, and maturation stage affect.

The majority of the known vascular anomalies' mutations are associated with the tyrosine kinase receptor-associated signaling pathway of RAS & PIK3CA [30, 31, 40]. Various somatic mutations affecting the MAP2K1 pathway can present as cutaneous malformations of several types of malignancies not related to vascular tissue but melanomas, lung cancer, and blood-related tumors.

2.7 Mutations and Vascular Lesions: *The Essentials*

Previously focal or multifocal and diffuse vascular lesions were defined with syndrome labeling. However, with the new molecular genetics and identification of somatic mutations, the diagnosis should be based on abnormal genetic pathways. Most of the vascular lesions have a single gene-related Mutation. Nevertheless, the mutation of a single gene may manifest in various forms of vascular anomalies with occasional multiple gene mutations. The identification of genetic mutations is ongoing research with at least close to a hundred publications in the last 25 years.

Mutations can be of broad two types -Germline and somatic (Table 2.1). Alterations in the genetic sequence involving all cells of the gamete organism are called a germline mutation. This type of altered genetic sequence is transmitted to future generations. Most of the vascular lesions are of somatic mutations, which occur after fertilization as variations of the post-zygotic DNA. They are random occurrences affecting the cell's genetic sequence and the derivative, but next generation does not inherit this Mutation type. Understanding these somatic mutations and their pathways may help in control with targeted pharmacotherapy in the future.

Other than that mutation type, alterations in the signaling pathway, the enriched cell type of the Mutation and Signaling pathways are also being understood in vascular anomalies' etiology pathogenesis. More the number of mutated alleles and their frequency of mutant varieties and wild types are also considered.

Gene signaling pathways and Cells enriched by the Mutation Are also being identified for novel therapeutic uses. RAS (phosphatidylinositol-4,5-bisphosphate 3-kinase) PIK3CA cell signaling pathways dependent on the tyrosine kinase receptor are the most common mutations identified in head and neck vascular anomalies.

2.8 Genetic Testing and Advances in the Diagnosis of Vascular Anomalies [3, 4, 26, 30, 31]

Advances in genomics with understanding and utilization of genetic sequencing, testing how provided various molecular basis approaches of pathophysiology in vascular anomalies.

2.8.1 Test Type and Reasons

Ideal genetic testing for vascular anomalies is with a purpose and undertaken with flow chart identification of the Mutation.

Blood, tissue sample of the lesion if obtained, or buccal mucosal scraping can detect Germline mutations. Tissue specimens are fixed in formalin if needed for transport. Simple D -dimer review of lesion activity with the specificities in mind can be performed.

2.9 Biopsy and Immunohistochemistry

2.9.1 GLUT-1 and the Importance of the Vascular Lesion Identification

Glucose transporter protein isoform -1 (GLUT-1) is a standard and ideal marker for hemangiomas.

2.9.2 GLUT 1 Receptor (Fig. 2.5)

Infantile hemangioma (IH) in all evolving stages of the lesion is positive for GLUT 1 (Fig. 2.5). This endothelial stain highlights the cytoplasm inside the vascular lesions' capillary endothelial cells in both the involuting and proliferative stages.

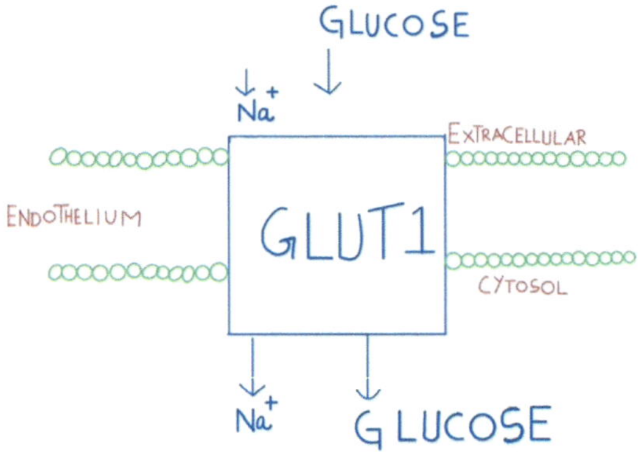

Fig. 2.5 Infantile hemangioma (IH) in all evolving stages of the lesion is positive for GLUT 1. Courtesy Dr Advaith Nair

Congenital Hemangioma (CH)—Rapidly involuting congenital hemangioma (RICH) has endothelial cells mostly GLUT 1 negative. Non-involuting congenital hemangioma (NICH) definitively is Immuno-negative for GLUT 1. Segmental hemangioma is positive for GLUT-1 staining.

2.10 VEGF -3, D2 -40, PROX 1, LYVE -1

These immune stains can differentiate arteries and veins from lymphatics.

Vascular endothelial growth factor receptor -3, Vascular immunostains for D2 -40 (podoplanin), Lymphatic vessels endothelial receptor–1 (LYVE –1 marker PROX 1 (Lymphatic endothelial markers).

2.11 CD31 and CD 34 Antibodies

2.11.1 Factor VIII Related Antigen

Antibodies of CD31 and CD 34 is a pan endothelial cells marker (low affinity for lymphatic endothelial affinity) [30, 31]. CD 31 is specific. These Vascular endothelial Immune peroxidase markers are commonly used along with Factor VIII-related antigen.

2.12 Next-generation Sequencing and Its Promise for Vascular Lesions

2.12.1 DNA Sequencing, What his Next-generation Sequencing?

Deoxyribonucleic acid sequencing, especially human genomic sequencing, has undergone a few generations of development since the early 1970s. Here is a brief review of some fundamentals to understand genetic testing for vascular lesion diagnosis and treatment.

Table 2.2 Table of Sanger and NGS

	Sanger (1977)	Next-Generation Sequencing (1996)
DNA sample	Cell DNA fragments; PCR clones in hotspot areas	DNA libraries; cell-free DNA
Sequencing	Linear read of single fragment	Parallel sequencing of million base pairs simultaneously
Utility	Unknown mutation diagnosis	Detection of unidentified mutations; complex and heterogenous phenotypes
Basic principle of DNA analysis	Chain termination PCR > ddNTPs label>fluorescent signal pick up of fragments	Sheared>tail adapters>DNA library>amplify>sequence> light density read
Cost	Cheap	Varies on the complexity
Sensitivity	Lower	High (lesion heterogeneity and contamination not a factor)
Data	Small storage capacity	Large data with bioinformatic systems

Next-generation sequencing (NGS) techniques are tools for mutation diagnosis. Targeted gene panel sequencing (TS) and Whole-Exome Sequencing and Whole-Genome sequencing are possible for an expressive phenotype's monogenetic disorder.

2.12.2 Sanger Method

The Sanger method took about 13 years for the human DNA genomics study of three million base pairs; NGS does this in a single day (Table 2.2).

Sanger with associates developed dideoxy synthesis with chain-terminating nucleotides at the 3-hydroxyl group. A Detailed nucleotide sequence review in the hundreds in the Sanger method. Sanger method sequences single strands of DNA.

Nevertheless, with the advances of next-generation sequencing (NGS), a whole-exome, genome, transcriptosome, mitochondrial DNA, or Target Gene panel sequencing is performed at a low cost.

2.13 Next-Generation Sequencing (NGS)

Commonly known as "NGS" is also "second generation" DNA sequencing, a significantly faster, low-cost development in the last ten years. This genome, exomes, and transcriptome sequencing will lead to paradigm changes in vascular lesion therapies.

Advances in genomics with understanding and utilization of genetic sequencing, testing how provided various molecular basis approaches of pathophysiology in vascular anomalies.

2.13.1 #1 Copy Number Variations (CNV)

Genome-wide CNV of more than 10,000 base sequence variations are detected done using high-resolution chromosomal microarray (CMA) and Whole-genome sequencing (WGS) methods.

2.13.2 #2 Single Nucleotide Variation (SNV)

This is the most common type of genomic variation affecting a single nucleotide of DNA base, causing short insertion and deletions. This alteration of Nucleotide can be detected using next-generation sequencing (NGS) methods of Whole-exome sequencing (WES) or whole-genome sequencing (WGS). In next Generation sequencing, unlike single-strand sequencing for DNA defects, it involves slicing of the DNA into numerous random strands before amplifying the fragments and then subjecting to Polymerase chain reaction (PCR)to align the exact 5′ and 3′ with attachments of adapters. In PCR, the genetic fragments get amplified to generate clonal clusters. Before that, DNA polymerase will be utilized for complementary; Nucleotide is created and attached to the strands. This stage utilizes Low-cost fluorescent technology and bioinformatics for Sequencing results.

Unlike vector cloning with the use of restriction enzymes and bacterial cells, the genetic sequencing by PCR aided Sanger and NGS are more accurate and do not use heat and anneal methods.

PCR is utilized for amplification and cloning DNA templates from a biopsy or liquid biopsy sources. The polymerase can rapidly produce a million copies of a single fragment.

NGS is a parallel sequencing of millions of fragmented DNA from a library, while the Sanger method does one fragment in a linear fashion.

The similarities between all the genetic sequencing methods

- Biopsy material for nucleic acid fragment.
- Adapter ligation.
- Multiplex Tag and clone amplification.
- Parallel sequencing.
- Data analysis.

The advances in the future with next impression sequencing technology are with the increase in signal detection, read length, costs, and run time. Exome analysis is by both the parents and the child for variations. Partial genomic hotspot testing or a complete gene panel testing.

The current platforms for next impression sequencing are primarily for research but have great potential for bedside therapeutics. Though the next impression's volume of sequencing is phenomenal for at least one million reads, the infrastructure is still expensive compared to the Sanger method.

2.14 Cell-free DNA (cfDNA) Testing in Prenatal Conditions for Vascular Anomalies

NGS can perform mutational analysis in a prenatal setting of cell-free DNA (cfDNA). Even though this technology has been in use for prenatal testing, tumor-derived cell-free DNA testing is possible with the NGS. The sensitivity of cfDNA may be less compared to actual lesion biopsies. However, it is a viable option in prepartum diagnosis and difficulty with repeated biopsies of highly vascular tissue and anatomically critical areas. cfDNA testing in vascular lesions can be applied to diagnoses, monitoring the evolution, therapeutic guidance, and follow-up. Cf DNA has helped monitor lung cancer therapy targeted at tyrosine kinase inhibitor response for epidermal growth factor activated mutations.

Exome analysis is by both the parents and the child for variations. Partial genomic hotspot testing or complete gene panel testing.

The current platforms for next generation sequencing are primarily for research but have great potential for bedside therapeutics. The sequencing by next generation is phenomenal for at least one million reads, the infrastructure is still expensive compared to the Sanger method (Fig. 2.6 and Table 2.3).

2.15 Therapeutic Hypotheses for the Treatment of Vascular Diseases [39–41, 46–48, 51] (Fig. 2.7)

2.15.1 Targeting the PI3K/AKT/mTOR Pathway

- **mTOR inhibitors, such as Rapamycin in VM, VMCM, MVM, BRBN, and LM; also HHT?**

  Targeting the RAS/BRAF/MAPK/ERK pathway
- Possible inhibitors could be the BRAF inhibitor vemurafenib or the MEK inhibitor trametinib.in CM, CM-AVM1 and 2, PG, NICH, RICH, and verrucous venous malformations.

  Targeting angiogenesis
- Antiangiogenic agents, such as bevacizumab in HHT, IH.

  Targeting TGF-ß pathway
- GVM?

Growth and differentiation of the vascular lesion and its endothelial cell proliferation or

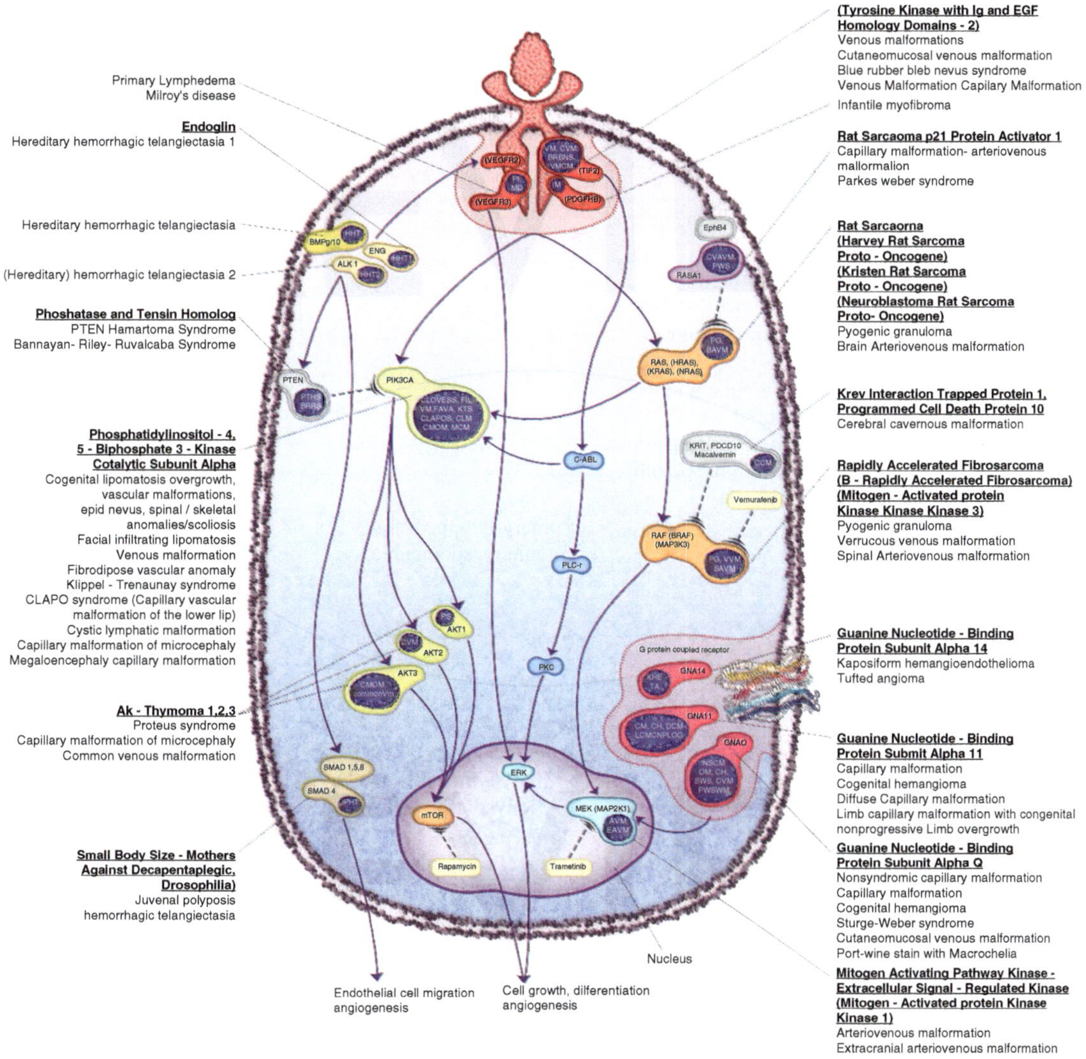

Fig. 2.6 Genetic basis of vascular lesions with Mutation and inheritance—Nair and Chandra [22, 39, 57, 60, 61]. Summary illustration of well-known genetic mutations based on that transmembrane tyrosine kinase MG protein-coupled signaling pathways. The protein mutations are abbreviated with the number's analogs. These vascular malformations caused by the mutations on the syndromic presentations are listed below the receptors which are mutated. The majority of these mutations are based on the well-known Ras-Raf-MEK-ERK and PIK3CA pathways. **Adapted from- International Society for the study of vascular anomalies 2014-classification scheme and associated genetic basis** (Table 2.3); Greene and Goss vascular anomalies: From a clinical histologically genetic framework, Plast Reconstr Surgery 2018 may; 141 (5): 709e–717e; Padia R, Zenner K, Bly R, Bennett J, Bull C, Perkins J. Clinical Application of Molecular Genetics in Lymphatic Malformations. Laryngoscope Investig Otolaryngol 2019, Feb:4(1):170–173

initiated at the cell membrane tyrosine kinase receptor with the RAS- RAF downstream to nucleus MAPK dependent gene transcription. The illustration demonstrates the potential therapy and inhibition of Src-tyrosine kinase family inhibitors; rapidly accelerated fibrosarcoma (RAF) inhibitors; mitogen activating pathway kinase-extracellular signal-regulated kinase (MEK) inhibitors; extracellular signal-regulated kinase is (ERK) inhibitors.

Table 2.3 Study of vascular anomalies 2014-classification scheme and associated genetic basis

Genetic basis of vascular lesion; Inheritance	Vascular tumors	Lymphatic malformations	Vascular malformations; arteriovenous malformation; additional syndromes and anomalies
Follicle-stimulating hormone; stem cell	Infantile hemangioma		
GNAQ GNA 11	Congenital hemangioma		
GNA 14	Kaposiform hemangioendothelioma		
KRAS; NRAS; GNA Q; B RAF	Pyogenic granuloma;		
PDPRB; PLCG; WWT R1-CAMTA 1 gene fusion; PDGF RB	Rare vascular tumors-epithelioid hemangioendothelioma; angiosarcoma; infantile myofibroma		
PIK3CA; VEGFR 3/ FLT-4; FOXC2; SOX 18; CCBE1; GJ C2, CX47;		Primary lymphedema-hereditary, sporadic	
VEGFR 3/FLT-4 dominant/recessive		Nonne–Milroy Syndrome	
FOXC2 dominant		Lymphedema-distichiasis	
SOX18 dominant/ recessive		Hyportrichosis–lymphedema-telangi ectasia	
GATA2		Primary lymphedema with myelodysplasia	
CCBE 1		Primary generalized lymphatic anomaly	
KIF11		Microcephaly with/without chorioretinopathy	
–		Lymphedema or mental retardation syndrome	
PTEN14		Lymphedema–choanal atresia	
PIK3CA somatic			Klippel–Trenaunay syndrome
RASA1/EPHB4 dominant			Parkes Weber syndrome
–			Servelle–Martorell syndrome
GNAQ			Sturge–Weber syndrome
			Capillary malformation & congenital nonprogressive overgrowth
IDH1/IDH2 somatic			Maffucci syndrome
PIK3CA			Megaloencephaly with capillary malformation
STAMBP			Microcephaly with capillary malformation
PIK3CA			CLOVES syndrome
AKT1 somatic			Proteus syndrome
PTEN			Bannayan_Riley_Ruvalcaba syndrome/Cowden syndrome
MAP2K1; RASA1; GDF2; VEGFR2;			Arteriovenous malformation; capillary AVM;

Table 2.3 (continued)

Genetic basis of vascular lesion; Inheritance	Vascular tumors	Lymphatic malformations	Vascular malformations; arteriovenous malformation; additional syndromes and anomalies
ENG (endoglin) ACVRL1/ ALK1(activating A receptor type 2-like 1) Autosomal dominant			Hereditary hemorrhagic telangiectasia (HHT 1 & 2)
SMAD4			Juvenile polyposis
PTEN- autosomal dominant			Hamartoma- tumor syndrome
TIE2 dominant			Cutaneomucosal venous malformation
KRIT1/malcavernin/ PDCD10 dominant			Cerebral cavernous malformation (CCM 1, 2 & 3)
Glomulin dominant			Glomuvenous malformation
TIE2 somatic			Sporadic venous malformation

2.15.2 Sirolimus (Rapamycin)

The literature on Sirolimus and its efficacy is equivocal. The best candidate for this therapeutic advantage is not clear. Strychowsky et al., in the 2018 phase 2 trial using Sirolimus in patients, evaluated the benefits of its empiric use complicated LM. They reported a reduction in cellulitis and incidence of hospitalizations with cellulitis-related complications. The adverse effects of therapy were—Metabolic toxicity (3%), gastrointestinal disturbance (3%), and blood/bone marrow abnormalities (27%). Not all the patients receiving therapy had a genetic test for the PIK3CA mutation confirmed. So, treatment was based on clinical considerations. Other studies have reported anecdotal success with Sirolimus. Sirolimus's current indications for therapy are for pain, lesion enlargement, vesicular ulcerations, bone erosion and expansion, bleeding, airway compression, hematologic abnormalities, and complex symptomatic cases [30–42, 55, 56].

There is significant crosstalk between pathways, which are not well understood. The targeted treatment therapies are focused on this receptor population pathway upregulation or downregulation. One such commonly used and established treatment is organ transplantation with immune suppression with Sirolimus (Rapamycin).

2.15.3 mTOR (Mammalian Target for Rapamycin) [30, 31, 39–45, 50, 52]

mTOR is a downstream enzyme in the PIK3CA pathway. Rapamycin is a chemotherapeutic agent derivative of *Streptomyces hygroscopicus* bacteria, a macrolide used for targeted therapy to block the PIK3CA pathway. Rapamycin (Sirolimus) inhibits cellular proliferation. Sirolimus has varied success in vascular malformations therapy, but clinical outcomes have not been consistent. Authors here present personal experiences in use with syndromic patients has been with adequate caution. Multiple centers have used Sirolimus empirically, and mutational tests before using the therapy have not been consistent.

Sirolimus as a B & T cell suppressor is very well studied in transplant patients, as mentioned with useful utility. Its use in head and neck vascular lesions has shown a qualitative reduction in size and side effects of bleeding and vesicular discharge. Nevertheless, Sirolimus therapy has documented side effects for its use with complicated LM throughout the body. A reduction in cellulitis and hospitalizations with cellulitis-related complications documented with case reports and lesion management publications.

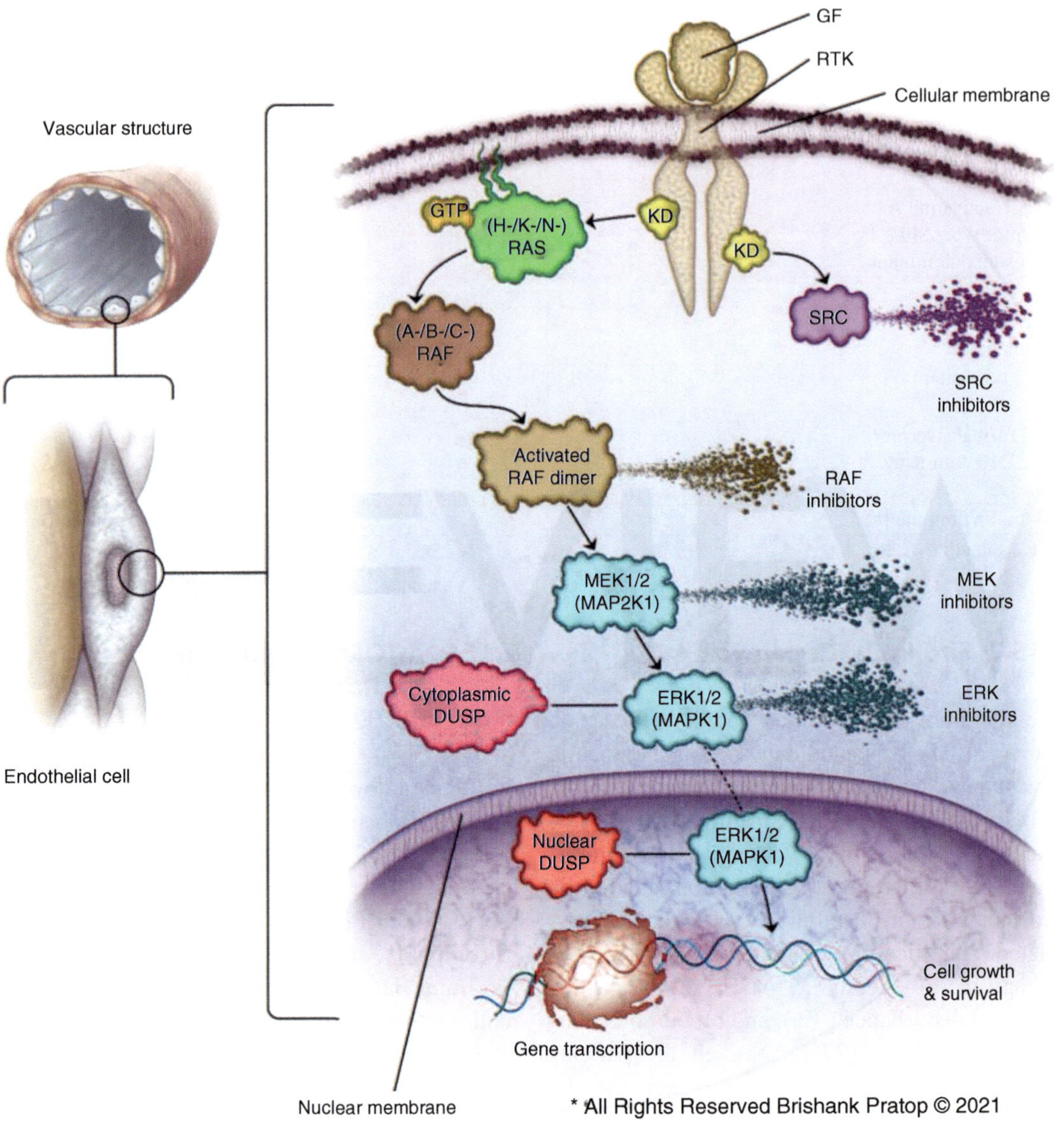

Fig. 2.7 MAPK/ERK pathway (well known as the Ras-Raf-MEK-ERK pathway) potential therapeutic inhibitors. Protein chain in a vascular cell that transmits signal from a cell surface receptor to the DNA in the cell nucleus

Gastrointestinal, general metabolic toxicity, blood dyscrasias, bone marrow suppression (even though one of the treatment indications is dyscrasias of hematological and marrow-derived cell function) were the reported adverse effects of the medications.

The literature on Sirolimus and its efficacy is equivocal. The best candidate for this therapeutic advantage is not clear. Strychowsky et al. [49], in the 2018 phase 2 trial using Sirolimus in patients, evaluated the benefits of its empiric use complicated LM. They reported a reduction in cellulitis and incidence of hospitalizations with cellulitis-related complications. The adverse effects of therapy were—Metabolic toxicity (3%), gastro-intestinal disturbance (3%), and blood/bone marrow abnormalities (27%). Not all the patients receiving therapy had a genetic test for the PIK3CA mutation confirmed. So, treatment was based on clinical considerations. Other studies have reported anecdotal success with Sirolimus. Sirolimus's current indications for therapy are for pain, lesion enlargement, vesicular ulcerations, bone erosion and expansion, bleeding, airway compression, hematologic abnormalities, and complex symptomatic cases [Refs. 2, 34].

2.16 Conclusion

Genetic testing and advances in the understanding of pathogenesis have provided more direct and targeted therapeutics. However, the molecular abnormalities similar to cancer mutations and the phenotypic presentation disparity is intriguing. Nevertheless, mutations provide an objective molecular etiology to educate patients, families, and researchers with HNLMS knowledge for further work with a group of pathologies. Clinical pathways for standardized outcome measures and building data banks for systematic collection in medical trials is needed.

Genetic testing for mutations is a very evolving topic with ongoing research. At the same time, many somatic mutations are not known even after the entire exome sequencing of the parents and the child. The causes for nondetection could be sampling the different hotspots in a different gene or low allele frequency for detection.

Aggressive therapy needs more close follow-up and reporting. HNLM research makes precision-based treatment a possibility. Precision therapy-based treatment decisions on specific molecular and genetic is the future. Biologic factors unique to an individual patient's rare conditions are always with meticulous risk–benefit ratio consideration.

Until now, therapeutic options to treat vascular tumors and malformations have is by classic approaches. To ablate or remove abnormal vessels by laser, sclerotherapy, embolization, and surgery. Detection of a genetic cause, inherited or somatic, has opened up understanding the underlying molecular mechanisms. Most genetic defects directly alter intracellular signaling activities and, subsequently, various downstream actions. Even if all the downstream effects are unknown, the identification of overt signaling opens these diseases to novel ideas to develop treatments.

Lesions caused by constitutively active PI3K/AKT/mTOR pathway (e.g., VMCM, MVM, VM, BRBN, and LM) may benefit from mTOR inhibitors as Rapamycin (see Fig. 2.1). A VM in vivo model is viable by injecting TIE2-L914F mutated human umbilical vein endothelial cells into nude mice. Treatment with Rapamycin prevented VM growth. Additionally, in vitro, Rapamycin significantly reduced mutant TIE2-induced AKT signaling [53–55]. Importantly, in a prospective clinical pilot study, six patients treated with Rapamycin had reduced pain, bleeding, lesional size, and intravascular coagulopathy.

In lesions where the RAS/RAF/MAPK/ERK pathway plays a significant role (e.g., CM, CMAVM1 and 2, PG, NICH, RICH, and verrucous venous malformation), other inhibitors are considered. There are conceivable tests of BRAF (vemurafenib) or MEK inhibitor (trametinib), which are used to treat metastatic BRAF-mutated melanoma (see Fig. 2.1) [30, 31, 57–60]. Because many kinase inhibitors have variable affinities to several intracellular proteins, and multiple crosstalks occur between signaling pathways, numerous studies are needed to characterize the most efficient modalities.

In HHT, receptor mutations lead to decreased BMP signaling, and this may lead in turn to an increase in angiogenic response. Thus, these patients could benefit from antiangiogenic agents, such as bevacizumab. However, diminished ALK activity also leads to increased PTEN phosphorylation and inactivation. There is subsequent PI3K/AKT activation. Rapamycin and other PI3K/AKT inhibitors may thus prove to be efficacious [51].

Other general angiogenesis inhibitors, such as thalidomide or bevacizumab, the anti-VEGF antibody, may also be useful [60–63]. They can inhibit VEGF action, whatever the underlying cause for expression may be. For example, they reduce nosebleeds in patients with HHT. The pathophysiology of GVMs is a little unclear. If earlier data hold, the TGF-ß pathway might serve as a target, in addition to modulation of mTOR.

References

1. Brouillard P, Vikkula M. Vascular malformations: localized defects in vascular morphogenesis. Clin Genet. 2003;63:340.
2. Lohela M, Bry M, Tammela T, et al. VEGFs and receptors involved in angiogenesis versus lymphangiogenesis. Curr Opin Cell Biol. 2009;21:154.
3. Holmes LB. Chorionic villus sampling and hemangiomas. J Craniofac Surg. 2009;1(20 Suppl):675.
4. Pocock B, Boon LM, Vikkula M. Molecular basis of vascular birthmarks. Sem Plast Surg. 2006;20:149.
5. Jinnin M, Medici D, Park L, et al. Suppressed NFAT-dependent VEGFR1 expression and constitutive VEGFR2 signaling in infantile hemangioma. Nat Med. 2008;14:1236.
6. Bischoff J. Progenitor cells in infantile hemangioma. J Craniofac Surg. 2009;20(Suppl 1):695.
7. Mulliken JB, Glowacki J. Hemangiomas and vascular malformations in infants and children: a classification based on endothelial characteristics. Plast Reconstr Surg. 1982;69:412.
8. Chang LC, Haggstrom AN, Drolet BA, et al. Growth characteristics of infantile hemangiomas: implications for management. Pediatrics. 2008;122:360.
9. Enjolras O, Mulliken JB. The current management of vascular birthmarks. Pediatr Dermatol. 1993;10:311.
10. Martinez-Perez D, Fein NA, Boon LM, et al. Not all hemangiomas look like strawberries: uncommon presentations of the most common tumor of infancy. Pediatr Dermatol. 1995;12:1–6.
11. Nair SC, Spencer NJ, Nayak KP, Balasubramaniam K. Surgical management of vascular lesions of the head and neck: a review of 115 cases. Int J Oral Maxillofac Surg. 2011;40(6):577–83.
12. Boon LM, Mulliken JB, Enjolras O, et al. Glomuvenous malformation (glomangioma) and venous mal- formation: distinct clinicopathologic and genetic entities. Arch Dermatol. 2004;140:971.
13. Dompmartin A, Acher A, Thibon P, et al. Association of localized intravascular coagulopathy with venous malformations. Arch Dermatol. 2008;144:873.
14. Dompmartin A, Bailleux F, Thibon P, et al. Elevated D-dimer level is diagnostic for venous malformations. Arch Dermatol. 2009;145:1239–44.
15. Wouters V, Limaye N, Uebelhoer M, et al. Hereditary cutaneomucosal venous malformations are caused by TIE2 mutations with widely variable hyper- phosphorylating effects. Eur J Hum Genet. 2010;18(4):414–20.
16. Boon LM, Mulliken JB, Vikkula M, et al. Assignment of a locus for dominantly inherited venous malformations to chromosome 9p. Hum Mol Genet. 1994;3:1583.
17. Vikkula M, Boon LM, Carraway KL 3rd, et al. Vascular dysmorphogenesis caused by an activating mutation in the receptor tyrosine kinase TIE2. Cell. 1996;87:1181.
18. Mulliken JB. Vascular anomalies. In: Aston SJ, Beasley RW, Thorne CHM, editors. Grabb and Smith's plastic surgery. Philadelphia: Lippincott-Raven; 1997. p. 191–204.
19. Marler JJ, Fishman SJ, Upton J, et al. Prenatal diagnosis of vascular anomalies. J Pediatr Surg. 2002;37:318–26.
20. Tunc M, Sadri E, Char DH. Orbital lymphangioma: an analysis of 26 patients. Br J Ophthalmol. 1999;83:76–80.
21. Mulliken JB, Young A. Vascular birthmarks: hemangiomas and malformations. Philadelphia: WB Saunders; 1988.
22. Brouillard P, Vikkula M. Genetic causes of vascular malformations. Hum Mol Genet. 2007;16(Spec No. 2):R140.
23. Jacobs AH, Walton RG. The incidence of birthmarks in the neonate. Pediatrics. 1976;58:218–22.
24. Enjolras O, Riche MC, Merland JJ. Facial port-wine stains and Sturge-Weber syndrome. Pediatrics. 1985;76:48–51.
25. Limaye N, Wouters V, Uebelhoer M, et al. Somatic mutations in angiopoietin receptor gene TEK cause solitary and multiple sporadic venous malformations. Nat Genet. 2009;41:118.
26. Boon LM, Brouillard P, Irrthum A, et al. A gene for inherited cutaneous venous anomalies ("glomangiomas") localizes to chromosome 1p21-22. Am J Hum Genet. 1999;65:125.
27. Gault J, Shenkar R, Recksiek P, et al. Biallelic somatic and germ line CCM1 truncating mutations in a cerebral cavernous malformation lesion. Stroke. 2005;36:872.
28. Pagenstecher A, Stahl S, Sure U, et al. A two-hit mechanism causes cerebral cavernous malformations: complete inactivation of CCM1, CCM2 or CCM3 in affected endothelial cells. Hum Mol Genet. 2009;18:911.
29. Shendure J, Balasubramanian S, Church GM, et al. DNA sequencing at 40: past, present and future. Nature. 2017;550:345–53.
30. Padia R, Zenner K, Bly R, Bennett J, Bull C, Perkins J. Clinical application of molecular genetics in lymphatic malformations. Laryngoscope Investig Otolaryngol. 2019;4(1):170–3.
31. Greene AK, Goss JA. Vascular anomalies: from a clinicohistologic to a genetic framework. Plast Reconstr Surg. 2018;141:709e–17e.
32. Kinross KM, Montgomery KG, Kleinschmidt M. An activating PIK3CA mutation coupled with Pten loss is sufficient to initiate ovarian tumorigenesis in mice. J Clin Invest. 2012;122:553–7.
33. Samuels Y, Wang Z, Bardelli A. High frequency of mutations of the PIK3CA gene in human cancers. Science. 2004;304:554.
34. Samuels Y, Ericson K. Oncogenic PI3K and its role in cancer. Curr Opin Oncol. 2006;18:77–82.
35. Luks VL, Kamitaki N, Vivero MP. Lymphatic and other vascular malformative/overgrowth disorders are caused by somatic mutations in PIK3CA. J Pediatr. 2015;166(1048–1054):e1041–5.

36. Keppler-Noreuil KM, Rios JJ, Parker VE. PIK3CA-related overgrowth spectrum (PROS): diagnostic and testing eligibility criteria, differential diagnosis, and evaluation. Am J Med Genet A. 2015;167A:287–95.
37. Balakrishnan K, Menezes MD, Chen BS, Magit AE, Perkins JA. Primary surgery vs primary sclerotherapy for head and neck lymphatic malformations. JAMA Otolaryngol Head Neck Surg. 2014;140:41–5.
38. Odeyinde SO, Kangesu L, Badran M. Sclerotherapy for vascular malformations: complications and a review of techniques to avoid them. J Plast Reconstr Aesthet Surg. 2013;66:215–23.
39. Vignot S, Faivre S, Aguirre D, Raymond E. mTOR-targeted therapy of cancer with rapamycin derivatives. Ann Oncol. 2005;16:525–37.
40. Sasongko TH, Ismail NF, Zabidi-Hussin Z. Rapamycin and rapalogs for tuberous sclerosis complex. Cochrane Database Syst Rev. 2016;7:CD011272.
41. Alemi AS, Rosbe KW, Chan DK, Meyer AK. Airway response to sirolimus therapy for the treatment of complex pediatric lymphatic malformations. Int J Pediatr Otorhinolaryngol. 2015;79:2466–9.
42. Cramer SL, Wei S, Merrow AC, Pressey JG. Gorham-Stout disease success- fully treated with Sirolimus and zoledronic acid therapy. J Pediatr Hematol Oncol. 2016;38:e129–32.
43. Dvorakova V, Rea D, O'Regan GM, Irvine AD. Generalized lymphatic anomaly successfully treated with long-term, low-dose Sirolimus. Pediatr Dermatol. 2018;35(4):533–4.
44. Lackner H, Karastaneva A, Schwinger W, et al. Sirolimus for the treatment of children with various complicated vascular anomalies. Eur J Pediatr. 2015;174:1579–84.
45. Laforgia N, Schettini F, De Mattia D, Martinelli D, Ladisa G, Favia V. Lymphatic malformation in newborns as the first sign of diffuse lymphangiomatosis: successful treatment with sirolimus. Neonatology. 2016;109:52–5.
46. Lagreze WA, Joachimsen L, Gross N, Taschner C, Rossler J. Sirolimus-induced regression of a large orbital lymphangioma. Orbit. 2018;38:1–2.
47. Yesil S, Tanyildiz HG, Bozkurt C, Cakmakci E, Sahin G. Single-center experience with sirolimus therapy for vascular malformations. Pediatr Hematol Oncol. 2016;33:219–25.
48. Yesil S, Bozkurt C, Tanyildiz HG, et al. Successful treatment of macroglossia due to lymphatic malformation with sirolimus. Ann Otol Rhinol Laryngol. 2015;124:820–3.
49. Strychowsky JE, Rahbar R, O'Hare MJ, Irace AL, Padua H, Trenor CC 3rd. Sirolimus as treatment for 19 patients with refractory cervicofacial lymphatic malformation. Laryngoscope. 2018;128:269–76.
50. Czechowicz JA, Long-Boyle JR, Rosbe KW, Mathes EF, Frieden IJ, Shimano KA. Sirolimus for management of complex vascular anomalies - A proposed dosing regimen for very young infants. Int J Pediatr Otorhino Laryngol. 2018;105:48–51.
51. Venot Q, Blanc T, Rabia SH. Targeted therapy in patients with PIK3CA-related overgrowth syndrome. Nature. 2018;558:540–6.
52. Balakrishnan K, Bauman N, Chun RH, et al. Standardized outcome and reporting measures in pediatric head and neck lymphatic malformations. Otolaryngol Head Neck Surg. 2015;152:948–53.
53. Mulliken JB, Fishman DJ. Mulliken and Young's vascular anomalies: hemangiomas and malformations. 2nd ed. New York: Oxford University Press; 2013.
54. Queisser A, Boon LM, MD, Vikkula M. Etiology and genetics of congenital vascular lesions. Otolaryngol Clin N Am. 2018;51:41–53.
55. Boscolo E, Limaye N, Huang L, et al. Rapamycin improves TIE2-mutated venous malformation in murine model and human subjects. J Clin Invest. 2015;125(9):3491–504.
56. Adams DM, Trenor CC 3rd, Hammill AM. Efficacy and safety of Sirolimus in the treatment of complicated vascular anomalies. Pediatrics. 2016;137(2):e20153257.
57. Welsh SJ, Corrie PG. Management of BRAF and MEK inhibitor toxicities in patients with metastatic melanoma. Ther Adv Med Oncol. 2015;7(2):122–36.
58. Tillet E, Bailly S. Emerging roles of BMP9 and BMP10 in hereditary hemorrhagic telangiectasia. Front Genet. 2014;5:456.
59. Ola R, Dubrac A, Han J, et al. PI3 kinase inhibition improves vascular malformations in mouse models of hereditary haemorrhagic telangiectasia. Nat Commun. 2016;7:13650.
60. Ardelean DS, Letarte M. Anti-angiogenic therapeutic strategies in hereditary hemorrhagic telangiectasia. Front Genet. 2015;6:35.
61. Peng HL, Yi YF, Zhou SK. Thalidomide effects in patients with hereditary hemorrhagic telangiectasia during therapeutic treatment and in Fli-EGFP trans- genic zebrafish model. Chin Med J. 2015;128(22):3050–4.
62. Thompson AB, Ross DA, Berard P, et al. Very low dose bevacizumab for the treatment of epistaxis in patients with hereditary hemorrhagic telangiectasia. Allergy Rhinol (Providence). 2014;5(2):91–5.
63. Uebelhoer M, Boon LM, Vikkula M. Vascular anomalies: from genetics toward models for therapeutic trials. Cold Spring Harb Perspect Med. 2012;2(8):a009688.

Syndromes Associated with Vascular Anomalies

3

Madanagopalan Ethunandan and Sanjiv C. Nair

Vascular anomalies encompass a spectrum of disorders that unfortunately continues to be plagued by incorrect nomenclature and misdiagnosis. Recent advances in clinical and basic research have led to better understanding of these lesions and their more appropriate categorisation. The international society for the study of vascular anomalies (ISSVA) has recently updated the classification that provides a sound framework and clarification of terminology, which can be used across the various clinical specialities [1].

Vascular anomalies are often sporadic, though in a small proportion of patients they can be associated with underlying diseases or systemic conditions. Some of the associated syndromes are well recognised, but other associations are not as well known [1–4]. Vascular lesions associated with syndromes can be difficult to treat and require long-term management plans and perspectives. In this chapter, the associated syndromes are discussed according to the presenting vascular lesion, as either vascular tumours or malformations, in accordance with the recently updated ISSVA classification.

M. Ethunandan (✉)
Oral & Maxillofacial Surgery, University Hospital Southampton, Southampton, UK

S. C. Nair
Department of Maxillofacial Surgery, B.M. Jain Hospital, Bangalore Institute of Dental Science, Bangalore, Karnataka, India

3.1 Syndromes Associated with Vascular Tumours

3.1.1 PHACE Syndrome (Fig. 3.1)

Pascual-Castroveijo in 1978, described a series of seven patients with vascular and non-vascular intracranial malformations associated with external capillary haemangiomas [5]. Freiden et al. in

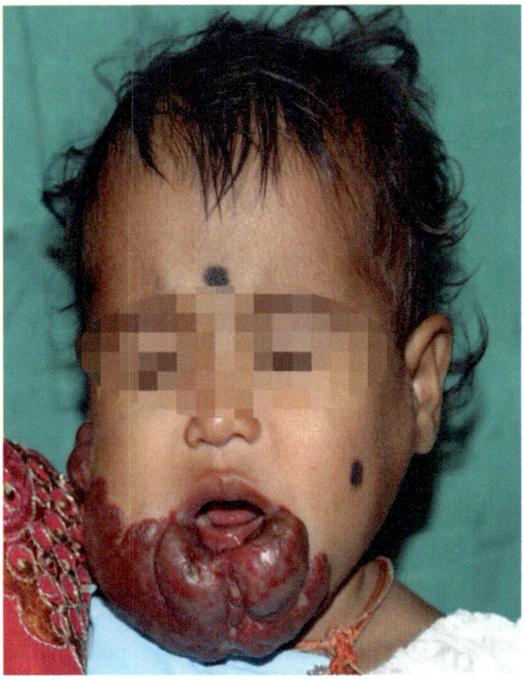

Fig. 3.1 Phace syndrome - Large segmental facial haemangioma

S. C. Nair, S. R. Chandra (eds.), *Management of Head and Neck Vascular Lesions*,
https://doi.org/10.1007/978-981-15-2321-2_3

1996 reported PHACE syndrome, an acronym that encompassed posterior fossa malformations, haemangiomas, arterial anomalies, cardiovascular anomalies, eye anomalies, and sternal defects [6]. The haemangiomas are infantile haemangiomas, often occurring in the face and neck, segmental in distribution and over 5 cm in diameter. Posterior fossa anomalies include Dandy-Walker malformations and ventricular dilatation. Cardiac anomalies include coarctation of the aorta, atrial septal defect, and ventricular septal defects. Eye anomalies include cataract, glaucoma, microphthalmos, and optic nerve hypoplasia. A recent multi-specialty consensus document (Table 3.1) provides updated diagnostic criteria and care recommendations [7]. In patients with a large head and neck/face haemangiomas more than 5 cm should be evaluated for PHACE. Patients with smaller haemangiomas with characteristic/major criteria and those without haemangiomas, but with major cri-

Table 3.1 PHACE syndrome—Revised diagnostic criteria [7]

Organ system	Major criteria	Minor criteria
Arterial anomalies	Anomaly of major cerebral or cervical arteries* Dysplasia of the large cerebral arteries# Arterial stenosis or occlusion with or without moyamoya collaterals Absence or moderate–severe hypoplasia of the large cerebral and cervical arteries Aberrant origin or course of the large cerebral or cervical arteries except common variants such as bovine arch Persistent carotid–vertebrobasilar anastomosis (proatlantal segmental, hypoglossal, otic and/or trigeminal arteries)	Aneurysm of any of the cerebral arteries
Structural brain	Posterior fossa brain anomalies Dandy-Walker complex Other hypoplasia/dysplasia of the mid and/or hindbrain	Midline brain anomalies Malformation of cortical development
Cardiovascular	Aortic arch anomalies Coarctation of the aorta Dysplasia Aneurysm Aberrant origin of the subclavian artery with or without a vascular ring	Ventricular septal defect Right aortic arch/double aortic arch Systemic venous anomalies
Ocular	Posterior segment abnormalities Persistent hyperplastic primary vitreous Persistent foetal vasculature Retinal vascular anomalies Morning glory disc anomaly Optic nerve hypoplasia Peripapillary staphyloma	Anterior segment abnormalities Microphthalmia Sclerocornea Coloboma Cataracts
Ventral/midline	Anomaly of the midline chest and abdomen Sternal defect Sternal pit Sternal cleft Supraumbilical raphe	
Definite PHACE		
Haemangioma >5 cm in diameter of the head including scalp PLUS 1 major criteria or 2 minor criteria Haemangioma of the neck, upper trunk or trunk and proximal upper extremity PLUS 2 major criteria		
Possible PHACE		
Haemangioma >5 cm in diameter of the head including the scalp PLUS 1 minor criteria Haemangioma of the neck, upper trunk or trunk and proximal upper extremity PLUS 1 major or 2 minor criteria No haemangioma PLUS 2 major criteria		

*Internal carotid artery, middle cerebral artery, anterior cerebral artery, posterior cerebral artery or vertebrobasilar system

#Includes kinking, looping, tortuosity and/or dolichoectasia teria, should also be evaluated. Screening tests include a thorough physical examination, echocardiogram, MRI/MRA of the brain, neck and aortic arch and ophthalmological examination.

3.1.2 Kasabach–Merritt Syndrome/ Phenomenon

Kasabach and Merritt in 1940 reported a case of capillary haemangioma with extensive purpura [8]. It was associated with coagulation abnormalities, reduced platelets and anaemia, causing haemorrhage, infection and multi-organ failure, leading to death in 12–24% of patients. It is now recognised that patients with Kaposiform hemangioendothelioma or tufted angiomas, but not infantile haemangiomas or malformations develop Kasabach–Merritt phenomenon (KMP) [9]. Abnormal platelet activation and aggregation may occur secondary to interaction with the abnormal tumour endothelium resulting in localised trapping of the platelets and consumption of clotting factors [10]. Kaposiform hemangioendothelioma involving more than one anatomic site, invading underlying muscle, bone, retroperitoneum and thoracic cavity are more often associated with increased incidence of KMP [11]. Outcomes have significantly improved and current management includes excision of the lesion, steroids, interferon, vincristine and radiotherapy.

3.2 Syndromes Associated with Capillary Malformations

3.2.1 Sturge–Weber Syndrome (Fig. 3.2a, b)

Sturge–Weber Syndrome (SWS) is characterised by a dermal capillary malformation occurring in association with vascular malformations of the

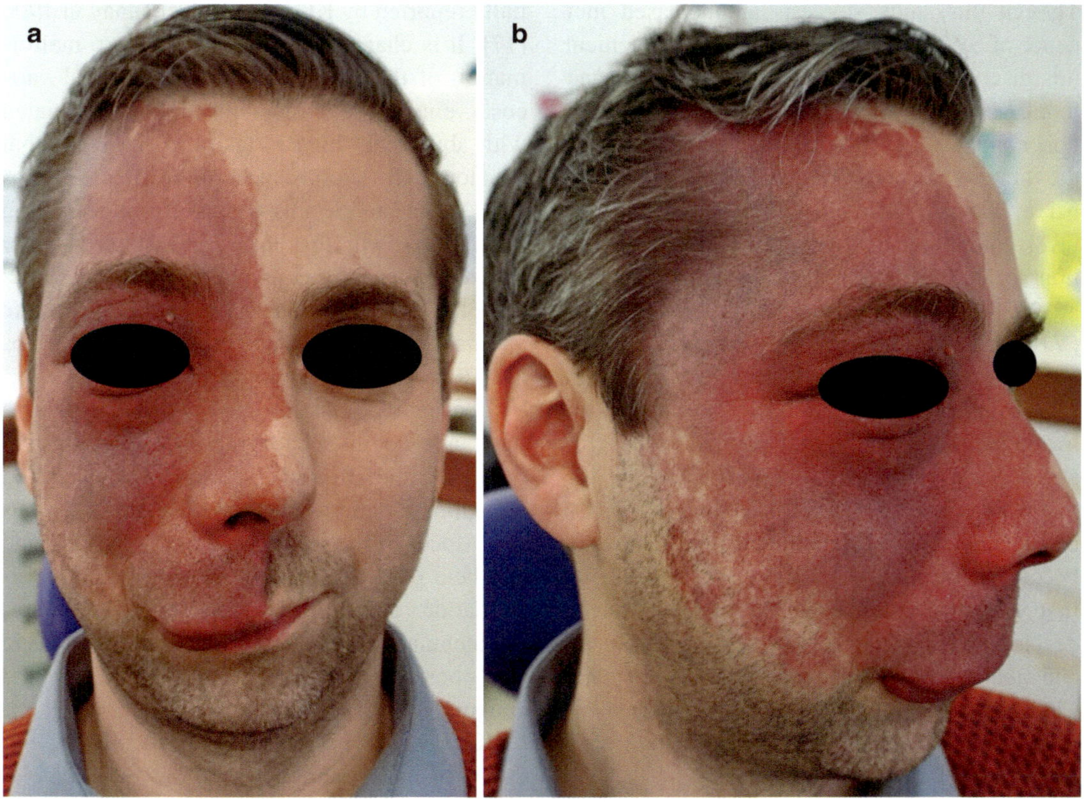

Fig. 3.2 (**a, b**) Sturge Weber Syndrome Frontal and lateral view- Capillary malformation affecting dermatomes supplied by the first and second divisions of the trigeminal nerve. Tissue hypertrophy in long standing lesions

leptomeninges and the eye. It was initially described by Sturge in 1879 and further characterised by Weber in 1922 [12, 13]. It typically includes a triad of facial dermal capillary malformation, ipsilateral central nervous syndrome vascular malformations (leptomeningeal angiomatosis), and vascular malformations of the choroid of the eye associated with glaucoma. Partial forms with eye and meningeal lesions without skin lesions and skin and eye lesions without meningeal lesions have been described, but all three features are required to be considered as having SWS [14].

The risk of SWS is determined by the distribution of the capillary malformations. SWS occurs exclusively in patients whose capillary malformations are located in the distribution of the first division (ophthalmic) of the trigeminal nerve. Talman et al. [15] found ocular and CNS abnormalities occurred exclusively in patients with capillary malformations involving the upper and lower eyelids (91%) or lower eyelids (9%). Though this study suggests an increased incidence of SWS with second division involvement, this discrepancy could be attributed to the anatomic variability of the "watershed" area of the upper and lower eyelids that can be innervated by the first or second division of the trigeminal nerve. The overall incidence of ocular or CNS involvement in patients with capillary malformation located in the first or second division is around 8%, but higher when multiple dermatomes (V1, V2, V3) or bilateral involvement (24%).

Leptomeningeal vascular malformations are most often present over the occipital lobes, followed by the temporal and parietal lobes [16]. Seizures are the most common neurologic abnormality associated with SWS and occur in 55–90% of patients. They are frequently focal but can become generalised and often occur within the first year of life. Most patients achieve normal developmental milestones in the first year of life and about 50% continue to develop normally. Those with extensive leptomeningeal involvement and seizures refractory to treatment are at a higher risk of developmental delay.

Glaucoma is the most common ophthalmologic abnormality seen in patients with SWS. It is associated with ipsilateral vascular malformation of the choroidal vasculature of the eye, though it can present on the contralateral side. Glaucoma is often present at birth in about two-thirds of patients, though it can arise at a later date. All patients with capillary malformations of the eyelids should be evaluated periodically for glaucoma, as early identification and management may prevent blindness.

SWS should be suspected in all patients with capillary malformations affecting the first division of the trigeminal nerve. Regular ophthalmological examination should be carried out to evaluate and manage glaucoma. Neurological development should also be monitored and seizures managed appropriately. Cutaneous capillary malformations can be managed by pulsed dye laser.

3.2.2 Klippel–Trenaunay Syndrome

Klippel–Trenaunay Syndrome (KTS) was initially reported by Klippel and Trenaunay in 1900 [17]. It is characterised by (1) capillary malformation of the lower limbs, (2) congenital varicose veins or venous malformations associated with abnormal, dilated "lateral megaveins" that develop in the lateral aspect of the affected limbs and (3) bone and soft tissue hypertrophy resulting from overgrowth. Just one limb is affected in over 75% of patients, though in a few the upper limb or both lower limbs can be affected. Lymphatic anomalies can also occur in the affected limbs [18–20].

The capillary malformation may be distributed in a confluent geographic pattern or randomly on the affected limb and adjacent trunk. Geographic patterns are often located in the lateral aspect of the thigh, knee and lower leg and can be a predictor of associated lymphatic malformation and complications of KTS. Life-threatening complications include deep vein thrombosis, pulmonary embolism, sepsis and coagulopathy [18–20].

KTS should be suspected in all infants with capillary malformations involving the limbs. If KTS is diagnosed, regular monitoring of the leg length is mandatory. It is important to look out for a high-flow arteriovenous malformation, to rule out Parkes Weber syndrome. The venous anomalies are often managed conservatively with elastic support garments. Surgery may be required in selected patients.

3.2.3 Rubinstein–Taybi Syndrome (Fig. 3.3a, b)

Rubinstein and Taybi in 1963 reported a condition characterised by mental retardation, growth retardation, broad thumbs, large toes and a typical facial appearance [21]. Though no specific diagnostic criteria have been established, a variety of additional features have been reported [22]. Skin manifestations included capillary malformations, hirsutism, keloid and excessive scar formation, and café au lait macules. Oral manifestations include thin upper lip, small oral opening, retro/micrognathia and high arched narrow palate. Cleft uvula and palate can be part of the syndrome. Dental anomalies include hypodontia, hyperdontia and natal teeth. Talon cusps were present in 73% of patients and 92% of permanent teeth. Two or more talon cusps are rarely found in the normal population and this finding supports the diagnosis of Rubinstein–Taybi syndrome, when this is suspected [23].

3.2.4 Beckwith–Wiedemann Syndrome (Fig. 3.4a, b, c)

Beckwith–Wiedemann syndrome is characterised by gigantism, omphalocele (exomphalos) and macroglossia [24, 25]. Predisposition to tumours in childhood (Wilms', rhabdomyosarcoma, hepatoblastoma, adrenal tumours) posterior helical pits, hypoglycaemia / hyperinsulinism and facial capillary malformations also occur as a part of the syndrome. Many of the cases are sporadic, though a familial autosomal dominant inheritance has been associated with this syndrome. A recent international consensus document has set out recommendations (Table 3.2) for clinical and molecular diagnoses, screening and management [26]. It is the most common (epi)genetic overgrowth-cancer predisposition disorder. An understanding of the genetic inheritance and specific mechanisms for tumorigenesis will assist in genetic counselling, early tumour detection and prognostic determination.

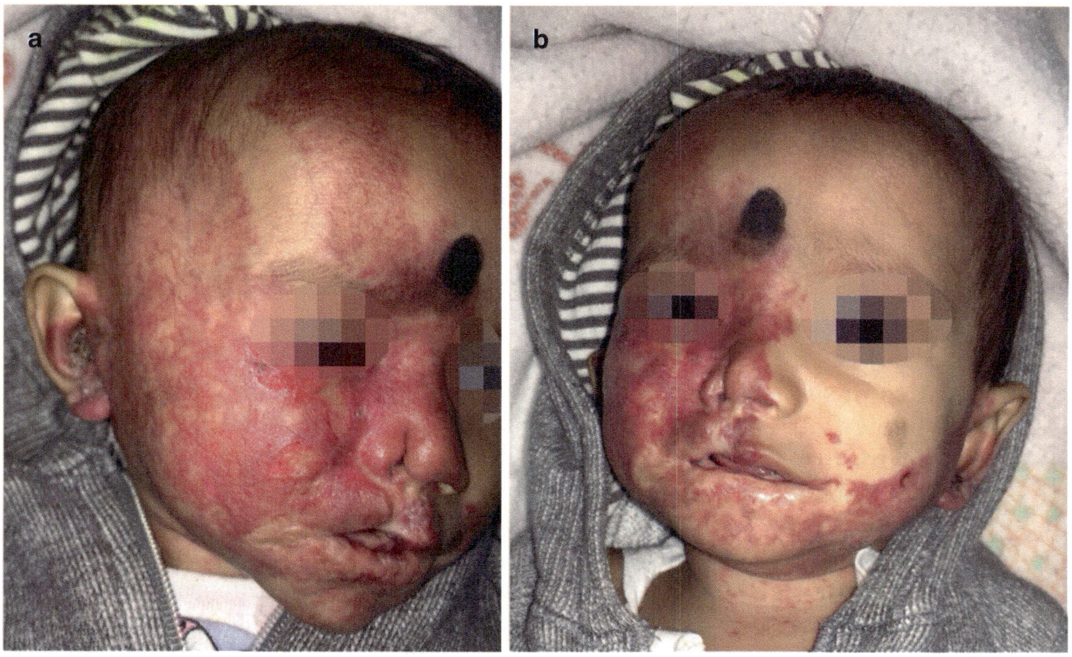

Fig. 3.3 (**a, b**) Rubinstein-Taybi syndrome - Infantile hemangioma involving V1, V2, V3 divisions of trigeminal nerve with cleft lip and nose

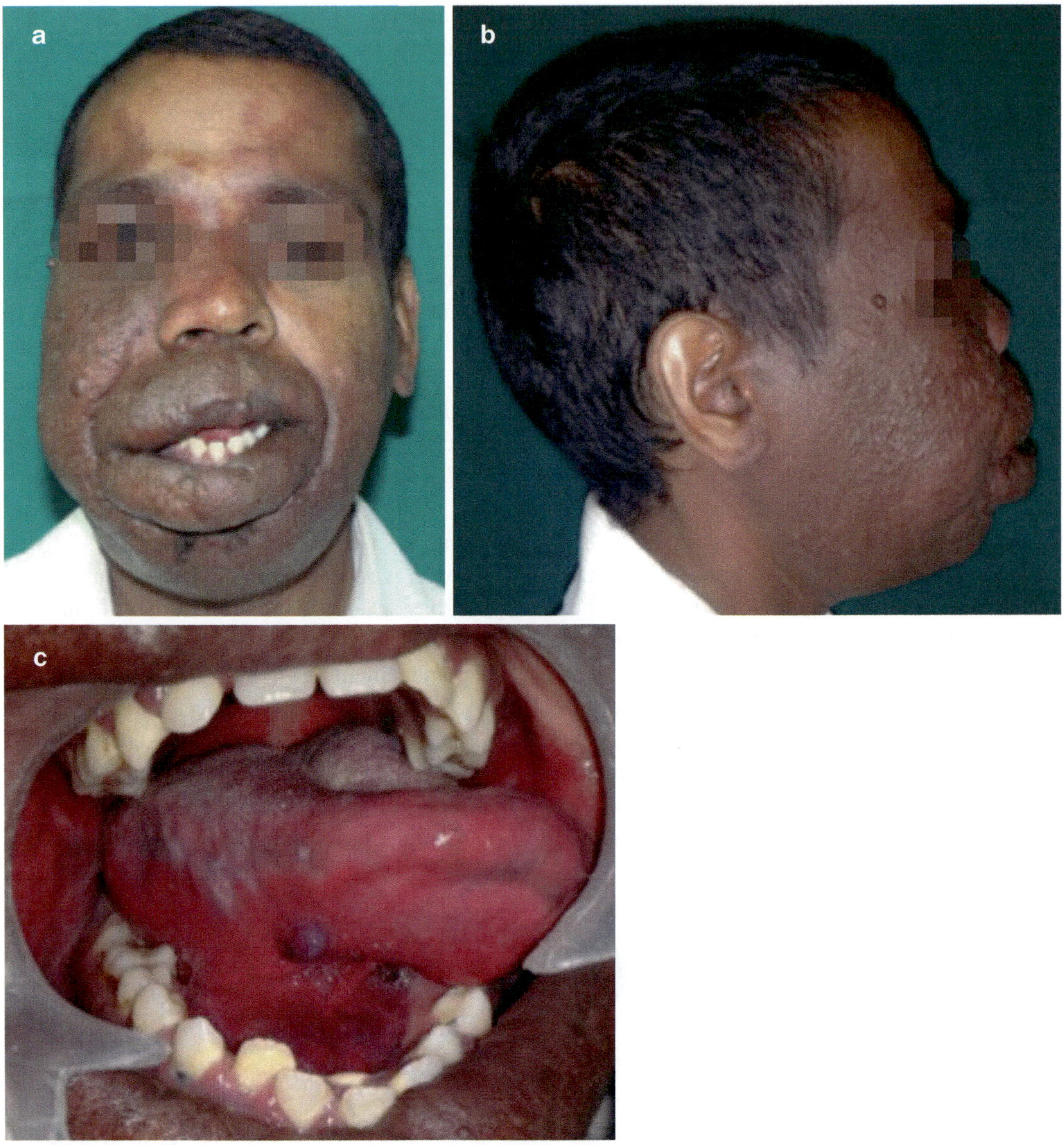

Fig. 3.4 Beckwith - Wiedmann Syndrome - Capillary malformation with tissue hypertrophy and macroglossia

3.3 Syndromes Associated with Low-flow Venous Malformations, Lymphatic Malformations or Mixed Malformations

3.3.1 Blue Rubber Bleb Nevus Syndrome (Fig. 3.5)

Gascoyne in 1860 reported a vascular malformation in the parotid region complicated by haemorrhage of the gastrointestinal (GI) tract [27]. Bean in 1958 reported additional cases and reviewed the literature and coined the term "blue rubber bleb nevus syndrome" to describe the classical skin and gastrointestinal tract findings [28].

The typical findings are compressible blue subcutaneous venous malformations ranging in size from 0.1 cm to 5.0 cm. They are often present at birth or early childhood and become more obvious and numerous as the patients become older. They can be present in any part of the skin

Table 3.2 Beckwith–Wiedemann syndrome—diagnostic criteria [26]

Cardinal features (2 points per feature)
Macroglossia
Exomplalos
Lateralised overgrowth
Multifocal and /or bilateral Wilms' tumour or nephroblastomatosis
Hyperinsulinism (lasting >1 week and requiring escalated treatment)
Pathology findings: Adrenal cortex cytomegaly, placental mesenchymal dysplasia or pancreatic adenomatosis
Suggestive features (1 point per feature)
Birth weight > 2 SDS above mean
Facial naevus simplex
Polyhydramnios and /or placentomegaly
Ear creases and/or pits
Transient hypogylcaemia (lasting <1 week)
Typical BWSp tumours (neuroblastoma, rhabdomyosarcoma, unilateral Wilms' tumour, hepatoblastoma, adrenocortical carcinoma or phaeochromocytoma)
Nephromegaly and/or hepatomegaly
Umbilical hernia and / or diastasis recti

For clinical diagnosis of classical Beckwith–Wiedemann syndrome (BWS), a patient requires a score of ≥4 (this clinical diagnosis does not require the molecular confirmation of an 11p15 anomaly). Patients with a score of ≥2 (including those with classical BWS with a score of ≥4) merit genetic testing for investigation and diagnosis of BWS. Patients with a score of <2 do not meet the criteria for genetic testing. Patients with a score of ≥2 with negative testing should be considered for an alternative diagnosis and/or referral to a BWS expert for further evaluation

BWSp Beckwith–Wiedemann spectrum, *SDS* standard deviation scores

and mucosa, including the scalp, but are more commonly located in the trunk and extremities.

Gastrointestinal venous malformations most commonly affect the small intestine and colon, though the entire bowel may be affected. Lesions may also be found in the orbit, genitourinary tract and central nervous system. GI lesions may present as chronic anaemia, abdominal pain, rectal bleeding and intussusception.

Blue rubber bleb syndrome should be considered in patients who present with multiple cutaneous venous malformations and patients should undergo evaluation for GI tract involvement and anaemia. Cutaneous lesions can be managed by carbon dioxide lasers, sclerotherapy and surgical excisions. GI lesions may be treated by endoscopic Argon or Nd:YAG lasers or surgical excision.

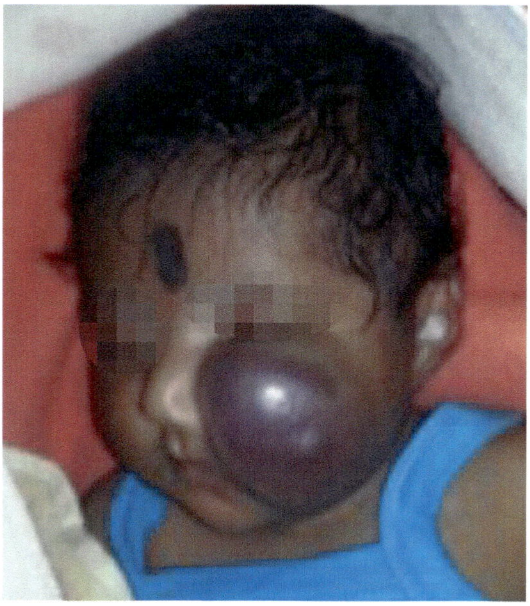

Fig. 3.5 Blue Rubber Bleb Nevus Syndrome (Compressible blue subcutaneous venous malformation from birth)

3.3.2 Parkes Weber Syndrome

Parkes Weber in 1907 described a vascular lesion with hemihypertrophy. It is characterised by overgrowth of the limb (usually lower) with diffuse arteriovenous fistulas and shunts. The arteriovenous fistulas often develop around puberty and can be complicated by high-output congestive cardiac failure. Lymphatic anomalies and lymphoedema may be present. It should be differentiated from Klippel–Trenaunay syndrome, the latter being associated with low-flow vascular malformations.

3.3.3 Proteus Syndrome (Figs. 3.6, 3.7)

Wiedemann et al. in 1983 described a disorder characterised by hypertrophy of the hands and feet, pigmented nevi, hemihypertrophy, skull and visceral abnormalities [29]. They named it Proteus syndrome after the Greek god, who could change his shape. Patients subsequently reported in the literature had very variable features, raising concerns about misdiagnosis. In 2004, specific

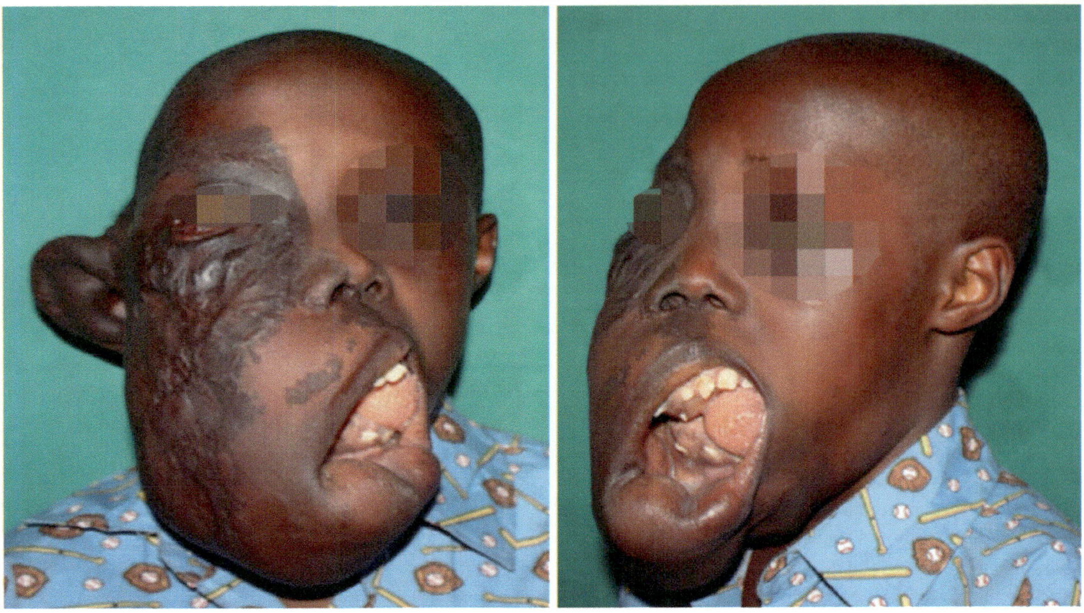

Fig. 3.6 Proteus syndrome - Typical facies - Hemihypertrophy of the face, lymhovenous malformations

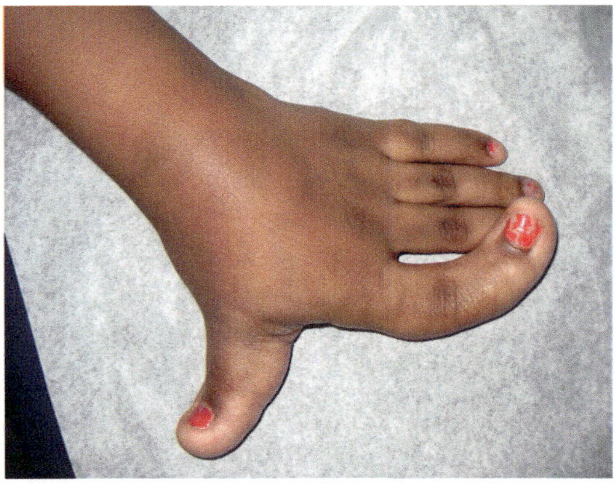

Fig. 3.7 Proteus syndrome - Asymmetric disproportionate growth of the digits. Adapted from

criteria (Table 3.3) were established for diagnosing Proteus syndrome [30]. The general characteristics of a sporadic occurrence, mosaic distribution of lesion, and a progressive clinical course are mandatory. Clinical features include connective tissue nevus of the palms and soles, epidermal nevus, disproportionate overgrowth, parotid monomorphic adenomas or ovarian cystadenomas before the second decade of life, lipomas or localised absence of fat and vascular malformations (venous, capillary, lymphatic). The characteristic facial features of dolichocephaly, long face, down slanting palpebral fissures, low nasal bridge and open bite have also been reported.

Joseph Merrick, who exhibited himself as the "elephant man" and whose story subsequently led to many medical articles, books and a movie by David Lynch, is now considered to have been affected by Proteus syndrome, rather than neurofibromatosis.

The diagnosis is currently based on satisfying the revised diagnostic criteria.

3.3.4 Maffucci Syndrome

Initially described by Maffucci in 1881, the disorder is characterised by enchondromatosis and multiple low flow vascular (mainly venous and rarely lymphatic) malformations [31].

It often manifests in early childhood with multiple superficial and deep venous malformations

Table 3.3 Proteus syndrome—Revised diagnostic criteria [30]

General criteria	Specific criteria
All the following: Mosaic distribution of lesions Sporadic occurrence Progressive course	Either category A (or) Two from category B (or) Three from category C A. 1. Cerebriform connective tissue nevus* B. 1. Linear epidermal nevus 2. Asymmetric, disproportionate growth# One or more (a) Limbs: Arms/legs Hands/feet/digits Extremities (b) Hyperostoses of the skull (c) External auditory meatus (d) Megaspondylodysplasia (e) Viscera Spleen/thymus 3. Specific tumours before the 2nd decade One of the following: (a) Ovarian cystadenoma (b) Parotid monomorphic adenoma C. 1. Dysregulated adipose tissue Either one: (a) Lipomas (b) Regional absence of fat 2. Vascular malformations One or more (a) Capillary malformation (b) Venous malformation (c) Lymphatic malformation 3. Lung cysts 4. Facial phenotypes+ All (a) Dolichocephaly (b) Long face (c) Down slanting palpebral fissures and/or minor ptosis (d) Low nasal bridge (e) Wide or anteverted nares (f) Open mouth at rest

To make a diagnosis of Proteus syndrome (PS), one must have all the general criteria and various specific criteria

*Cerebriform connective tissue nevi are skin lesions characterised by deep grooves and gyrations as seen on the surface of the brain

#Asymmetric, disproportionate overgrowth should be carefully distinguished from asymmetric proportionate overgrowth

+The facial phenotype has been found to date only in PS in patients who have mental deficiency and in some cases seizures and/or brain malformations

in the extremities. Oral and intra-abdominal venous and lymphatic malformations have also been reported [32, 33]. Simultaneously, endochondromas present as hard nodules in the fingers and long bones. About 30%–40% of these lesions undergo malignant transformation into chondrosarcomas. Breast, ovarian, pancreatic, parathyroid and pituitary tumours have also been reported in patients with Maffucci syndrome. Spindle cell hemangioendothelioma is commonly found beside venous nodules or intermingled with the venous malformations on pathologic sections in these patients.

Diagnosis is based on the clinical features and regular follow-up is mandatory to monitor the endochondromas and detect malignant transformation. The venous malformations are managed conservatively, unless symptomatic.

3.3.5 Gorham–Stout Syndrome (Fig. 3.8a, b)

Initially reported by Jackson in 1838 [34], Gorham and Stout in 1955 reported 24 cases characterised by vascular malformations, intraosseous vascular malformations and osteolysis [35]. This syndrome has also been termed as disappearing bone disease, phantom bone disease and diffuse skeletal haemangiomatosis. Lymphatic malformations are most common, though capillary and venous malformations have been reported. Cutaneous malformations are uncommon. Truncal bone and upper extremities are most commonly affected. Patients often present in early childhood with a pathological fracture following minor trauma. The degree of bone resorption is variable and complete resorption has been reported in several cases.

The cause has not been established and pathological analysis demonstrates a proliferation of dilated lymph channels communicating with blood vessels in the bone. When osteolytic lesion of unknown is identified, Gorham–Stout syndrome should be considered. Surgery, radiotherapy and bisphosphonates have been used in its management [36].

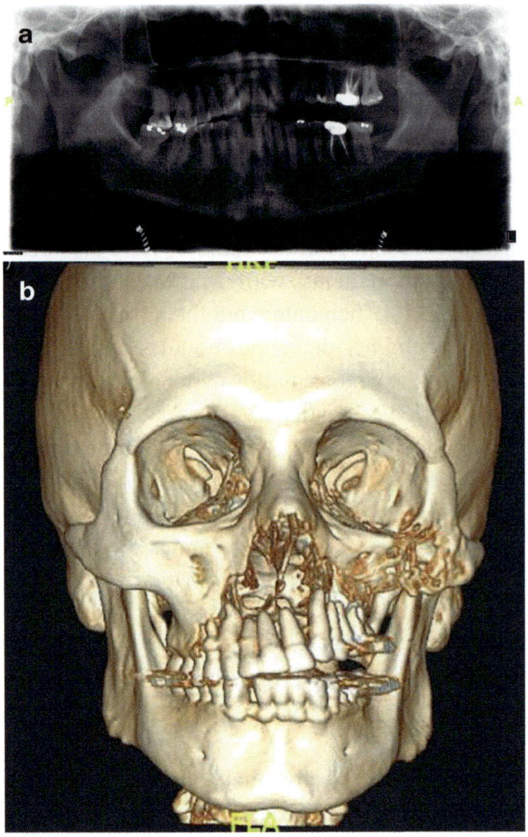

Fig. 3.8 Gorham Stout syndrome—Left facial skeleton with maxillary and zygomatic bone osteolysis. (**a**) Orthopantomograph (**b**) 3D reconstruction of the CT scan

3.4 Syndromes Associated with High-flow Vascular Malformations

3.4.1 Rendu-Osler-Weber Syndrome (Hereditary Haemorrhagic Telangiectasia)

Rendu (1896) [37], Osler 1901) [38] and Weber (1907) [39]described a hereditary disorder characterised by dilated skin and mucosal blood vessels leading to epistaxis and haemorrhage into the digestive tract (hereditary haemorrhagic telangiectasia—HHT). It is an autosomal dominant disorder affecting one to two per 100,000 people and belongs to the group of diseases with abnormal transforming growth factor-beta. Clinically it is classified into five phenotypes based on ENG, ALK or SMAD4 abnormalities: HHT1, HHT2, HHT3, HHT4 and juvenile polyposis and hereditary haemorrhagic telangiectasia (JPHT). HHT1 is the most common and is caused by the ENG mutation [40].

Telangiectasia in the nose, leading to recurrent epistaxis is often the initial presentation and occurs before the appearance of cutaneous lesions. Telangiectases are also present in the lips, oral mucosa, upper extremities, fingers and trunk. Arteriovenous malformations and fistulas in the lung, liver and central nervous system are also found in these patients. Criteria have been established for the diagnosis of HHT (Table 3.4) and people with three criteria receive a "definitive" diagnosis and those with two a "possible" diagnosis [41].

HHT should be suspected in children with multiple skin and mucosal lesions. Once established, they should be evaluated for pulmonary and other site involvement. Management of local lesions has included cautery, laser photocoagulation and sclerotherapy. Bevacizumab, when injected submucosally has also been shown to be of benefit [42].

Table 3.4 Hereditary Haemorrhagic Telangiectasia—Diagnostic criteria [41]

Criteria	Definition
Epistaxis	Spontaneous, recurrent nose bleeds
Telangiectasia	Multiple characteristic sites (lips, oral cavity, nose, fingers)
Arteriovenous malformations (AVM)	Any of the following: 1. Cerebral AVM 2. Spinal AVM 3. Pulmonary AVM 4. Hepatic AVM 5. Gastrointestinal telangiectasia (with or without bleeding)
Family history	A first-degree relative with HHT according to criteria
Definite HHT—If 3 criteria are present Possible HHT—If 2 criteria are present Unlikely HHT—If fewer than 2 criteria are present	

HHT Hereditary haemorrhagic telangiectasia

3.4.2 Bonnet–Dechume–Blanc Syndrome or Wyburn–Mason Syndrome

Bonnet et al. [43] in 1937 and Wyburn et al. [44] in 1943 reported a disorder characterised by cerebral arteriovenous malformation usually involving the midbrain, ipsilateral retinal vascular malformation and a red stain in the face, often misinterpreted as a capillary malformation. Bonnet–Dechume–Blanc syndrome and Wyburn–Mason syndrome are generally considered to be synonymous.

The cutaneous vascular malformation is not a consistent feature and when present can be unilateral and involves the skin innervated by the trigeminal nerve or central involving the mid-forehead, glabella, nose and upper lip. Patients can present with headaches and seizures. Fundoscopy and MRI can be helpful in delineating the extent of the lesions.

3.5 Summary

Recent advances have enabled this complex group of patients to be more accurately diagnosed, enabling tailored management plans. Some of these patients are at a greater risk of developing tumours and serious complications. Identifying the varying elements of syndrome complex, recognising the potential complications and liaising with the various specialities is essential to improve the management of these patients.

References

1. Wassef M, Blei F, Adams D, Alomari A, Baselga E, et al. Vascular anomalies classification: recommendations from the International Society for the Study of Vascular Anomalies. Pediatrics. 2015;136(1):1–12.
2. Garzon M, Huang J, Enjolras O, Frieden I. Vascular malformations part II: associated syndromes. J Am Acad Dermatol. 2007;56(4):541–64.
3. Nozaki T, Nosaka S, Miyazaki O, Makidono A, Yamamoto A, Niwa T, et al. Syndromes associated with vascular tumours and malformations: a pictorial review. Radiographics. 2013;33(1):175–96.
4. Blei F, Bittman M. Congenital vascular anomalies: current perspective on diagnosis, classification and management. J Vasc Diagn Interv. 2016;4:23–37.
5. Pascual-Castroviejo I. Vascular and nonvascular intracranial malformation associated with external capillary hemangiomas. Neuroradiology. 1978;16:82–4.
6. Frieden IJ, Reese V, Cohen D. PHACE syndrome: the association of posterior fossa brain malformations, hemangiomas, arterial anomalies, coarctation of the aorta and cardiac defects and eye abnormalities. Arch Dermatol. 1996;132(3):307–11.
7. Garzon MC, Epstein LG, Heyer GL, Frommet PC, Orbach DB, et al. PHACE syndrome: consensus-derived diagnosis and care recommendations. J Pediatr. 2016;178:24–33.
8. Kasabach HH, Merritt KK. Capillary hemangiomas with extensive purpura: report of a case. Am J Dis Child. 1940;59:1063–70.
9. Sarkar M, Mulliken JB, Kozakewich HP, Robertson RL, Burrows PE. Thromboctopenic coagulopathy (Kasabach-Merritt phenomenon) is associated with Kaposiform hemangioendothelioma and not with common infantile hemangioma. Plast Reconstr Surg. 1997;100(6):1377–86.
10. Hall GW. Kasabach-Merritt syndrome: pathogenesis and management. Br J Haematol. 2001;112:851–62.
11. Croteau SE, Liang MG, Kozakewich HP, Alomari AI, Fishman SJ, et al. Kaposiform hemangioendothelioma: atypical features and risks of Kasabach-Merritt phenomenon in 107 referrals. J Pediatr. 2013;162(1):142–7.
12. Sturge WA. A case of partial epilepsy apparently due to a lesion of one of the vasomotor centers of the brain. BMJ. 1879;1:704.
13. Weber FP. Right sided hemi-hypotrophy resulting from right-sided congenital spastic hemiplegia with a morbid condition of the left side of the brain revealed by radiograms. J Neurol Psychopathol. 1922;3(10):134–9.
14. Sudarsanam A, Arden-Holmes SL. Sturge-Weber syndrome: from the past to the present. Eur J Pediatr Neurol. 2014;18(3):257–66.
15. Tallman B, Tan OT, Morelli JG, Pienbrink J, Stafford TJ, Trainor S, et al. Location of port-wine stains and the likelihood of ophthalmic and/or central nervous system complications. Pediatrics. 1991;87:323–7.
16. Griffiths PD. Sturge-Weber syndrome revisited: the role of neuroradiology. Neuropediatrics. 1996;27:284–94.
17. Klippel M, Trenaunay D. Du naevus variqueux osteohypertrophique. Arch Gen Med (Paris). 1900;3:641.
18. Oduber CE, Van der Horst CM, Hennekam RC. Klippel-Trenaunay syndrome: diagnostic criteria and hypothesis on etiology. Ann Plast Surg. 2008;60(2):217–23.
19. Baskerville PA, Ackroyd JS, Lea Thomas M, Browse NL. The Klippel-Trenaunay syndrome: clinical,

radiological and haemodynamic features and management. Br J Surg. 1985;72:232–6.
20. Gloviczki P, Hollier LH, Telander RL, Kaufman B, Bianco AJ, Stickler GB. Surgical implications of Klippel-Trenaunay syndrome. Ann Surg. 1983;197:353–62.
21. Rubinstein JH, Taybi H. Broad thumbs and toes and facial abnormalities. A possible mental retardation syndrome. Am J Dis Child. 1963;105:588–608.
22. Milani D, Manzoni FMP, Pezzani L, Ajmone P, Gervasini C, et al. Rubinstein-Taybi syndrome: clinical features, genetic basis, diagnosis and management. Ital J Pediatr. 2015;41:4.
23. Hennekam RC, Van Doorne JM. Oral aspects of Rubinstein- Taybi syndrome. Am J Med Genet Suppl. 1990;6:42–7.
24. Beckwith JB. Extreme cytomegaly of the adrenal fetal cortex, ompholocele, hyperplasia of the kidneys and pancreas and Leydig-cell hyperplasia? Another syndrome in Annual Meeting of Western Society of Pediatric Research, Los Angles, California, 1963.
25. Wiedemann HR. Familial malformation complex with umbilical hernia and macroglossia – a new syndrome? J Genet Hum. 1964;13:223–32.
26. Brioude F, Kalish J, Mussa A, Foster A, Bliek J, Ferrero GB, et al. Clinical and molecular diagnosis, screening and management of Beckwith_Wiedemann syndrome: an international consensus statement. Nat Rev Endocrinol. 2018;14:229–49.
27. Gascoyen M. Case of naevus involving the parotid gland and causing death from suffocation: naevi of the viscera. Trans Pathol Soc. 1860;11:267.
28. Bean WB. Blue rubber bleb nevi of the skin and gastrointestinal tract. In: Vascular spiders and related lesions of the skin. Springfield, IL: Charles Thomas; 1958. p. 178–85.
29. Wiedemann HR, Burgio GR, Aidenhoff P. The proteus syndrome. Eur J Pediatr. 1983;140:5–12.
30. Turner JT, Cohen MM Jr, Biesecker LG. Reassessment of the proteus syndrome literature: application of diagnostic criteria to published cases. Am J Med Genet A. 2004;130:111–22.
31. Maffucci A. Di un caso di encondroma ed angioma multiplo. Mov Med Chir Nap. 1881;3:399–412.
32. McDermott AL, Dutt SN, Chavda SV, Morgan DW. Maffucci's syndrome: clinical and radiographic features of a rare condition. J Laryngol Otol. 2001;15:845–7.
33. Lee NH, Choi EH, Choi WK, Lee SH, Ahn SK. Maffucci's syndrome with oral and intestinal haemangioma. Br J Dermatol. 1999;140:968–9.
34. Jackson JB. A singular case of absorption of bone (a boneless arm). Boston Med Surg J. 1838;18:368.
35. Gorham LW, Stout AP. Massive osteolysis (acute spontaneous absorption of bone, phantom bone, disappearing bone): its relation to hemangiomatosis. J Bone Joint Surg Am. 1955;37:985–1004.
36. Liu Y, Zhong DR, Zhou PR, Lv F, Ma DD, et al. Gorham-Stout disease. Radiological, histological and clinical features of 12 cases and review of literature. Clin Rhematol. 2016;3593:813–23.
37. Rendu M. Epistaxis repetees chez un sujet porteur de petiis angiomes cutanes et muqueux. Bull Mem Soc Med Hop Paris. 1896;13:731.
38. Osler W. On a family form of recurring epistaxis associated with multiple telangiectasis of skin and mucous membranes. Bull Johns Hopkins Hosp. 1901;12:333.
39. Weber FP. Multiple hereditary developmental angiomata (telagiectases) of the skin and mucous membranes associated with recurring hemorrhages. Lancet. 1907;2:160.
40. McDonald J, Bayrak-Toydemir P, Pyeritz RE. Hereditary hemorrhagic telangiectasia: an overview of diagnosis, management and pathogenesis. Genet Med. 2011;13(7):607–16.
41. Shovlin CL, Guttmacer AE, Buscarini E, Faughnan ME, Hyland RH, et al. Diagnostic criteria for hereditary hemorrhagic telagiectasis (Rendu-Osler-Weber syndrome). Am J Med Genet. 2000;91(1):66–7.
42. Lupa MD, Wise SK. Comprehensive management of hereditary hemorrhagic telangiectasia. Curr Opin Otolaryngol Head Neck Surg. 2017;25(1):64–8.
43. Bonnet P, Dechaume J, Blanc E. L'aneurysme cirsoide de la retine (aneurysme vasemeaux). J Med Lyon. 1937;18:165–78.
44. Wyburn-Mason R. Arteriovenous aneurysm of midbrain and retina, facial nevi and mental changes. Brain. 1943;66:163–203.

Radiological Diagnosis of Head and Neck Vascular Anomalies

4

Srinivasa R. Chandra, Lei Yu, and Basavaraj Godhke

Objectives

- Review ideal sequencing of imaging in a head and neck vascular lesion.
- Variations in presentations of the lesion in head and neck.
- Lesion and anatomical appropriate imaging of a vascular lesion guidelines.
- Outlines of imaging characteristics of each vascular anomaly.

4.1 Introduction

Radiographic evaluation is useful to elucidate the locations, extent, and flow dynamics of lesions. With the advancement of diagnostic radiology, imaging is frequently and widely utilized for the diagnosis and management of vascular anomalies. Among different imaging modalities, ultrasound (US), magnetic resonance imaging (MRI), and magnetic resonance angiography (MRA) are most frequently used, especially in the pediatric population.

Computed tomography (CT) and conventional radiographs are also, though less commonly, used in certain situations compared to MRI and MRA.

Due to its invasive nature, angiogram is now often reserved for interventional planned procedures only.

4.2 Variations in the Radiological Presentations of Vascular Lesions of the Head and Neck Region

Most sporadic lesions may be different in clinical presentation compared to lesions associated with syndromes.

The senior author and editor (Chandra and Ghodke) undertook a retrospective study for reviewing medical and neuroradiology interventional records of all patients with head and neck vascular anomalies, diagnosed and/or surgically treated at the University of Washington medical system from 2006 to 2016. The exclusion criteria were patients with segmental lesions, those associated with syndromes such as Sturge-Weber, and

S. R. Chandra (✉)
Oral & Maxillofacial- Head & Neck Oncology Reconstructive Surgery, Oregon Health & Science University Portland, Portland, OR, USA
e-mail: chandrsr@ohsu.edu

L. Yu
Radiology, University of Nebraska Medical Center, Omaha, NE, USA
e-mail: Lei.yu@unmc.edu

B. Godhke
Neuroradiology and Neurosurgery, University of Washington, Seattle, WA, USA
e-mail: bggodhke@uw.edu

S. C. Nair, S. R. Chandra (eds.), *Management of Head and Neck Vascular Lesions*,
https://doi.org/10.1007/978-981-15-2321-2_4

patients with intracranial tissues or viscera involved. A total of 102 patients (Male = 52 and Female = 50) were included in the study. There were 62 patients in the vascular tumor group, and 40 patients in the vascular malformation group. The radiologic appearances varied from unilocular to multilocular, regular to irregular, and well defined to poorly defined margins. Lesion location varied with involvement of the scalp, orbits, nose, maxilla, mandible, and neck regions. Seventy-five patients were symptomatic. Forty-seven patients were surgically treated. Vascular anomalies have varied symptomatic and radiological presentations. So, it is prudent to understand based on the findings from this large study, we should be minimizing unnecessary interventions, biopsies, and therapies. We describe the most salient features of vascular anomalies in Tables 4.1 and 4.2 with ultrasound and magnetic resonance imaging. Ultrasound and MRI are the most frequently used initial review investigational procedures. Some vascular anomalies have a characteristic appearance as described in Table 4.2.

4.3 Imaging Modalities

4.3.1 Ultrasound

- Ultrasound is the first choice for an initial evaluation in most cases. It has a good spatial resolution for superficial lesions. Other advantages include lack of ionizing radiation, wide availability, and relatively low cost. Doppler study can measure blood flow direction and volume in real time, and essential for differentiating low flow from high-flow vascular malformations. High-frequency linear array transducer is preferred in most cases, however,

Table 4.1 US and MRI features of major vascular anomalies [1–8]

Vascular anomalies	US features	MRI features
Vascular tumor		
Infantile hemangioma	Heterogeneous soft tissue mass with mixed echogenicity. Proliferative phase: high vascularity (more than 5 vessels/cm^2) and low RI. Involuting phase: decreased vascularity and high RI	Proliferative phase: well-defined mass with low SI on T1WI, high SI on T2WI, intense contrast enhancement, and flow-voids on gradient echo (GRE) sequence. Involuting phase: high SI on T1WI
Congenital hemangioma	Similar to infantile hemangioma; often contains internal foci of calcifications or hemorrhage	
Low-flow vascular anomalies		
Venous	Hypoechoic cystic lesion with sinusoidal chambers and hyperechoic foci (phleboliths)	Lobulated mass with iso-to-low SI on T1WI, high SI on T2WI, delayed contrast enhancement, lack of flow voids on GRE sequence, and signal voids (phleboliths)
Lymphatic	Macrocystic: anechoic, multiloculated cystic mass, echogenic hemorrhage. Microlytic: Hyperechoic soft tissue thickening. No intracity vascular signals on Doppler	High SI on T2WI with fluid–fluid level and hypodense septations. Macrocystic: rim and septal enhancement; microcystic: no enhancement
Capillary	Clinical diagnosis only; no imaging necessary	
High-flow vascular anomalies		
AVM	Enlarged feeding arteries and dilated draining veins without soft tissue mass	Large flow voids on SE sequences. Early arterial washout and early venous enhancement

RI resistant index, *SI* signal intensity, *T1WI* T1 weighted image, *T2WI* T2 weighted image, *SE* spin echo

Table 4.2 Key features of most common vascular lesions of head and neck. Adapted from Nair et al. JMOS 2016

	US with CDUS	MRI
IH	Hyperechoic or hypoechoic Hypervascular on CDUS	Iso to intermediate signal on T1W, bright signal on T2W, high-intensity flow enhancement on gradient echo, internal flow voids, vigorous enhancement after contrast administration
RICH	Central, non-enhancing, hypodense, hypoechoic, more robust feeding vessels with large diameter than IH	T2W hyperintense component is quite prominent
NICH	Almost similar to IH	Almost similar to IH
VMs	Solid echogenic mass with phleboliths, often multispatial and compressible. Low flow or monophasic or no flow on CDUS	T1W heterogenous intermediate signal, no flow voids, T2 fast spin-echo fat-saturated or short T1 inversion recovery high signal intensity, T1W spin-echo postgadolinium enhancement
LM	Variable multicystic, multispatial masses, with or without fluid or debris levels. No flow pattern on CDUS	T1W low to intermediate signal intensity, T2W high signal intensity, T1W postgadolinium, no enhancement except within septa
AVM	Clusters of vessels with no intervening well-defined mass. High flow (arterial flow) on CDUS. Arterial and venous signals from vessels in the lesions with arterializations of venous structure	T1W and T2W sequences show serpiginous signal voids without a focal mass

US ultrasound, *CDUS* color Doppler ultrasound, *MRI* magnetic resonance imaging, *T1W* T1 weighted, *T2W* T2 weighted, *IH* infantile hemangioma, *RICH* rapidly involuting congenital hemangioma, *NICH* non-involuting congenital hemangioma, *VM* venous malformation, *LM* lymphatic malformation, *AVMs* arteriovenous malformations

depending on the size and depth of the lesion, a combination of different transducers might be required. Limited penetration of ultrasound makes it difficult to evaluate deep structures and the extension of lesions. Also, ultrasound findings are highly dependent on operator experience and thus can vary between different examiners.

4.3.2 Magnetic Resonance Imaging

- When ultrasound findings are equivocal, MRI is the next step. MRI is a favorable exam for most clinicians when evaluating very large lesions or lesions within specific locations (infraorbital or intracranial lesion, etc.) [1]. MRI not only provides valuable information about extension of disease, the depth of lesions, and internal organ involvement, but also guide treatment planning and posttreatment evaluation. MRI does not use ionizing radiation and is preferred in pediatric population. However, sedation is often required for pediatric patients during lengthy MRI exam. Spin Echo sequences and contrast enhancement patterns often provide useful information for diagnosis. MRA can provide hemodynamic information of vascular malformation and is helpful in differentiating high flow from low-flow lesions [2].

4.4 Major Imaging Finding of Vascular Tumors

4.4.1 Infantile Hemangioma

- Most infantile hemangiomas are diagnosed clinically and only a few cases require image studies. The findings vary depending on the clinical phases. In the proliferative phase, it presents as a well-defined lobular mass with high vascular activity. In the involuting phase, fatty replacement occurs with decreased vascular activity.
- Ultrasound demonstrates a well-defined soft tissue mass with variable internal echogenicity. Calcifications are rare. Color Doppler is very helpful in showing the characteristic

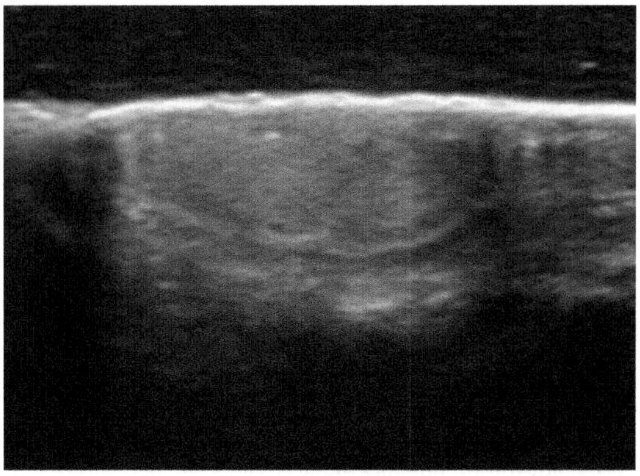

Fig. 4.1 Grayscale ultrasound shows hyperechoic subcutaneous soft tissue mass overlying the right lambdoid suture

high vascularity with both arterial and venous flow. Hypervascularity in proliferative phase is defined as more than **5 vessels per square centimeter with low resistive index** (Figs. 4.1 and 4.2). The involuting phase, on the contrary, has decreased vascularity and increased resistive index.
- MRI is mainly used for lesions involving critical organs (i.e., infraorbital or intracranial extension) or treatment planning. In the proliferative phase, lesions are well-defined with low signal intensity on T1-weighted image (T1WI), high signal intensity on T2-weighted image (T2WI), and intense contrast enhancement. In the involuting phase, there is high signal intensity on T1WI due to fatty replacement.

4.4.2 Congenital Hemangioma

- Both ultrasound and MRI findings of congenital hemangioma are similar to infantile hemangioma, characterized by soft tissue mass with hypervascularity. It often contains internal foci of calcifications or hemorrhage [1–3].

4.4.3 Kaposiform Hemangioendothelioma

- Ill-defined, infiltrating soft tissue mass with diffuse enhancement involving multiple tissue planes. Calcifications are common. Perilesional edema makes it difficult to define tumor margins. On MRI, diffuse high signal intensity on T2WI mix with foci of intermediate to low signal intensity. Feeding/draining vessels are usually smaller and along the tumor margin other than within the lesion.

4.5 Low-flow Vascular Malformations

4.5.1 Venous Malformation

- Venous malformation usually presents as an asymptomatic soft tissue mass. In imaging study, it appears as a well-defined lobulated lesion.
- Ultrasound is very useful for the evaluation of superficial lesions. It shows a characteristic hypoechoic cystic lesion with sinusoidal chambers and hyperechoic foci (phleboliths). It is compressible with low-velocity venous flow or less commonly no flow on color Doppler which confirms the venous component.
- One of the few lesions that CT could be helpful for diagnosis. The presence of phleboliths within a soft tissue mass on CT is characteristic of venous malformation (Fig. 4.3). However, CT utilizes ionizing radiation which limits the use in pediatric patients.
- MRI demonstrates a lobulated mass with iso-to-low signal intensity on T1WI, high signal intensity on T2WI due to its cystic nature, delayed contrast enhancement, and signal voids suggestive of phleboliths.

4.5.2 Lymphatic Malformation

- There are two main subtypes of lymphatic malformation, macrocystic and microcystic. Each subtype has distinguished radiologic appearances. Macrocystic lymphatic malformation is a well-defined lobulated soft tissue mass with multiple septations and fluid–fluid level. Microcystic lesion is typically an

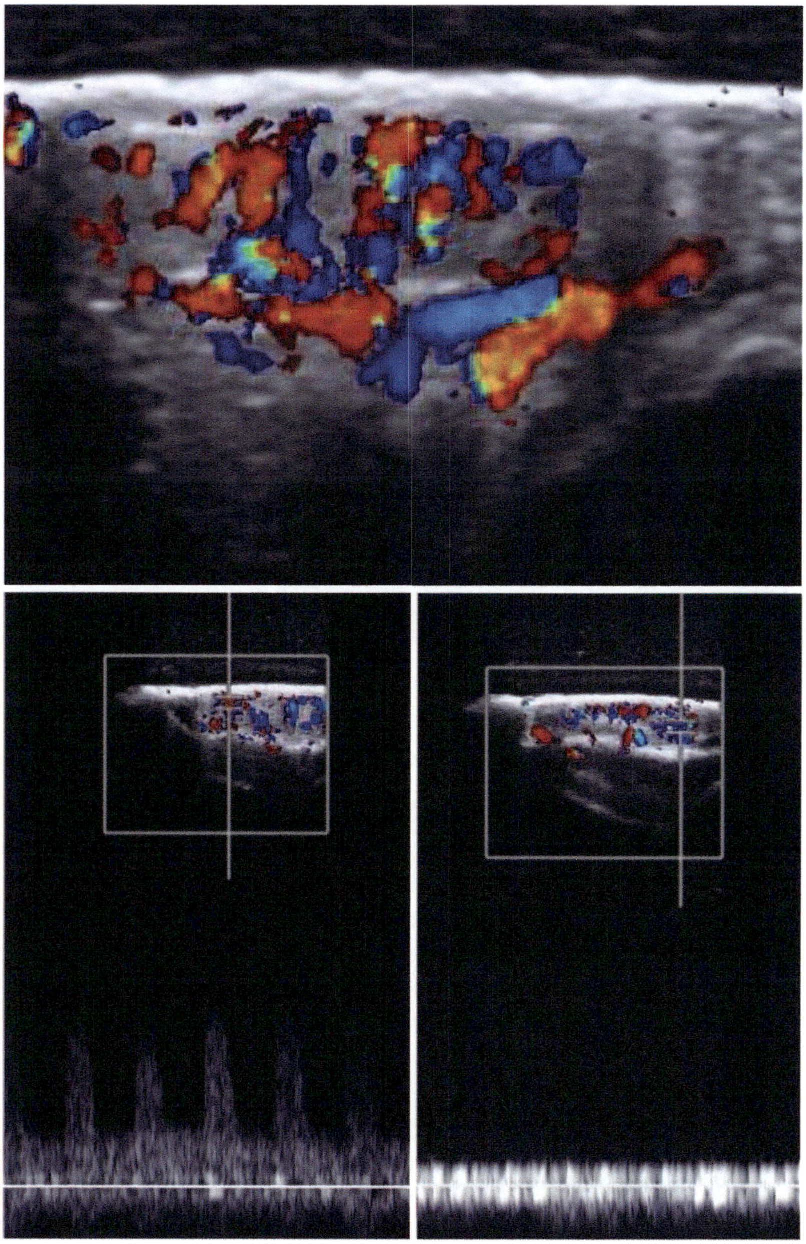

Fig. 4.2 Doppler study shows intralesional hypervascularity with both arterial and venous flow, compatible with infantile hemangioma

ill-defined, infiltrative, solid mass that involves multiple tissue planes [4, 5].

- On US, macrocystic lymphatic malformation is presented as an anechoic, multiloculated cystic mass, often with echogenic intralesional hemorrhage (Fig. 4.4). However, US often cannot show the extent of large lesions. Microcystic lymphatic malformation is often presented as an ill-defined hyperechoic soft tissue thickening. No intra-lesions vascular signals were seen on Doppler.
- On MRI, lymphatic malformation has high SI on T2WI with fluid–fluid level and hypodense thin septations (Fig. 4.5). Macrocystic and microcystic lesions have different contrast enhancement patterns. Macrocystic lesions have rim and septal enhancement while microcystic lesions have no enhancement.

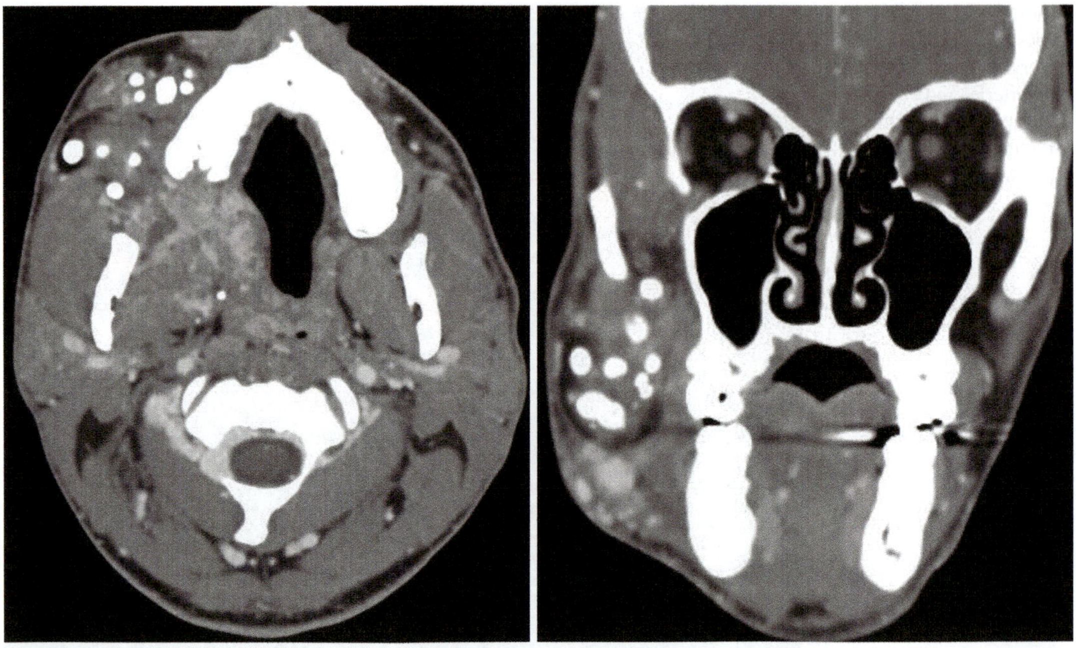

Fig. 4.3 Contrast-enhanced axial and coronal CT images show soft tissue mass with serpiginous enhancement and numerus phleboliths involving multiple compartments of the right face, suggestive of low flow lympho-venous malformation

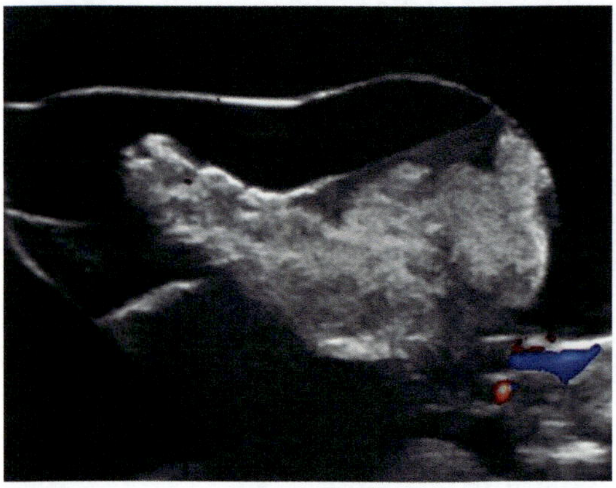

Fig. 4.4 Large multiloculated left neck mass on ultrasound with fluid–fluid level and echogenic debris from recent hemorrhage. No internal flow on color Doppler. Findings are characteristics of a macrocystic lymphatic malformation

4.5.3 Capillary Malformation

- Capillary malformation is a clinical diagnosis. Imaging is not necessary for diagnosis [4].

4.6 High-flow Vascular Malformations

4.6.1 Arteriovenous Malformation (AVM)

- Ultrasound is usually the first choice for diagnosis. Tangles of enlarged feeding arteries and dilated draining veins without discrete soft tissue mass suggest the diagnosis. The feeding arteries have low resistant waveform on color Doppler due to shunting.
- On MRI, the enlarged feeding arteries and draining veins are shown as large flow voids on echo spin sequences. AVM has a characteristic contrast enhancement pattern due to shunting. Early arterial washout and early venous enhancement are typically for AVM. Figure 4.6 depicted a T2WI MRI and CT angiogram of a large arterial venous malformation within the right frontal parasagittal white matter with tangles of enlarged feeding arteries and a large draining vein [6–8].

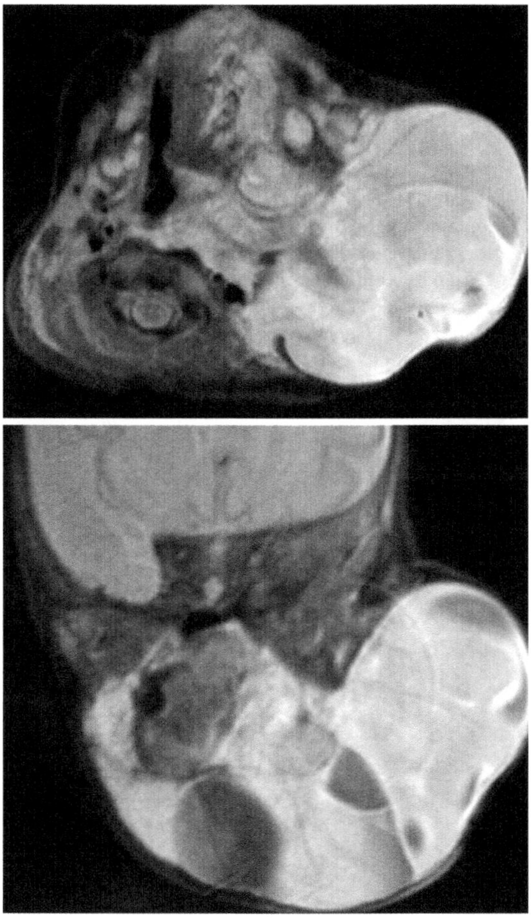

Fig. 4.5 Axial and Coronal T2-weighted MR images show a large multiloculated and multispatial left neck mass with fluid–fluid levels and associated mass effect, compatible with lymphatic malformation with recent hemorrhage

- CT Angiography or MR Angiography shows details of feeding arteries, nidus, and draining veins, and are often used for treatment planning.

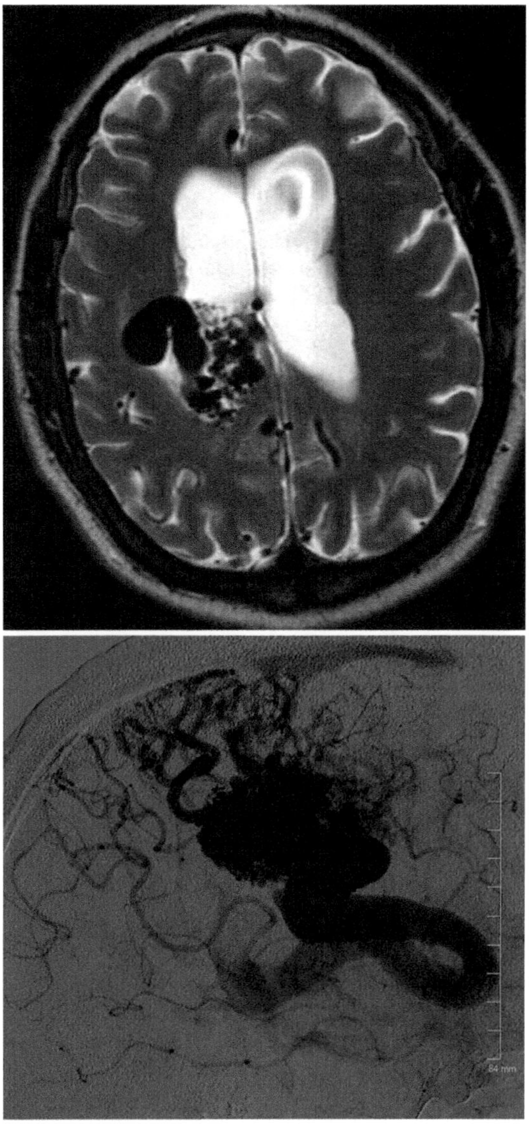

Fig. 4.6 T2WI MRI and CT angiogram show a large arterial venous malformation within the right frontal parasagittal white matter with tangles of enlarged feeding arteries and a large draining vein

References

1. Flors L, et al. MR imaging of soft-tissue vascular malformations: diagnosis, classification, and therapy follow-up. Radiographics. 2011;31(5):1321–40.
2. Navarro OM, Laffan EE, Ngan B-Y. Pediatric soft-tissue tumors and pseudo-tumors: MR imaging features with pathologic correlation: part 1. Imaging approach, pseudotumors, vascular lesions, and adipocytic tumors. Radiographics. 2009;29(3):887–906.
3. Paltiel HJ, et al. Soft-tissue vascular anomalies: utility of US for diagnosis. Radiology. 2000;214(3):747–54.
4. Merrow AC, et al. 2014 revised classification of vascular lesions from the international society for the study of vascular anomalies: radiologic-pathologic update. Radiographics. 2016;36(5):1494–516.
5. Steinklein JM, Shatzkes DR. Imaging of vascular lesions of the head and neck. Otolaryngol Clin N Am. 2018;51(1):55–76.
6. Hyodoh H, et al. Peripheral vascular malformations: imaging, treatment approaches, and therapeutic issues. Radiographics. 2005;25(suppl_1):S159–71.
7. Masand P. Radiographic findings associated with vascular anomalies. Semin Plast Surg. 2014;28(2) Thieme Medical Publishers:069–78.
8. StatDX. https://my.statdx.com

Medical Management of Vascular Lesions: Current and the Future

5

Srinivasa R. Chandra, Jagadeesh Kumar, and Sanjiv C. Nair

5.1 General Approach for Treatment

The treatment of hemangiomas should be individualized, based upon the size of the lesion(s), morphology, location, presence or possibility of complications, the potential for scarring or disfigurement, the age of the patient, and the rate of growth or involution at the time of evaluation [1, 2]. The potential risk(s) of treatment against the potential benefits is a consideration as detailed below. Medical management of infantile hemangiomas.

Consultation with a pediatric maxillofacial specialist, pediatric ophthalmologist, pediatric dermatologist, vascular anomalies team, or other knowledgeable specialists in pediatric hemangiomas with actual or potential risk for complications and when therapy is being considered [3]. Such children should be referred to as early as possible during the early proliferation phase (i.e., during the first few months of life).

S. R. Chandra (✉)
Oral & Maxillofacial- Head & Neck Oncology Reconstructive Surgery, Oregon Health & Science University Portland, Portland, OR, USA
e-mail: chandrsr@ohsu.edu

J. Kumar
Elkton Dermatology, Elkton, MD, USA

S. C. Nair
Department of Maxillofacial Surgery, B.M. Jain Hospital, Bangalore Institute of Dental Science, Bangalore, Karnataka, India

After clinical examination of the hemangioma, the family may need education regarding the natural course, potential complications; treatment indications; and risks, benefits, and expectations of available treatment options. Depending upon the type of lesion and the parents' level of concern, the patient may need to be re-evaluated frequently during the proliferative phase and again before school entry. Serial photographs of the lesion can help to monitor the clinical course.

The family's education should include information about the natural course, potential complications, treatment indications, and risks, benefits, and expectations of available treatment options for hemangiomas. Families can have realistic expectations about the duration of involution and the possibility of residual changes. The involution phase may continue up to the age of 10 years, although in some studies, complete involution has been known at a median age of 4 years [4, 5]. However, this timeline is highly variable and dependent on hemangioma size, morphology, and location. In many cases, involution does not result in normal-appearing skin. More than one-half of children with untreated hemangiomas experience residual changes such as scarring, atrophy, redundant skin, discoloration, and telangiectasia [6].

Finally, the family should have anticipatory guidance regarding responding to comments and queries from family members and strangers. Parents are commonly subject to inappropriate

S. C. Nair, S. R. Chandra (eds.), *Management of Head and Neck Vascular Lesions*,
https://doi.org/10.1007/978-981-15-2321-2_5

comments from strangers, including accusations of child abuse [7]. Other children, who are usually extremely curious about the hemangioma, are often satisfied to know that "It is a birthmark, it does not hurt, and it will get better" [7]. Addressing the psychosocial aspects of care and providing the parents' anticipatory guidance, emotional support, and reassurance is essential for the effective management of hemangiomas [1, 7].

Treatment modality depends upon the above factors and the availability of specific choices and treating clinicians' experience.

Indications for Intervention Intervention required for complicated lesions can interfere with a vital structure or function.

These include, but are not limited to:

- Very large, rapidly growing cutaneous hemangiomas.
- Lesions in the periorbital region.
- Lesions in the airway, liver, or gastrointestinal tract.

Besides, intervention indicated for lesions associated with other complications such as ulceration and increased risk of scarring or disfigurement [8]:

- Large, plaque-like segmental or nodular hemangiomas, especially in trauma-prone locations, can ulcerate, which invariably leads to scarring (Fig. 5.1a, b).
- Any lesion of the face, especially when large or segmental; hemangiomas of the lip), nose ("Cyrano nose"), and auricle are particularly prone to disfigurement.
- Large, nodular, superficial hemangiomas, especially those that exhibit a sharp, "cliff-like" border or pedunculated lesions (hemangiomas extending from a small base), have the

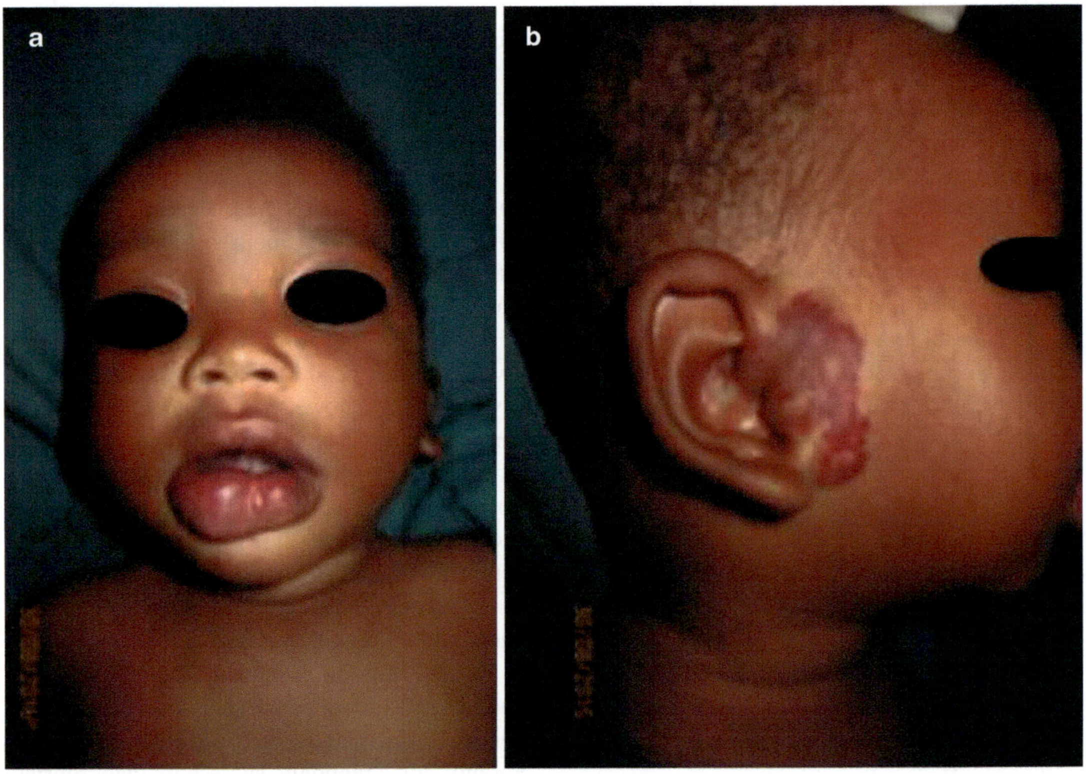

Fig. 5.1 (**a, b**) Lesions of the ear, lip, and nasal regions can cause significant deformity, including airway and vision compromise. These lesions can be amenable to medical management before surgical management. Courtesy: Dr. Amol Kulkarni, Senior Consultant OMF Surgeon, MDS, MOMS RCSEd, FIBCSOMS—ONC Kigali, Rwanda

most significant scarring risk. These lesions are also at risk for leaving residual fibrofatty tissue that may require surgical revision.

5.2 Goals of Treatment [1]

- Prevention or reversal of life-threatening or function-threatening complications.
- Prevention or minimization of a disfigurement from residual skin changes.
- Minimization of psychosocial distress for the patient and family.
- Adequate treatment of ulceration to minimize scarring, bleeding, infection, and pain.

5.3 Uncomplicated Hemangiomas

Serial observation is the mainstay of therapy for many uncomplicated, localized hemangiomas because hemangiomas involute spontaneously after the first year of life. The decision not to pursue medical and surgical therapy may not be necessarily a passive intervention since the growth and involution of the hemangiomas are monitored and the psychosocial implications, particularly facial hemangiomas, anticipated addressed [7]. Serial photographs of the lesion may be helpful to monitor the involution process and outcome.

Local Therapies Local pharmacotherapy is primarily used to treat small or superficial infantile hemangiomas and is not ideal for treating complex lesions. Data on topical therapies' efficacy, including topical beta-blockers, corticosteroids, and imiquimod, are limited.

Topical Beta-blockers Reports of successful treatment of hemangiomas with systemic propranolol led to the investigation of topical beta-blocker therapy to treat infantile hemangiomas [9, 10]. Topical beta-blockers in the treatment of small superficial hemangiomas (e.g., hemangiomas of minor cosmetic concern located on the face, small lesions in the anogenital area) as an alternative to observation, particularly if parents desire treatment.

Topical timolol gel-forming solution, 0.5%, can be used to treat lesions. One drop is applied two to three times per day for 6 to 12 months or until stable improvement.

A systemic review has espoused topical propranolol 1% or topical timolol 0.5% efficacy. And meta-analysis and a large retrospective cohort study [11, 12]. Topical timolol is generally well tolerated. However, data on its safety are limited.

- A retrospective study of 22 high-risk infants (young or preterm infants, infants were receiving more than two drops/day, or infants receiving application to a site with potential increased systemic absorption) with hemangiomas predominantly located in the periocular area treated with topical timolol. They received continuous cardiac monitoring for at least 24 hours [13]. Two infants developed symptomatic bradycardia associated with apnea or hypothermia requiring discontinuation of timolol; both were preterm (weighing <2500 grams) and had a history of symptomatic bradycardia before the initiation of timolol treatment.

High-potency topical corticosteroids (e.g., clobetasol propionate cream) have been used in the past for small, superficial hemangiomas at risk for ulceration or small periocular lesions [14]. They are now infrequently used since the introduction of topical timolol. Topical corticosteroids may be helpful for the treatment of minor but recurrent ulcerations. Adverse effects of long-term use of topical corticosteroids include skin atrophy, hypopigmentation, and hypertrichosis.

The use of intralesional corticosteroids such as triamcinolone acetonide 10 to 40 mg/mL is limited to small, well-localized, deep hemangiomas [15]. Individual doses should not exceed 3 mg/kg. A response usually is noted within two weeks, with the continued response over the ensuing six to eight weeks [16]. Serial injections administered at four-week intervals are sometimes needed.

Adverse effects of intralesional corticosteroids most commonly include local skin atrophy from leaks or inadvertent application to the normal surrounding skin. Adrenal suppression from systemic absorption is also possible, even with localized use [17–19].

5.3.1 Orbital, Mucosal and Maxillofacial Vascular Tumors/Infantile Hemangiomas

Orbital, mucosal, airway, and maxillofacial vascular lesions with rapid growth can cause significant ulceration, bleeding, pain, secondary infection, significant anatomical asymmetry, and psychological effects on the infant and the parents. Many of these infants and children need an inpatient setting. Especially considering cardiovascular or syndromic correlations need care too. Adequate care is taken as the skin is thin in infants. Desiccated mucosa can ulcerate, and topical medication absorption is high along with a further propensity to ulcerate.

5.3.1.1 Beta-blockers

The anti-angiogenic effect of Beta-blockers is a documented therapeutic. In the British journal of dermatology, 2010, Storch et al., espoused the inhibition of signal transduction pathway by beta-blockers in the proliferative vascular endothelial cells. Other actions of propranolol and beta-blockers have been reported to suppress beta FGF, VEGF, MMP-o2, MMP-9 through adrenoreceptor blockade. As we have alluded to in the chapter about etiopathogenesis, the mutational makeup of vascular lesions and oncologic mutational pathways are similar but produce a varied effect. An increased level of matrix metalloproteinases (MMP) is seen in sinonasal malignancy. The MMP levels seen a decrease with beta-blocker therapy compared to an increase with beta-adrenergic receptor agonist norepinephrine.

Propranolol at an Oral dose of 1.0–1.5 mg/kg per day- deep-seated lesions, multiple periodic doses with monitoring of cardiovascular and systemic effects as mentioned below during the proliferative phase (Fig. 5.2a, b).

Timolol maleate 0.5% ophthalmic solution, 25 mg per five mL-effective for topical superficial hemangiomas; applied as coats twice daily to minimize systemic absorption or peripheral runoff loss.

Beta-adrenergic nonselective blocker (propranolol) was a serendipitous therapy intervention for infantile hemangiomas, including orbital lesions. Leaute- Labreze et al., a French group,

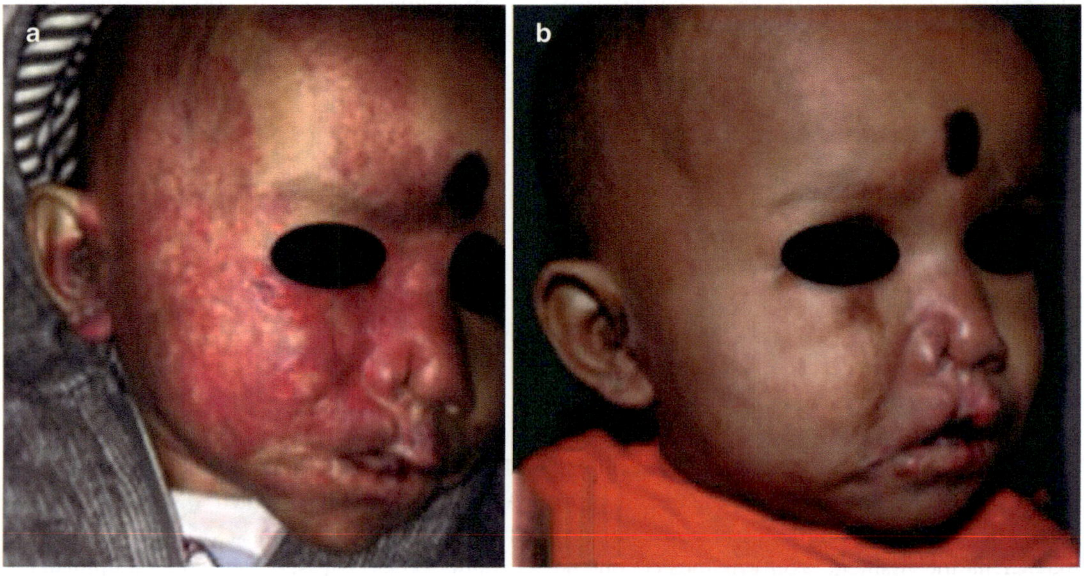

Fig. 5.2 Rapidly involuting congenital Hemangioma (RICH) of right face treated with propranolol therapy ((**a**) pre-treatment, (**b**) post-treatment)

unwittingly utilized propranolol in a couple of infantile maxillofacial hemangioma patients with impending cardiac failure. There was a significant resolution of the rate of growth and size regression of hemangiomas in these children while being used for cardiac symptoms. The group's findings are published in the New England Journal of Medicine in 2008. The use of topical timolol was reviewed by Puttgen et al. in the "Pediatrics" in 2016. Similar studies are in the maxillofacial literature.

The mechanism is poorly understood; the current literature reports growth factors (fibroblast growth factor- FGF, especially betaFGF) and matrix metalloproteinases (MMP 2 & 9) upregulation in these rapidly growing hemangiomas of the maxillofacial and periorbital areas. The beta-blocker therapy can be monitored with a reduction in urine excretion of the FGF and MMP as detected by enzyme-linked immunosorbent assay (ELIZA) and zymography tests.

Beta-blocker adverse reaction of hypoglycemia, hypotension, bradycardia, bronchial constriction, peripheral cyanosis, EKG changes, gastrointestinal symptoms (anorexia, diarrhea, vomiting), sleep changes, drowsiness, skin erythema, and exfoliation are all cared for appropriately, especially in infants. Cardiovascular and vital sign monitoring must be undertaken in an inpatient setting (3–7 days), especially when therapy is at the proliferative phase. Duration of the entire treatment can last between 1 and 8 weeks during the proliferative phase. Low doses of oral beta-blocker are advised during combination therapy with topical beta-adrenergic therapy in mitigating adverse effects.

Complicated Hemangiomas Complicated hemangiomas that require treatment include large hemangiomas at increased risk of scarring or disfigurement, life-threatening hemangiomas (e.g., airway hemangiomas), hemangiomas carrying operational risks (e.g., periocular hemangiomas), or hemangiomas with severe ulceration.

Propranolol Propranolol, a nonselective beta-blocker, is the first-line agent for hemangiomas with the potential to impair function or cause permanent disfigurement if there are no cardiac or neurovascular concerns [20].

Propranolol inhibits the growth and induces the regression of infantile hemangiomas [21] (Fig. 5.2a, b).

Efficacy In 2008, the serendipitous observation that propranolol to treat heart failure in two young children with infantile hemangiomas was associated with a color change, softening, and decrease in size hemangiomas led to the initiation of more extensive observational studies and randomized trials. All studies demonstrated improvement with propranolol [21–28].

Pretreatment Evaluation Treatment with propranolol should undertake in consultation with a pediatric dermatologist or another specialist with expertise in diagnosing and treating pediatric vascular tumors and using propranolol in children.

The pretreatment evaluation should include:

- History should focus on cardiovascular and respiratory abnormalities and family history of heart block or arrhythmia.
- Physical examination is with a cardiac and pulmonary assessment with measurement of heart rate and blood pressure.
- Electrocardiogram.
- Imaging studies, including cardiac ultrasound or cardiac magnetic resonance imaging (MRI), should be obtained in children with large facial hemangiomas at risk for PHACE to rule out the possibility of severe aortic coarctation, which is a contraindication to propranolol use.

5.3.1.2 Contraindications

- Cardiogenic shock.
- Documented chronic and significant sinus bradycardia.
- Documented chronic and significant hypotension.
- Greater than first-degree heart block.
- Heart failure.
- History of bronchospasm or wheezing.

- Hypersensitivity to propranolol.
- Preterm infants with corrected age < 5 weeks (postnatal age in weeks minus number of weeks preterm).

Treatment is usually started with oral propranolol at 0.5–1 mg/kg per day in two or three divided doses with feeds. If tolerated, the dose is then gradually increased (i.e., in increments of 0.5 mg/kg per day) over one to two weeks to the target dose of 2 mg/kg per day, given in two or three divided doses with feeds. Administering propranolol with feeds reduces the risk of hypoglycemia.

Monitoring Parents are educated about recognizing signs of serious adverse effects, including hypotension, bradycardia, wheezing, and hypoglycemia [29]. Early clinical signs of hypoglycemia include:

- Sweating.
- Jitteriness.
- Irritability.
- Cyanosis.
- Poor feeding.
- Hypothermia.
- Lethargy.

All these clinical signs, which are masked by beta-blockers except sweating, are paramount in treatment. Thus, sweating may be the most reliable early sign of hypoglycemia to watch.

Assessment of response and treatment duration — Children with infantile hemangiomas treated with propranolol should be followed up at one- to three-month intervals for response assessment and dose adjustment for weight gain. The treatment duration typically ranges between 6 to 12 months (or until the child is a 12- to 18-month-old) but maybe longer, depending upon the hemangioma's size and location, and response to treatment. Lack of response to treatment with propranolol is rare.

Rebound Growth Rebound growth after propranolol discontinuation was noted in approximately 14–25% of children [30–32]. The factors associated with the risk of relapse are not entirely understood. Some children with rebound growth may need a second course of propranolol. Topical beta-blockers may be used to treat mild to moderate relapses. However, mild relapses do not require treatment in most cases, and parents should be educated about the lesion's eventual involution.

Adverse Effects Serious adverse effects of propranolol therapy for hemangiomas, including hypotension, bradycardia, hyperkalemia, bronchospasm, and hypoglycemia, are infrequent [28, 33, 34]. Restless sleep, constipation or diarrhea, and cold extremities are more commonly reported [34]. Thus, children treated with this drug need close monitoring.

Of the potentially severe adverse effects, hypoglycemia is the most worrisome—risk reduction by daytime administration of propranolol with a feeding shortly before or after administration. Propranolol is discontinued during periods of illness or inadequate oral intake [20, 29, 35].

Other Beta-blockers A few small trials suggest that nadolol and Atenolol may be as effective as propranolol for the treatment of proliferative hemangiomas, potentially with a lower rate of adverse effects such as Broncho reactivity and sleep disturbances [36, 37]. However, these findings are preliminary and need to be confirmed by more extensive trials.

Systemic Corticosteroids Treatment with systemic corticosteroids remains a treatment option for patients with complicated hemangiomas, in whom treatment with beta-blockers is contraindicated.

Systemic corticosteroids were as effective as propranolol in a small randomized trial [38].

Dosing The starting dose for prednisolone is 2 to 3 mg/kg per day. A single, morning dose is preferred to minimize adrenal suppression. A response is usually seen within the first few weeks [39, 40]. Treatment is generally continued for several months or more, depending upon the indications for treatment, the response, and the child's age at initiation.

Prednisone should be slowly discontinued since abrupt discontinuation or rapid tapering of glucocorticoids while a hemangioma is still in its active growth phase may result in rebound proliferation.

Adverse Effects Adverse effects of systemic corticosteroids are more likely to develop with higher doses and courses of six months or longer, and they resolve with drug tapering.

Cushingoid facies, personality changes, delayed skeletal growth, gastric upset occurs in some cases. Serious corticosteroid complications, such as aseptic necrosis of the femoral head, hypertension, osteoporosis, and cataracts, are infrequent in children [41].

Other Systemic Therapies Vincristine and interferon alfa are alternative systemic agents for treating complicated hemangiomas but are rarely used since the advent of propranolol.

STEROID THERAPY
SYSTEMIC STEROIDS—Prednisolone in proliferative phase
FOCAL STEROIDS—Triamcinolone (40 mg/ml),
Betamethasone (6 mg/ml)
VINCRISTINE FOR LIFE-THREATENING LESIONS
INTERFERON THERAPY- ALPHA 2a and BETA (serious side effects)
Beta-blockers – 2 mg/kg body wt. (propranolol)

Surgical Therapies When a hemangioma poses primarily cosmetic concerns, therapeutic interventions are tailored individually. In addition to systemic, topical, and intralesional medications, therapeutic options include laser therapy and surgery.

5.4 Special Situations

Periocular Hemangiomas Periocular hemangiomas can compromise vision and cause amblyopia, astigmatism, or strabismus. These hemangiomas can be evaluated by an ophthalmologist experienced with hemangiomas and their treatment [16]. Surgical excision also may be an option for small, localized lesions [42–45].

5.4.1 Ulcerated Hemangiomas (Fig. 5.3a, b)

Wound Care Gentle and meticulous local wound care is the mainstay of ulcer therapy and is particularly important for lesions in locations subject to trauma and infection, such as the perineum. Local wound care reduces pain and helps to prevent secondary infection [46]. Commonly used therapies include topical antibiotics, barrier creams, and non-stick dressings [47]. Very gentle debridement of crusted wounds with saline soaks two to three times daily may also be helpful since crusting prevents re-epithelization and favors infection.

Topical metronidazole gel, often used in combination with topical mupirocin, has proved to be safe and efficacious for ulceration, particularly in intertriginous or moist areas such as the lip and perineum [46]. When clinically indicated, broad-spectrum oral antibiotics are also occasionally used.

Oral Propranolol We suggest oral propranolol in addition to meticulous wound care and appropriate analgesia for the treatment of ulcerated hemangiomas.

A beneficial effect of propranolol on ulcerated hemangiomas has also been reviewed in several case series [48–51].

Analgesia The pain associated with ulceration can be severe. Affected infants commonly suffer from sleep disturbance and increased irritability. Use of oral acetaminophen (without codeine) or a topical anesthetic agent (i.e., lidocaine hydrochloride 2 to 5% ointment) may be warranted.

Airway Hemangiomas (Fig. 5.4a–c) Because of the infant airway's small caliber, a growing airway hemangioma can lead to life-threatening airway obstruction.

Systemic propranolol is generally the first line of therapy for children with symptomatic airway hemangiomas [22, 52]. Laser ablation is an occasional second-line therapy [53]. Rarely, a tracheotomy may be required. Adult hemangiomas of the airways are reviewed with flexible endoscopy (Fig. 5.4a–c) frequently if asymptomatic.

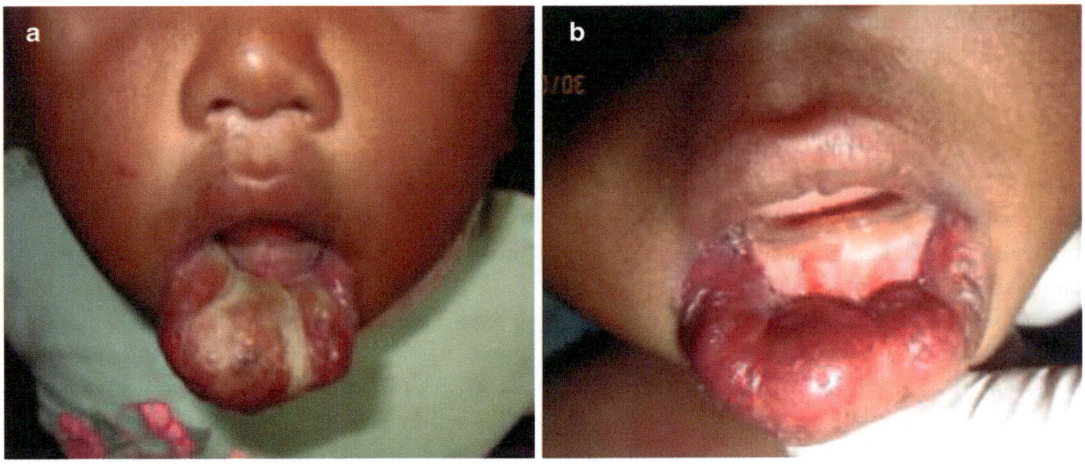

Fig. 5.3 (**a, b**) Pre- and post-op of lip with ulceration and progressive increase in the size and thickness. Therapy was with an intralesional Injection of Bleomycin 1 IU / Kg weight. There is no safe dosage for this useful and readily available chemotherapeutic agent called Bleomycin. It is known to cause pulmonary, hepatic dysfunction even in the smallest doses. (Pictures Courtesy: Dr. Amol Kulkarni, Senior Consultant OMF Surgeon, MDS, MOMS RCSEd, FIBCSOMS—ONC Kigali, Rwanda)

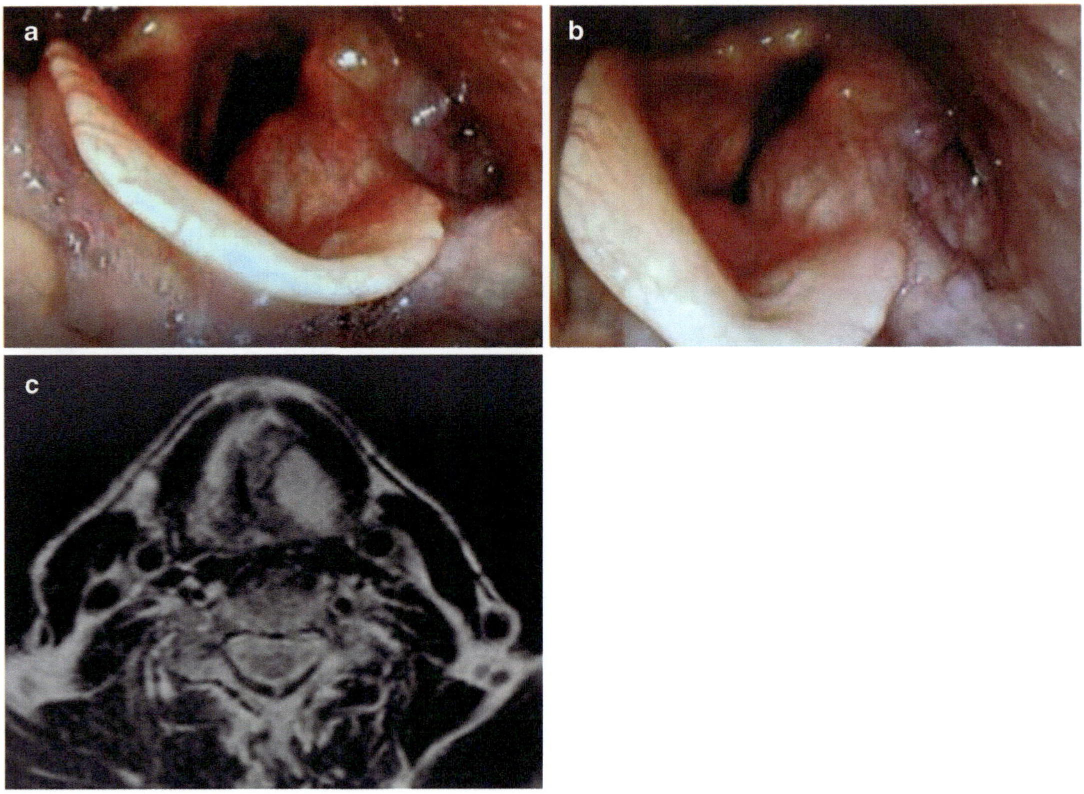

Fig. 5.4 (**a, b**) Endoscopic images of left laryngeal area showing low flow vascular lesion of the pyriform fossa, (**c**) MRI scan image of the same lesion with intense contrast uptake in left pyriform with vocal cord deviation in the laryngeal area

Surgical resection is a consideration in noted obstructive or bleeding episodes. Sclerotherapy as described can be utilized for management.

PHACE Syndrome The presence of severe arterial anomalies may restrict propranolol in some patients with PHACE syndrome [54]. In addition to large facial hemangiomas, patients with this disorder exhibit coarctation of the aorta and abnormalities of the aortic arch's cerebral and cervical vasculature and vessels. A small percentage of patients with severe cerebral or cervical anomalies develop acute arterial ischemic stroke, most often during infancy or toddlerhood [55].

Consensus guidelines recommend that infants with PHACE syndrome be thoroughly evaluated with magnetic resonance imaging/magnetic resonance angiography (MRI/MRA) of the head and neck and cardiac imaging to include the aortic arch before starting propranolol treatment [20].

The risks and benefits of propranolol treatment for patients with PHACE syndrome who have high-risk MRA features are reviewed for treatment and in consultation with neurology and cardiology specialists [20].

Lymphatic malformations are treated depending on the type and location in the head and neck. As mentioned previously, these lesions can cause pressure on the airway, aerodigestive tract, and enlarge due to repeated infection or hemorrhage into the lesion. In the majority of patients with macrocystic LMs, sclerotherapy with *Picibanil (OK-432)* has shown good results. Patients may develop inflammation at the site of injection and fever, which is managed symptomatically. Microcystic LMs may require systemic therapy with *Sirolimus* or surgery as they do not always respond to Picibanil. Sirolimus is a natural macrolide secluded from the Streptomyces genus (Streptomyces hygroscopicus). It causes a decrease in the vascular endothelial growth factor (VEGF) and is a key regulator in lymphangiogenesis and angiogenesis.

Algorithm for management of vascular anomalies (Adapted from: R. Mattassi, D.A. Loos and M. Vaghi for congenital vascular anomalies. Fonseca RJ, Turvey RD, Timothy A, Marciani RD, Turvey TA. Surgical pathology. Philadelphia: Saunders; 2000.)

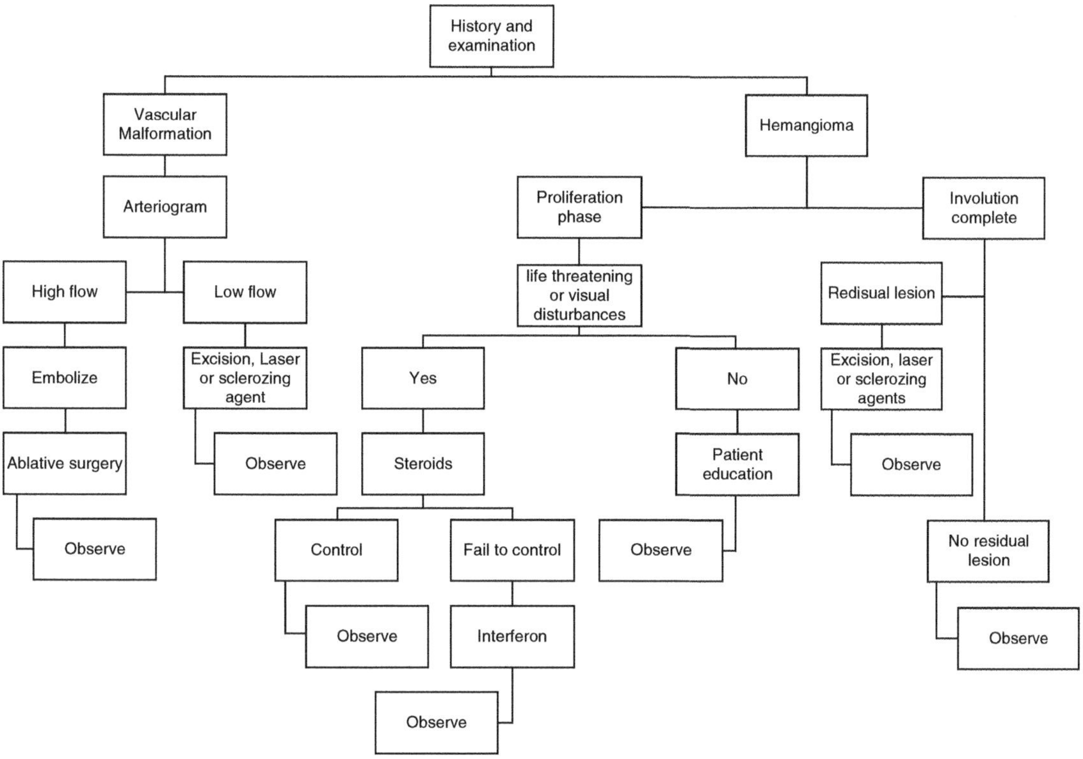

5.4.2 Sclerosing Agents (Table 5.1)

PYM, also known as Bleomycin A5, is the most used single-drug therapy for the treatment of cervicofacial malformations. Transient fever and swelling are commonly seen side effects. Skin ulceration and subcutaneous tissue atrophy are scarcely seen complications.

Absolute ethanol causes alteration in cellular proteins and hence damages the endothelium of the vascular wall leading to obliteration of its lumen. Common complications include nerve injury, necrosis, and ulceration of skin.

OK-432 is a lyophilized preparation of low-virulence bacteria, group- A Streptococcus pyogenes, incubated with benzylpenicillin. It causes,

Table 5.1 Table for use of medical therapy in vascular lesions (Adapted from: S.C.Nair, Vascular anomalies of the Head and Neck region. Journal of Maxillofacial and Oral Surgery. https://doi.org/10.1007/s12663-017-1063-2)

Sclerosing agent	Important facts	Advantage	Disadvantages
Bleomycin	First used by Yura and coworkers in 1977 [25]	Can absorb systemically at very low levels, even if administered locally [25]	Development of fatal pulmonary fibrosis even in low doses [26] hyperpigmentation
Pingyangmycin	Chemical structure similar to Bleomycin A5, this anticancer drug can be extracted from gram +ve streptococci	Most effective in treating vascular malformations of size less than 5.0 cm and for superficial lesions. Percutaneously, it is very simple and effective	Allergic reactions, cutaneous or mucosal necrosis and sensory nerve or motor nerve injuries
5% sodium morrhuate	Earlier, it was successfully used	May remain in lesion, causing sclerosis and involution for a longer duration	Irritating and has tendency for the induction of severe reactions like tissue necrosis
Absolute ethanol	Clinical application over the decades used globally, even in complicated and extensive lesions [27]	Low cost, remarkable results, quick metabolism and lower recurrence rates [28]	Ethanol sclerotherapy is painful and requires general anesthesia. Facial palsy and allergy
Lauromacrogol aethoxysklerol or polidocanol	Most effective sclerosing agents with low risk of complications and contains 95% hydroxyl polyethoxydodecane with 5% ethyl alcohol	Injection technique is simple, safe and time-saving, painless, rarely allergic, and well tolerated by patients	It may cause necrosis and ulceration, if solution leaks out into mucosa or skin
OK-432	OK-432, also called picibanil, is a biological preparation of lyophilized powder containing Streptococcus pyogenes Su strain cells (group A, type 3) treated with benzylpenicillin potassium [29]	No perilesional fibrosis [30]Possibility to perform multiple subsequent injections with additional shrinkage response Low complication rate Better esthetics results [30]	The main disadvantage of OK-432 is that some lesions require more than one injection to shrink satisfactorily. Other complications include fever, allergy, erythema and swelling [31]
Detergent sclerosants (sodium tetradecyl, the most commonly used sclerosant, ethanolamine and polidocanol	Detergents came into use in the 1930s they work by a mechanism known as protein theft denaturation	Addition of air results in a microfoam which is felt to be more effective than the bland solution. A reasonable dose limit for image-guided sclerotherapy is 0.5 ml/kg or 30.	It is painful to inject, but effective and relatively nontoxic

induction of various cytokines. The inflammatory response caused by this remains localized and causes endothelial damage. The complications include local swelling and transient facial nerve palsy.

Ethanolamine oleate is an emulsion of fatty acids, which induces thrombosis and damages the endothelium. Complications like ulceration and necrosis of skin are known but infrequently observed.

Polidocanol is a non-ionic detergent, causes absorption at the cell membrane and leads to lysis of endothelial lining. Superficial necrosis of skin or mucosa is a known complication with Polidocanol.

Doxycycline belongs to the tetracycline group of antibiotics. Its mode of action is not yet clear, but its effects are known to be due to inhibition of matrix metalloproteinases and cell proliferation. It also causes suppression of vascular endothelial growth factors during angiogenesis and lymphangiogenesis. This further leads to dense adhesions and fibrosis due to collagen and fibrin deposition. Macrocystic LM's show a better response to treatment with doxycycline in comparison to microcystic LMs. Hemorrhage, cellulitis, pain, and transient edema are commonly seen complications. Scarring, skin excoriation, and Horner syndrome are seen less commonly. These adverse effects are self-limiting and likely to be related to the sclerosing effect rather than a side effect of the medication itself.

STS, also known as *sotradecol*, causes denaturation of proteins like clotting factors due to disruption of the normal architecture of the lipid bilayer in cell membranes of endothelial cells. This causes fibrosis and occlusion of vessels. It is not known to have any major complications so far.

5.4.3 Bleomycin

As it is available and inexpensive this drug has been effectively used for cystic lymphatic lesions to scar them to reduce the volume of macrocyctic lesions.

Bleomycin is used widely for the treatment of VMs and microcystic lesions too.

It inhibits DNA synthesis and has a non-specific inflammatory reaction on the endothelial cells. Adverse effects of bleomycin are minimal and transient (Fig. 5.5a, b), mostly being localized pain and swelling. Skin infections around injection are seen less commonly. Some people report occasionally severe nausea.

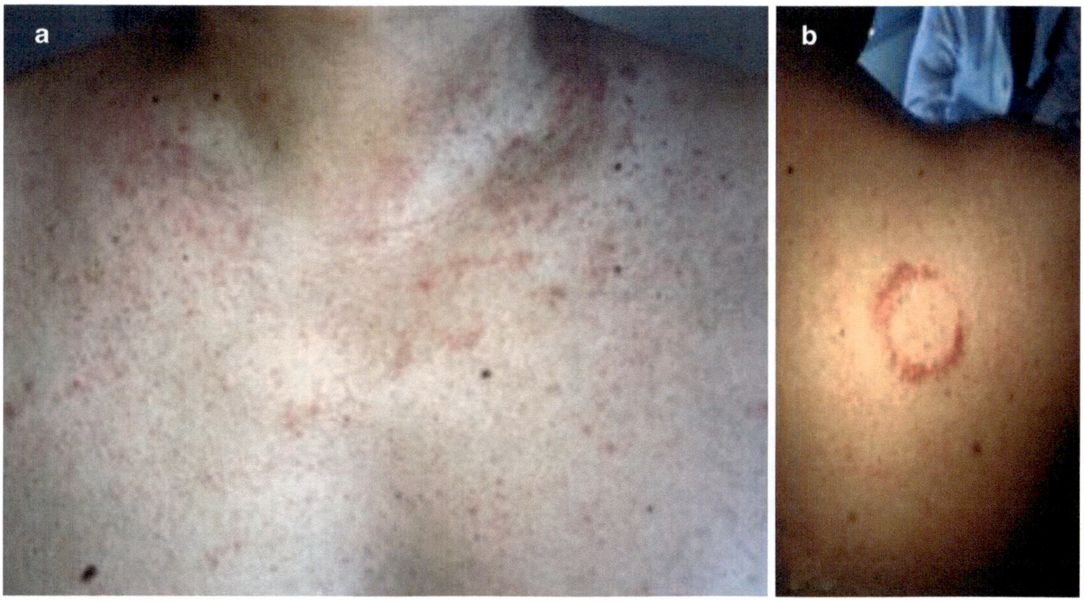

Fig. 5.5 (**a**) Koebner phenomenon after bleomycin injection for a vascular cystic lesion, with rash around the neck due to friction irritation of clothing. (**b**): shows annular or ring-like erythema of the area of electrocardiogram lead sticker

It has been used along with OK-432 and alone. Large lymphatic lesions treated with intralesional Injection of Bleomycin 1 I.U / Kg weight. There is no safe dosage for this effective and readily available chemotherapeutic agent called Bleomycin. It is known to cause pulmonary hepatic dysfunction even in the smallest doses.

mechanism of action on microcystic disease is not completely understood and may involve derangement of tight junctions between endothelial cells or induction of endothelial mesenchymal transition. The overall response is a favorable but complete response is seen in only about 20–57%.

The authors follow a protocol of intralesional injection of 15 IU Bleomycin in 5 ml of fresh normal saline, administered every 15 days. Most patients show a response in 3–4 sittings (Fig. 5.6a–c).

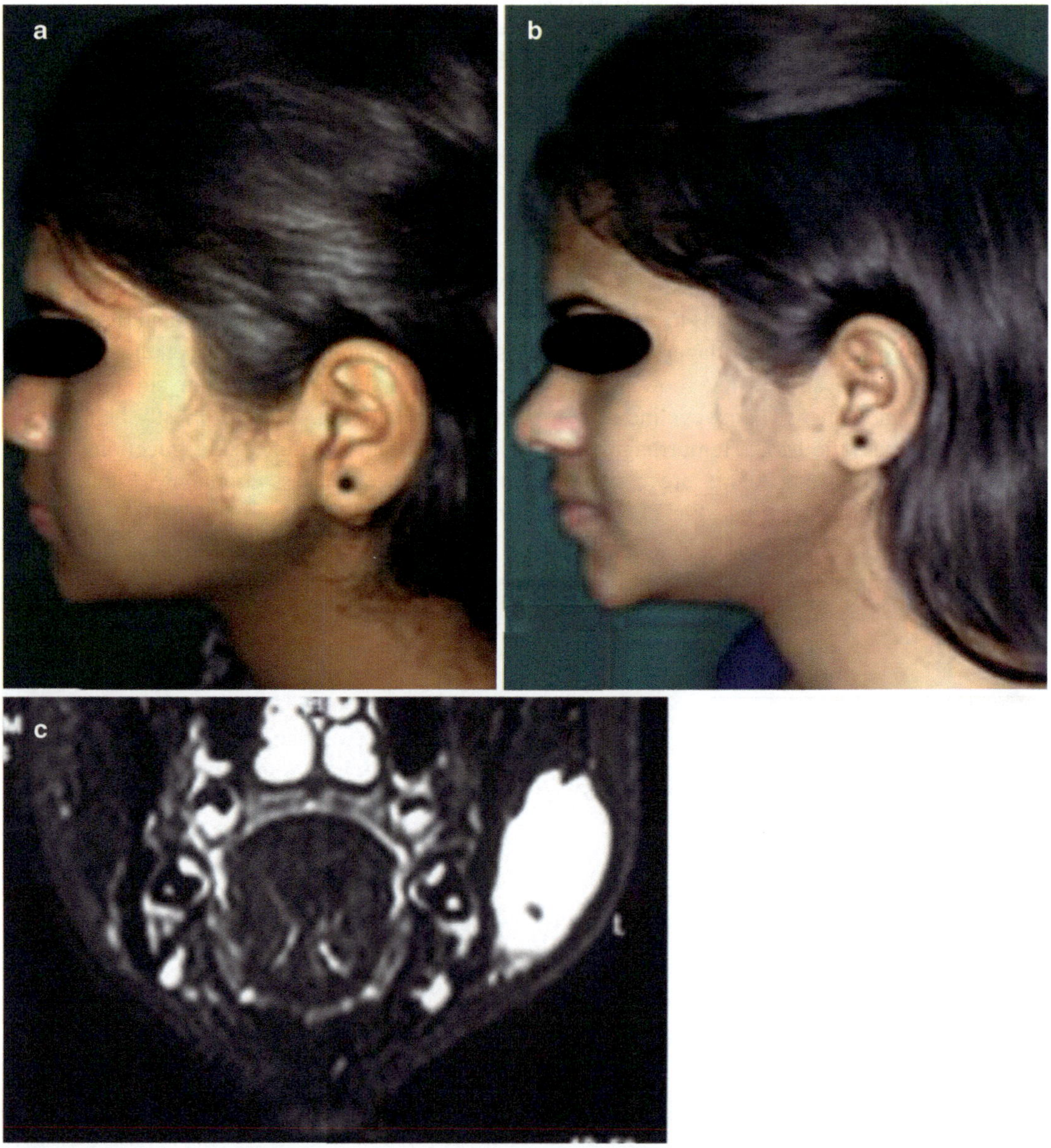

Fig. 5.6 Venous malformation-Left cheek (**a**) before sclerotherapy, (**b**) after sclerotherapy, (**c**) pretreatment T2-weighted MRI image

5.4.4 Protein Chain in a Vascular Cell that Transmits Signal from a Cell Surface Receptor to the DNA in the Cell Nucleus

Growth and differentiation of the vascular lesion and its endothelial cell proliferation or initiated at the cell membrane tyrosine kinase receptor with the RAS- RAF downstream to nucleus MAPK dependent gene transcription. The illustration demonstrates the potential therapy and inhibition of Src-tyrosine kinase family inhibitors; rapidly accelerated fibrosarcoma (RAF) inhibitors; mitogen activating pathway kinase-extracellular signal-regulated kinase (MEK) inhibitors; extracellular signal-regulated kinase is (ERK) inhibitors (Fig. 5.7).

5.4.5 Sirolimus/Rapamycin

Rapamycin is a chemotherapeutic agent derivative of *Streptomyces hygroscopicus* bacteria, a macrolide used for targeted therapy to block the PIK3CA

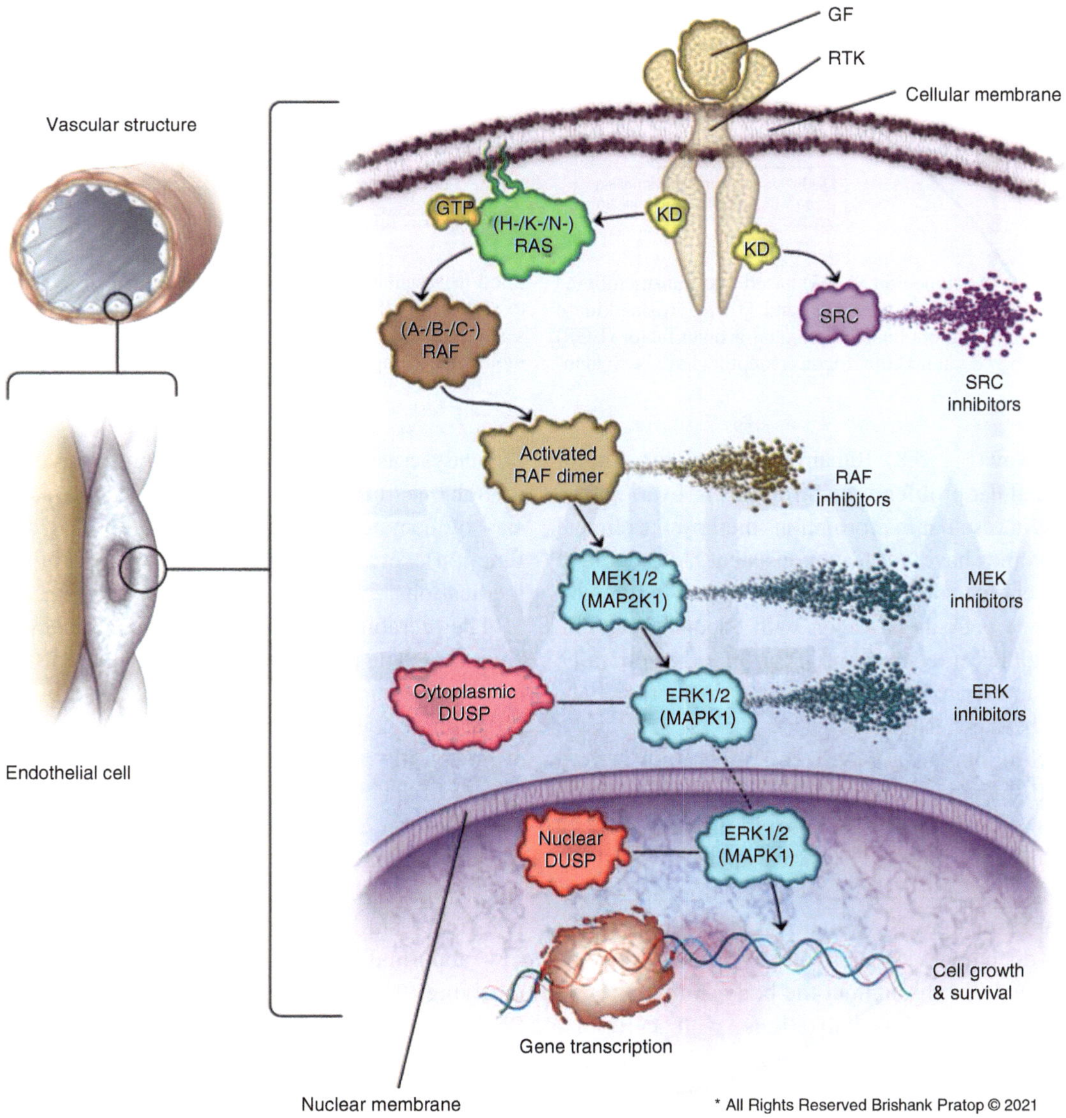

Fig. 5.7 MAPK/ERK pathway (well known as the Ras-Raf-MEK-ERK pathway) potential therapeutic inhibitors

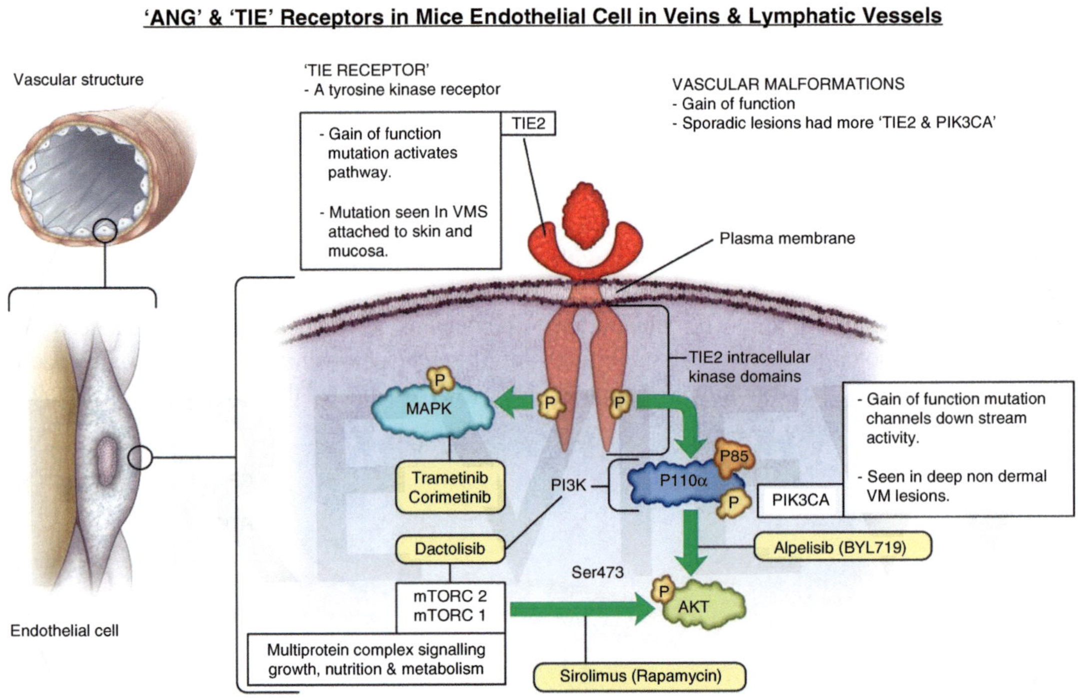

Fig. 5.8 Angiopoeitin (ANG) based two transmembrane tyrosine kinase receptors-TIE1 and TIE 2 (tyrosine kinase with immunoglobulin and epithelial growth factor (EGF) homology domain) homologous receptors have been identified in vascular and lymphatic endothelial cells leading to vascular malformations. This picture illustration represents the identified pathway and the potential therapeutic molecular therapies

pathway (Fig. 5.8). Rapamycin (Sirolimus) inhibits cellular proliferation. Sirolimus has varied success in vascular malformations therapy, but clinical outcomes have not been consistent. Authors here present personal experiences in use with syndromic patients has been with adequate caution. Multiple centers have used Sirolimus empirically, and mutational tests before using the therapy have not been consistent.

Sirolimus as a B & T cell suppressor is very well studied in transplant patients, as mentioned with useful utility. Its use in head and neck vascular lesions has shown a qualitative reduction in size and side effects of bleeding and vesicular discharge. Nevertheless, Sirolimus therapy has documented side effects for its use with complicated LM throughout the body. A reduction in cellulitis and hospitalizations with cellulitis-related complications documented with case reports and lesion management publications. Gastrointestinal, general metabolic toxicity, blood dyscrasias, bone marrow suppression (even though one of the treatment indications is dyscrasias of hematological and marrow-derived cell function) were the reported adverse effects of the medications.

The literature on Sirolimus and its efficacy is equivocal. The best candidate for this therapeutic advantage is not clear. Strychowsky et al., in the 2018 phase 2 trial using Sirolimus in patients, evaluated the benefits of its empiric use complicated LM. They reported a reduction in cellulitis and incidence of hospitalizations with cellulitis-related complications. The adverse effects of therapy were—Metabolic toxicity (3%), gastrointestinal disturbance (3%), and blood/bone marrow abnormalities (27%). Not all the patients receiving therapy had a genetic test for the PIK3CA mutation confirmed. So, treatment was based on clinical considerations. Other studies have reported on anecdotal success with Sirolimus. Sirolimus's current indications for therapy are for pain, lesion enlargement, vesicular ulcerations, bone erosion and expansion, bleeding, airway compression, hematologic abnormalities, and complex symptomatic cases. Please also review the pathways of this therapy and references in Chap. 2 on mutational basis and etiopathogenesis of vascular lesions.

Many medications like interferons, bisphosphonates, and chemotherapeutic agents have been used by various groups of physicians with anecdotal evidence and with a lack of large clinical trials. Many of the patients have suffered long-term hepatic and renal impairment with such aggressive therapy in benign lesions. The molecular basis as being investigated (Fig. 5.9), will channel better therapeutic modalities for benign vascular lesions.

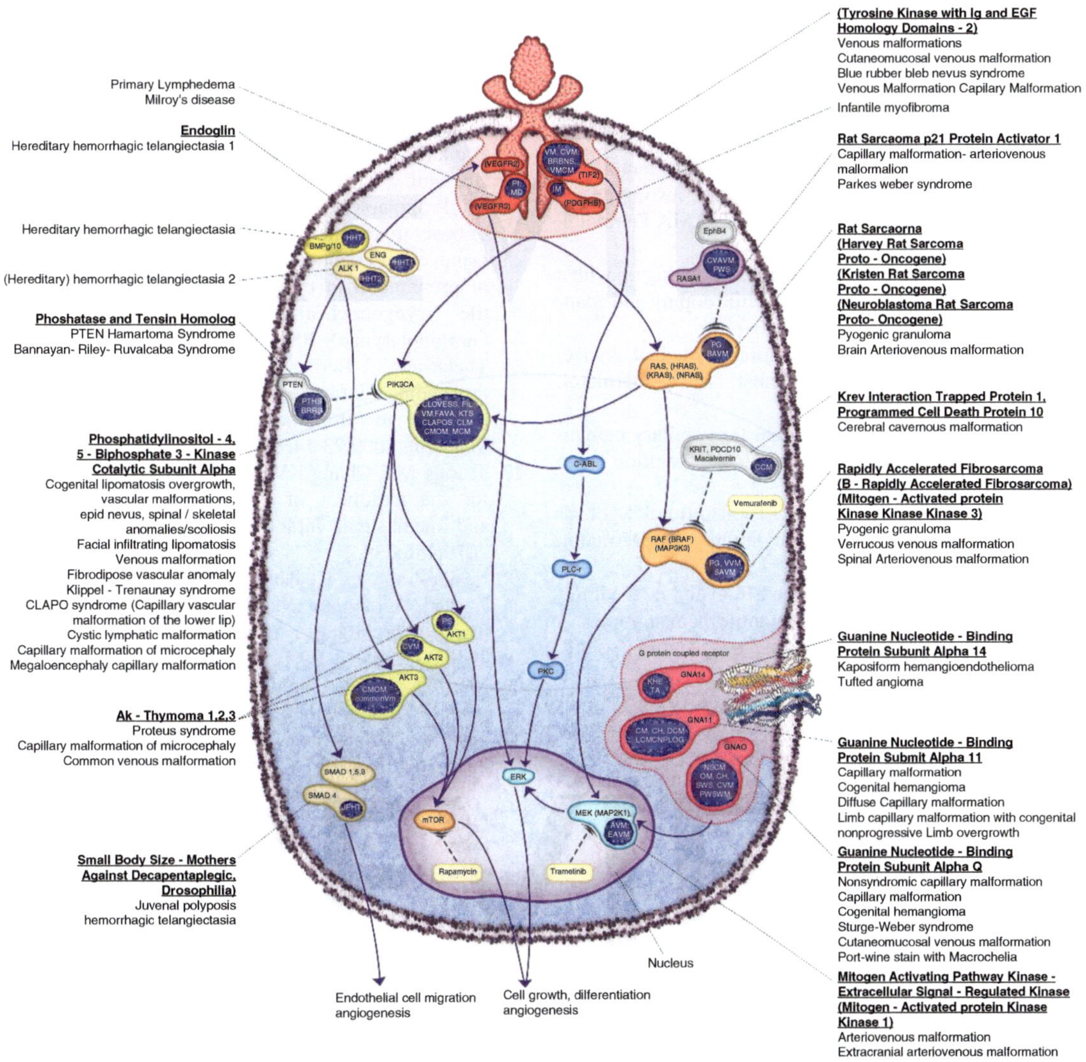

Fig. 5.9 Summary illustration of well-known genetic mutations based on that transmembrane tyrosine kinase MG protein-coupled signaling pathways. The protein mutations are abbreviated with the number's analogs. These vascular malformations caused by the mutations on the syndromic presentations are listed below the receptors which are mutated. Majority of these mutations are based on the well-known Ras-Raf-MEK-ERK and PIK3CA pathways. Adapted from Refs. [56–58]

References

1. Frieden IJ, Eichenfield LF, Esterly NB, et al. Guidelines of care for hemangiomas of infancy. American Academy of Dermatology Guidelines/ Outcomes Committee. J Am Acad Dermatol. 1997;37:631.
2. Frieden IJ. Which hemangiomas to treat-and how? Arch Dermatol. 1997;133:1593.
3. Chang LC, Haggstrom AN, Drolet BA, et al. Growth characteristics of infantile hemangiomas: implications for management. Pediatrics. 2008;122:360.
4. Couto RA, Maclellan RA, Zurakowski D, Greene AK. Infantile hemangioma: clinical assessment of the involuting phase and implications for management. Plast Reconstr Surg. 2012;130:619.
5. Bauland CG, Lüning TH, Smit JM, et al. Untreated hemangiomas: growth pattern and residual lesions. Plast Reconstr Surg. 2011;127:1643.
6. Baselga E, Roe E, Coulie J, et al. Risk factors for degree and type of sequelae after involution of untreated hemangiomas of infancy. JAMA Dermatol. 2016;152:1239.
7. Tanner JL, Dechert MP, Frieden IJ. Growing up with a facial hemangioma: parent and child coping and adaptation. Pediatrics. 1998;101:446.
8. Luu M, Frieden IJ. Haemangioma: clinical course, complications and management. Br J Dermatol. 2013;169:20.
9. Guo S, Ni N. Topical treatment for capillary hemangioma of the eyelid using beta-blocker solution. Arch Ophthalmol. 2010;128:255.
10. Pope E, Chakkittakandiyil A. Topical timolol gel for infantile hemangiomas: a pilot study. Arch Dermatol. 2010;146:564.
11. Ovadia SA, Landy DC, Cohen ER, et al. Local administration of β-blockers for infantile hemangiomas: a systematic review and meta-analysis. Ann Plast Surg. 2015;74:256.
12. Püttgen K, Lucky A, Adams D, et al. Topical timolol maleate treatment of infantile hemangiomas. Pediatrics. 2016;138:e20160355.
13. Frommelt P, Juern A, Siegel D, et al. Adverse events in young and preterm infants receiving topical timolol for infantile hemangioma. Pediatr Dermatol. 2016;33:405.
14. Garzon MC, Lucky AW, Hawrot A, Frieden IJ. Ultrapotent topical corticosteroid treatment of hemangiomas of infancy. J Am Acad Dermatol. 2005;52:281.
15. Chen MT, Yeong EK, Horng SY. Intralesional corticosteroid therapy in proliferating head and neck hemangiomas: a review of 155 cases. J Pediatr Surg. 2000;35:420.
16. Ceisler EJ, Santos L, Blei F. Periocular hemangiomas: what every physician should know. Pediatr Dermatol. 2004;21:1.
17. Mills CM, Marks R. Side effects of topical glucocorticoids. Curr Probl Dermatol. 1993;21:122.
18. Gilbertson EO, Spellman MC, Piacquadio DJ, Mulford MI. Super potent topical corticosteroid use associated with adrenal suppression: clinical considerations. J Am Acad Dermatol. 1998;38:318.
19. Olsen EA, Cornell RC. Topical clobetasol-17-propionate: review of its clinical efficacy and safety. J Am Acad Dermatol. 1986;15:246.
20. Drolet BA, Frommelt PC, Chamlin SL, et al. Initiation and use of propranolol for infantile hemangioma: report of a consensus conference. Pediatrics. 2013;131:128.
21. Léauté-Labrèze C, Dumas de la Roque E, Hubiche T, et al. Propranolol for severe hemangiomas of infancy. N Engl J Med. 2008;358:2649.
22. Hogeling M, Adams S, Wargon O. A randomized controlled trial of propranolol for infantile hemangiomas. Pediatrics. 2011;128:e259.
23. Sans V, de la Roque ED, Berge J, et al. Propranolol for severe infantile hemangiomas: follow-up report. Pediatrics. 2009;124:e423.
24. Buckmiller L, Dyamenahalli U, Richter GT. Propranolol for airway hemangiomas: case report of novel treatment. Laryngoscope. 2009;119:2051.
25. Denoyelle F, Leboulanger N, Enjolras O, et al. Role of propranolol in the therapeutic strategy of infantile laryngotracheal hemangioma. Int J Pediatr Otorhinolaryngol. 2009;73:1168.
26. Theletsane T, Redfern A, Raynham O, et al. Life-threatening infantile haemangioma: a dramatic response to propranolol. J Eur Acad Dermatol Venereol. 2009;23:1465.
27. Truong MT, Chang KW, Berk DR, et al. Propranolol for the treatment of a life-threatening subglottic and mediastinal infantile hemangioma. J Pediatr. 2010;156:335.
28. Léauté-Labrèze C, Hoeger P, Mazereeuw-Hautier J, et al. A randomized, controlled trial of oral propranolol in infantile hemangioma. N Engl J Med. 2015;372:735.
29. Martin K, Blei F, Chamlin SL, et al. Propranolol treatment of infantile hemangiomas: anticipatory guidance for parents and caretakers. Pediatr Dermatol. 2013;30:155.
30. Shah SD, Baselga E, McCuaig C, et al. Rebound growth of infantile hemangiomas after propranolol therapy. Pediatrics. 2016;137:e20151754.
31. Wedgeworth E, Glover M, Irvine AD, et al. Propranolol in the treatment of infantile haemangiomas: lessons from the European propranolol in the treatment of complicated haemangiomas (PITCH) taskforce survey. Br J Dermatol. 2016;174:594.
32. Ahogo CK, Ezzedine K, Prey S, et al. Factors associated with the relapse of infantile haemangiomas in children treated with oral propranolol. Br J Dermatol. 2013;169:1252.
33. Lawley LP, Siegfried E, Todd JL. Propranolol treatment for hemangioma of infancy: risks and recommendations. Pediatr Dermatol. 2009;26:610.
34. de Graaf M, Breur JM, Raphaël MF, et al. Adverse effects of propranolol when used in the treatment of

hemangiomas: a case series of 28 infants. J Am Acad Dermatol. 2011;65:320.
35. Holland KE, Frieden IJ, Frommelt PC, et al. Hypoglycemia in children taking propranolol for the treatment of infantile hemangioma. Arch Dermatol. 2010;146:775.
36. Pope E, Chakkittakandiyil A, Lara-Corrales I, et al. Expanding the therapeutic repertoire of infantile haemangiomas: cohort-blinded study of oral nadolol compared with propranolol. Br J Dermatol. 2013;168:222.
37. Ábarzúa-Araya A, Navarrete-Dechent CP, Heusser F, et al. Atenolol versus propranolol for the treatment of infantile hemangiomas: a randomized controlled study. J Am Acad Dermatol. 2014;70:1045.
38. Kim KH, Choi TH, Choi Y, et al. Comparison of efficacy and safety between propranolol and steroid for infantile Hemangioma: a randomized clinical trial. JAMA Dermatol. 2017;153(6):529.
39. Dinehart SM, Kincannon J, Geronemus R. Hemangiomas: evaluation and treatment. Dermatol Surg. 2001;27:475.
40. Mulliken JB, Fishman SJ, Burrows PE. Vascular anomalies. Curr Probl Surg. 2000;37:517.
41. Boon LM, MacDonald DM, Mulliken JB. Complications of systemic corticosteroid therapy for problematic hemangioma. Plast Reconstr Surg. 1999;104:1616.
42. Slaughter K, Sullivan T, Boulton J, et al. Early surgical intervention as definitive treatment for ocular adnexal capillary haemangioma. Clin Exp Ophthalmol. 2003;31:418.
43. Schneider D, Lee MS, Harrison AR, Sidman J. Excision of periorbital hemangiomas to correct visual abnormalities. Arch Facial Plast Surg. 2011;13:195.
44. Frank RC, Cowan BJ, Harrop AR, et al. Visual development in infants: visual complications of periocular haemangiomas. J Plast Reconstr Aesthet Surg. 2010;63:1.
45. Claude O, Picard A, O'Sullivan N, et al. Use of ultrasonic dissection in the early surgical management of periorbital haemangiomas. J Plast Reconstr Aesthet Surg. 2008;61:1479.
46. Kim HJ, Colombo M, Frieden IJ. Ulcerated hemangiomas: clinical characteristics and response to therapy. J Am Acad Dermatol. 2001;44:962.
47. Morelli JG, Tan OT, Yohn JJ, Weston WL. Treatment of ulcerated hemangiomas infancy. Arch Pediatr Adolesc Med. 1994;148:1104.
48. Saint-Jean M, Léauté-Labrèze C, Mazereeuw-Hautier J, et al. Propranolol for treatment of ulcerated infantile hemangiomas. J Am Acad Dermatol. 2011;64:827.
49. Hermans DJ, van Beynum IM, Schultze Kool LJ, et al. Propranolol, a very promising treatment for ulceration in infantile hemangiomas: a study of 20 cases with matched historical controls. J Am Acad Dermatol. 2011;64:833.
50. Kim LH, Hogeling M, Wargon O, et al. Propranolol: useful therapeutic agent for the treatment of ulcerated infantile hemangiomas. J Pediatr Surg. 2011;46:759.
51. Hong E, Fischer G. Propranolol for recalcitrant ulcerated hemangioma of infancy. Pediatr Dermatol. 2012;29:64.
52. Peridis S, Pilgrim G, Athanasopoulos I, Parpounas K. A meta-analysis on the effectiveness of propranolol for the treatment of infantile airway haemangiomas. Int J Pediatr Otorhinolaryngol. 2011;75:455.
53. Rahbar R, Nicollas R, Roger G, et al. The biology and management of subglottic hemangioma: past, present, future. Laryngoscope. 2004;114:1880.
54. Metry DW, Garzon MC, Drolet BA, et al. PHACE syndrome: current knowledge, future directions. Pediatr Dermatol. 2009;26:381.
55. Siegel DH, Tefft KA, Kelly T, et al. Stroke in children with posterior fossa brain malformations, hemangiomas, arterial anomalies, coarctation of the aorta and cardiac defects, and eye abnormalities (PHACE) syndrome: a systematic review of the literature. Stroke. 2012;43:1672.
56. Kangas J, Nätynki M, Eklund L. Development of molecular therapies for venous malformations. Basic Clin Pharmacol Toxicol. 2018;123(Suppl 5):6–19. https://doi.org/10.1111/bcpt.13027. Epub 2018 May 29
57. Kim JS, Hwang SK, Chung HY. The molecular pathophysiology of vascular anomalies: genomic research. Arch Plast Surg. 2020;47(3):203–8. https://doi.org/10.5999/aps.2020.00591. Epub 2020 May 15
58. Greene AK, Goss JA. Vascular anomalies: from a clinicohistologic to a genetic framework. Plast Reconstr Surg. 2018;141(5):709e–17e. https://doi.org/10.1097/PRS.0000000000004294.

6 The Role of Interventional Radiology

Jack Burt, Jose Rodriguez-Vasquez, Basavraj Ghodke, and Srinivasa R. Chandra

Objectives
(a) Provide an overview of Interventional Radiology in the Maxillofacial & Head and Neck Surgery
(b) Discuss the role of Interventional Radiology in the Management of Head and Neck Vascular Lesions

6.1 Outline

6.1.1 Section 1: Diagnostic Imaging of the Head and Neck

1. General Imaging [1–14]
   (a) The Head and Neck (H&N) is a complex anatomical region divided into both anatomic and functional sections and spaces.
   (b) The role of imaging in the H&N is to detect, characterize, and delineate lesions, while also determining involved surrounding structures and lymph nodes.
   (c) Imaging is also used for interventional procedure guidance, distant metastasis detection, therapy planning, monitoring response, and surveillance.
   (d) Commonly employed cross-sectional modalities include magnetic resonance imaging (MRI), computed tomography (CT), ultrasound (US), and positron emission tomography computed tomography (PET-CT).
   (e) The primary imaging modality will depend on the main clinical concern, availability, cost, reimbursement, and patient-specific factors such as contrast allergies or implanted metallic devices.
   (f) Most modalities will be complementary, but in any case, the initial study should be one that will both provide all the necessary information for proper management and being safe and cost-effective.
   (g) US is a reasonable first step in the evaluation of any H&N vascular pathology given its rapid deployment, cost-effectiveness, and safety; however, imaging should be tailored to best address the clinical concern.
   (h) MRI, as in other parts of the body, is superior to CT in the evaluation of soft

J. Burt (✉) · J. Rodriguez-Vasquez
Department of Radiology, University of Nebraska Medical Center, Omaha, NE, USA
e-mail: john.burt@unmc.edu; j.rodriguezvazquez@unmc.edu

B. Ghodke
Department of Neuroradiology and Neurosurgery, University of Washington, Seattle, WC, USA
e-mail: bggodhke@uw.edu

S. R. Chandra
Oral & Maxillofacial- Head & Neck Oncology Reconstructive Surgery, Oregon Health & Science University Portland, Portland, OR, USA
e-mail: chandrsr@ohsu.edu

S. C. Nair, S. R. Chandra (eds.), *Management of Head and Neck Vascular Lesions*,
https://doi.org/10.1007/978-981-15-2321-2_6

tissues, however there are certain caveats when imaging the H&N with MRI. MRI is typically employed to evaluate the suprahyoid neck, where it is less affected by artifact from dental amalgam or motion and is less suitable for the evaluation of the infrahyoid neck, a region that is sensitive to respiratory motion artifact from coughing or breathing.

   (i) Common indications for imaging of the H&N include lesion localization, tumor staging, and infection workup. When imaging the head and neck for the purpose of finding a lesion, contrast-enhanced CT (CECT) is generally the preferred initial modality. In some cases, CECT is also generally preferred for staging. For example, CECT is the best first step for staging of Squamous Cell Carcinoma. The same is true for the evaluation of a suspected infection, as CECT is excellent at distinguishing between cellulitis, phlegmon, or abscess.
   (j) MRI is the preferred modality in the evaluation of tumor extent, perineural tumor spread, and/or intracranial extension.
   (k) It is important to have a general approach to lesions that are found in the H&N. As mentioned before, the H&N is divided into many sections or spaces, and as such, the first step is to determine the space in which the lesion originated. This allows us to formulate a space-specific differential diagnosis.
   (l) It is also important to consider whether a lesion could represent a normal structure or variant, or whether the abnormal finding merits no further intervention.
2. Imaging of Vascular Lesions
   (a) Radiology plays a crucial role in the diagnosis and management of vascular lesions in the H&N.
   (b) Diagnostic imaging can confirm a diagnosis, precisely delineate a lesion, distinguish associated abnormalities from normal variation, and allow for the surveillance and monitoring of a lesion, pre- and post-therapy.
   (c) Interventional radiology provides several therapeutic options for vascular anomalies, which will be discussed in greater detail in later sections.
   (d) Ultrasound is often used to image vascular anatomy given its ability to demonstrate flow in real time, as well as its ability to quantify flow using Doppler technique.
   (e) As mentioned before, ultrasound may be used as the first step in the evaluation of H&N vascular lesions and may help characterize the lesion as having primarily venous or arterial flow.
   (f) Although typically not preferred for the evaluation of vascular lesions given the associated ionizing radiation, CT can be employed to assess bony anatomy, as well as to detect calcifications or phleboliths in venous malformations.
   (g) Vascular lesions are best assessed when enhanced following the administration of intravenous contrast.
   (h) Generally, MRI is the primary modality for the evaluation of vascular anomalies. Its superior soft tissue resolution makes it the preferred imaging tool.
   (i) When compared to other modalities, MRI is better able to identify aggressive imaging features that may suggest a more invasive or malignant diagnosis.
   (j) A basic MRI protocol of the H&N will at least include precontrast and fat-saturated postcontrast T1-weighted images, as well as T2-weighted images, and will require at least 30 min of scanning time.
   (k) MR angiography can be used to evaluate high-flow lesions during arterial and venous phase.
3. Overview of Non-Invasive Imaging Modalities
   (a) Ultrasound
      (i) General
         1. Based on the transmission, reflection, and reception of sound waves of variable frequencies.
         2. Higher frequencies (5–15 MHz) are used for the evaluation of superficial structures, such as the

H&N. Lower frequencies (2–4 MHz) are used for the evaluation of deeper structures, such as the abdomen and pelvis.
3. Non-contrast techniques include gray-scale, spectral Doppler, color Doppler, and power Doppler.
4. Contrast-enhanced US (CEUS), recently approved by the FDA, is modality used to evaluate lesion enhancement.

(ii) Techniques
1. Gray-scale
    (a) Used to evaluate anatomy and morphology.
2. Spectral Doppler
    (a) Used to evaluate spectral waveforms, as well as blood flow velocity, direction, and resistance.
3. Color Doppler
    (a) Assigns color to blood velocity and direction (red reflects flow towards the transducer and blue reflects flow away from the transducer).
4. Power Doppler
    (a) Detects slow flow, otherwise not seen on color Doppler. Does not provide information on velocity or direction.
5. CEUS
    (a) Consists of intravenous injection of highly echogenic microbubbles.
    (b) Used to evaluate lesion enhancement, blood flow dynamics, tissue vascularity, and stent grafts.

(iii) Advantages
1. US is widely available, portable, affordable, and entails no ionizing radiation risk.
2. It is excellent at evaluating tumors in real time, including the assessment of adjacent blood vessels and tumor vascularity.
3. CEUS can be used to evaluate lesion enhancement in patients with contraindications to MRI or CT contrast.
4. If the lesion is well visualized, US may be the preferred modality for image-guided interventions.

(iv) Disadvantages
1. Operator dependent.
2. Greatly limited by bone and air.
3. May not be able to fully evaluate larger lesions.

(b) Computed Tomography/Computed Tomography Angiography (CTA)

(i) General
1. CTA is useful in the evaluation of vascular lesions as it can provide information about the vessel wall and lumen, including information on atherosclerotic vascular disease and calcifications.

(ii) Technique
1. Images are acquired and reconstructed in thin sections typically measuring 1–2 mm.
2. For CTA, iodinated contrast is injected intravenously, and imaging is timed in order to obtain maximal arterial enhancement within the area of clinical concern.
3. Maximal arterial enhancement will depend on location and size of target vessel, vascular pathology, and cardiac function.
4. Arterial enhancement can be modified by adjusting contrast agent concentration, flow rate, and volume.

(iii) Advantages
1. Like US, CT is a reasonable first modality as it is also widely available, fast, and relatively affordable.
2. High spatial resolution.
3. Post-processing and 3D reconstruction capabilities.

4. Less sensitive to motion artifact than MRI (including vascular artifact from turbulent or slow flow).
5. Excellent at evaluating bone and calcifications.
6. Generally easier to interpret than MRI.

(iv) Disadvantages

1. Ionizing radiation exposure.
2. Susceptible to streak artifact from metallic material.
3. Risk of contrast-induced nephropathy.
4. Risk of contrast allergies.

(c) Magnetic Resonance Imaging/Magnetic Resonance Angiography (MRA)

(i) General

1. MRI excels at evaluating soft tissues.
2. As mentioned above, it is the preferred modality to evaluate for tumor extent, perivascular/perineural spread, and/or intracranial extension.
3. Imaging of vascular lesions with MRA can be performed using both contrast and non-contrast techniques.
4. Contrast-enhanced MRA (CEMRA) is less sensitive to artifacts and shows higher morphologic detail than non-contrast technique.
5. CEMRA is more technically challenging as it requires good bolus timing and patient cooperation (breath hold, staying still, etc.).
6. MRA without contrast still allows for the evaluation of vessel morphology, as well as blood flow and direction.

(ii) Advantages

1. Multiplanar scanning.
2. Ability to evaluate vasculature without contrast, which is particularly important in patients who are pregnant or have severe renal failure.
3. No ionizing radiation exposure.
4. MRI contrast allergies are rare.
5. Contrast agents are less nephrotoxic.
6. Ability to perform functional imaging (DWI, tissue perfusion, blood flow/volume, etc.)

(iii) Disadvantages

1. Cost.
2. Long acquisition times.
3. Technically more complex accounting for numerous different sequences.
4. More sensitive to artifact, particularly in the H&N region.
5. Less sensitive to small calcifications.
6. Ferromagnetic metal implants, devices, or fragments may prohibit the use of MRI.
7. May require sedation or anesthesia in the pediatric population.

(d) Positron Emission Tomography Computed Tomography

(i) Advantages

1. Whole body imaging.
2. Excellent at detecting distant metastases and nodal involvement.
3. Useful for therapy monitoring.

(ii) Disadvantages

1. Glucose uptake on 18FDG PET-CT can be nonspecific.
2. Cost.
3. Requires patient preparation and cooperation.
4. Radiation exposure.

6.1.2 Section 2: General Interventional Radiology [1–18]

1. Interventional radiology originally developed from diagnostic angiography and was officially

born on January 16, 1964 with the first percutaneous angioplasty of a superficial femoral artery (SFA) stenosis by a diagnostic angiographer, Dr. Charles Dotter, whom many consider to be the forefather of Interventional Radiology [1–6, 19]

2. Since that time, the specialty itself and the minimally invasive surgical techniques are increasing in popularity and have been ever-changing
   (a) As Dotter once said: "*The angiographic catheter can be more than a tool for diagnostic observation; used with imagination, it can become an important surgical instrument.*"
3. Many interventional radiology procedures have been shown to reduce cost, recovery time, pain, and risk as compared to conventional surgery
4. Interventional radiology procedures, as they relate to the head and neck as well as elsewhere in the body, can be divided into vascular and nonvascular procedures
   (a) Vascular
      (i) Major vascular procedures include diagnostic conventional angiography, angioplasty, atherectomy, thrombolysis, stenting, and embolization
   (b) Nonvascular
      (i) Major nonvascular procedures include percutaneous biopsy/drainage/injection, percutaneous ablation, nonvascular stenting, and pain management
   (c) Interventions within the head and neck are accomplished by a variety of proceduralists including interventional radiologists, neurointerventional radiologists, neurosurgeons, ENT surgeons, etc.
   (d) Specialty selection in regard to "procedural territory" often varies by institution
   (e) A few of the main vascular and nonvascular procedures pertaining to interventional radiologists are discussed below
   (f) Pre/peri-operative workup
      (i) Always thoroughly review history of present illness, labs, medications, and pertinent imaging
         1. If pertinent imaging or labs have not yet been obtained, recommend ordering prior to procedure
         2. Request patient be NPO for at least 6 h (or per hospital policy) if sedation is planned
      (ii) Risk stratify patient via the American Society of Anesthesiologists (ASA) Physical Status Classification System
         1. I: Normal healthy patient
         2. II: Mild to moderate systemic disease
            (a) Obesity, smoker
         3. III: Severe systemic disease that limits normal activity
            (a) ESRD
         4. IV: Severe systemic disease that is constant threat to life
            (a) Sepsis, recurrent variceal bleeds
         5. V: Not expected to survive without intervention
            (a) Ruptured AAA, large hemorrhage
         6. VI: Brain dead
      (iii) Assess bleeding risk [5]
         1. Desired INR < 1.5 and platelets > 50,000/μL for most interventional procedures
         2. Assess patient-specific and procedure-specific bleeding risk
         3. Hold antiplatelets and anticoagulants per procedure/hospital protocol
            (a) Clopidogrel: ideally held for 5 days prior to procedure
            (b) Aspirin: does not need to be withheld
            (c) Warfarin: desired INR for most procedures is <1.5
               (i) FFP or vitamin K for correction if needed
            (d) LMWH (therapeutic dose): held morning of procedure

(iv) Assess post-procedure contrast-induced nephropathy (CIN) risk [4–8]
1. Contrast-induced nephropathy (CIN) is defined by the Acute Kidney Injury Networks as an increase in serum creatinine >25% from baseline or serum creatinine increase of 0.3 mg/dL within 72 h after contrast administration
2. Risk factors for CIN include
   (a) Glomerular filtration rate <60 mL/min (particularly <30 mL/min) or baseline serum creatinine > 1.5 mg/dL
   (b) Age > 75
   (c) Diabetes
   (d) Medical conditions that decrease renal perfusion (i.e. heart failure)
   (e) Use of nephrotoxic medications (i.e. NSAIDS)
   (f) Procedure-related risk factors
      (i) Risk of CIN is dose dependent (procedures with a larger volume of intra-arterial contrast media use pose a greater risk)
3. CIN prevention
   (a) Pre/intra/post-procedural oral and/or IV hydration
      (i) Ideally 1 mL/kg/h of IV hydration 12 h prior to and after elective procedure
   (b) Minimize volume of intra-procedural arterial contrast
      (i) Consider other contrast agents, such as carbon dioxide (CO2) angiography
         1. An absolute contraindication to CO^2 angiography includes cerebral arteriography
      (ii) Note, a dose-toxicity direct relationship has only been shown for intra-arterial use of contrast, not intravenous
   (c) Temporal separation of contrast media procedures
   (d) Hold nephrotoxic medications
      (i) Patients taking metformin who develop CIN are at risk for lactic acidosis
4. Contrast reactions
   (a) Acute reactions to intravenous contrast can be divided into allergic-type and nonallergic-type; both of which can range in severity
   (b) Premedication
      (i) History of severe contrast reaction is considered a relative contraindication to receiving the same class of contrast
      (ii) In a patient with a known contrast allergy, any future administration of that class of contrast is likely to produce a similar reaction
         1. In fact, no evidence that premedication decreases the *incidence* of moderate or severe contrast reactions, it can however decrease the severity
         2. Therefore, if IV contrast is necessary for a patient who has had a previous reaction, a premedication regimen is recommended
      (iii) Premedication regimens vary by institution; those recommended by ACR include

1. Methylprednisolone 32 mg PO 12, 2 h prior ± diphenhydramine (Benadryl) 50 mg PO 1 h prior
2. **Or** prednisone 50 mg PO 13, 7, 1 h prior ± Benadryl 50 mg PO 1 h prior
3. **Or** hydrocortisone 200 mg IV 5 h and 1 h prior and Benadryl 50 mg IV 1 h prior
   (a) Note that IV steroids are only shown to be effective when given *at least* > *4 h* prior to administration of contrast (IV steroids given in emergent premedication < 4 h prior to contrast administration has not shown efficacy)

(v) Assess level of sedation needed
1. Local anesthetic
2. Minimal sedation/anxiolysis
3. Moderate sedation
   (a) Most interventional procedures are accomplished with moderate sedation
   (b) Level of sedation where patient can respond to verbal stimuli and protect their airway
   (c) Midazolam (Versed) is a benzodiazepine most commonly used for sedation
      (i) Typical starting dose is 1–2 mg IV with repeat doses 0.5–1 mg IV
      (ii) Onset of action is 1–5 min
      (iii) Lower doses should be considered in elderly patients and patients with liver or kidney failure due to impaired metabolism/clearance/excretion
      (iv) Can have paradoxical reaction whereby patient experiences hyper-agitation
   (d) Again, request patient be NPO for at least 6 h (or per hospital policy) if sedation is planned
4. Deep sedation
5. Monitored anesthesia care (MAC)
6. General anesthesia (endotracheal intubation)

(vi) Assess level of intra-/post-operative analgesia needed
1. Fentanyl (Sublimaze) is an opioid commonly used for analgesia in most IR procedures
   (a) Typical starting dose is ~50 μg IV with repeat doses 25–50 μg IV
   (b) Onset of action is within a minute
   (c) Higher doses may be needed for patients with high opiate tolerance
   (d) Hepatic or renal impairment has less effect and dose does not typically need to be lowered

5. Needles, wires, catheters, sheaths, balloons, and stents
   (a) Size
      (i) Needles are measured in gauge
         1. Gauge (g) refers to the outer diameter of the needle
         2. Higher the gauge, smaller the needle
         3. Typical needles encountered in IR include a 21 g needle to do micro puncture access and a 19 g needle to do direct access or transjugular liver biopsies

(ii) Wires are measured in inches
1. Typical wires encountered in IR include an 0.018″ wire used during microaccess and an 0.035″ guidewire
2. 19 g ~ 0.038″
(iii) Catheters and sheaths are measured in French
1. French (Fr) refers to the outer diameter of the catheter or sheath
2. 1 French = 0.33 mm
3. 3 French ~ 1 mm
4. The internal diameter of a catheter or sheath will vary with thickness of the wall of the device
(a) Thicker wall of device = smaller internal diameter
5. A 5 Fr sheath should accept a 5 Fr catheter
(iv) Balloons and stents are measured in millimeters
(v) It is essential to know the size relationships of these different measuring standards because inserting these devices into the body requires sliding one device through another device
(vi) The "size rule":
1. 19 g ~ 0.038″ ~ 3 Fr ~ 1 mm
(a) Note, these are all about the same size
(b) Also note, a 3 Fr catheter will not accept an 0.035″ wire due to catheter wall thickness
(i) Again, French is the *outer* diameter

6. Needles
(a) Divided into vascular access needles versus biopsy needles
(b) Vascular access needles are single-wall needles—have a single beveled (angled) edge with a small notch on the hub that corresponds to the bevel. They are more steerable than trocar needles because a beveled needle will bend toward the distal tip of the bevel
(c) Will often contain an inner stylet that is pulled out once the needle tip is confirmed, by ultrasound, to be within the vessel lumen
(i) A 21 g needle accepts a 0.018″ wire (which is what comes in most IR vascular microaccess kits)
1. Note—a 21 g needle does not accept a 0.035″ wire
(d) Biopsy needles are made to remove bodily tissue for pathologic analysis
(i) Biopsy needles come in various designs in regard to the shape of the needle tip
(ii) Trocar needle: two-part needle system with an outer cannula and a removable inner sharp three-sided trocar needle (*trois carre* = three sided).
1. Not steerable because of the three-sided tip
(iii) Chiba needle: two-part high-gauge needle system with a beveled edge that allows steering

7. Wires
(a) Wires have three main properties
(i) Size (diameter—typically 0.018″ or 0.035″)
(ii) Must have at least a 3 French catheter/sheath for an 0.018″ wire
(iii) Must have at least a 5 French catheter/sheath for an 0.035″ wire
1. Stiffness (determined by inner core and material constructed from)
2. Hydrophilic versus non-hydrophilic
(b) Three basic wire types (based on above properties)
(i) Microaccess wire: 0.018″ wire that used to get access and then quickly exchanged
(ii) Maneuver wire: floppy wire that is often hydrophilic ± curved tip to subselect vessels
1. Standard or stiff Glidewire (Terumo Medical, Somerset, NJ)
2. Fathom (Boston Scientific, Marlborough, MA)

(iii) Rail wire: stiff wire that provides a stability for catheter exchanges and during angioplasty/stenting
1. Amplatz (Boston Scientific, Marlborough, MA)
2. Rosen (Cook Medical, Bloomington, IN)
3. Lunderquist (Cook Medical, Bloomington, IN)

8. Catheters
   (a) Numerous catheter types available with different nuances
   (b) Divided into nonselective (flush) catheters and selective catheters
   (c) Nonselective flush catheters have multiple side holes which allow for high-flow injections into large arteries or veins and prevent vascular injury at the tip of the catheter during power injections
      (i) Commonly used for large vessel angiogram
   (d) Selective catheters usually have a single end hole and require lower flow rates injections than flush catheters but allow for more precise/selective injection
      (i) Commonly used for embolization and small vessel angiogram
      (ii) Microcatheters are typically 3F or smaller and allow for the subselection of small vessels advanced through a base or "parent" catheter

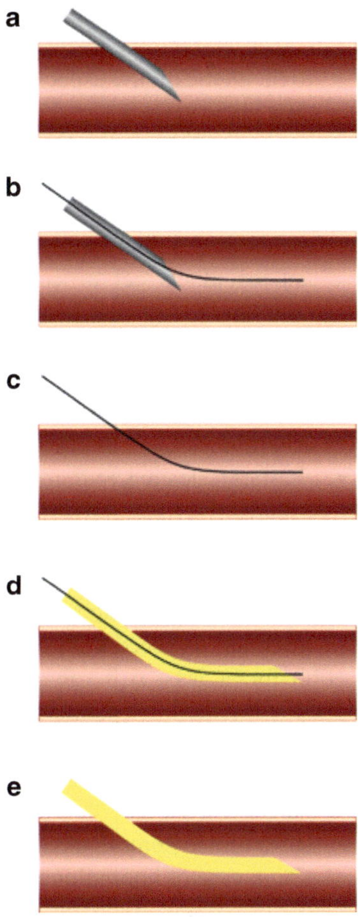

Fig. 6.1 (**a**) Under ultrasound guidance, a needle and stylet are introduced into the artery; (**b**) stylet removed and microwire introduced through needle; (**c**) needle removed; (**d**) catheter or sheath advanced over microwire; (**e**) microwire removed. (Image: wiki commons)

6.1.2.1 Vascular Access

- Proper vascular access is the foundation for all vascular interventional procedures
- The Seldinger puncture technique (Fig. 6.1a–e)
  - Fundamental interventional radiology maneuver whereby a guidewire/microwire is introduced through a needle puncture which is then exchanged for a sheath/catheter
  - A 21-g needle is needed for the 0.018″ microwire system
  - An 18-g needle is needed for the direct 0.035″ wire system
- Venous access
  - Most commonly accessed veins are the internal jugular and common femoral veins
  - Indications
    - Central venous access
    - Procedural access (i.e., transjugular intrahepatic portosystemic shunt [TIPS] or IVC filter placement/removal)
    - Diagnostic venography
  - Pre-procedural
    - Check history and review appropriate imaging
      - Patients with numerous prior venous access procedures or those with longstanding central venous access catheters may be challenging due to stenotic central venous system

Check labs and medications

- Check eGFR and potential nephrotoxic medications, especially if contrast planned
- Desired INR < 1.5 and platelets > 50,000/μL
- Assess patient and procedural risk of bleeding; holding antiplatelets and anticoagulants per procedure/hospital protocol
- Clopidogrel: ideally held for 5 days prior to procedure
- Aspirin: does not need to be withheld
- Warfarin: desired INR for most procedures is <1.5
  - FFP or vitamin K for correction if needed
- LMWH (therapeutic dose): held morning of procedure

NPO for at least 6 h (or per hospital policy) if sedation is planned

- Procedural

  Patient supine on table, sterile prepped, ± analgesia/sedation

  - Head turned contralaterally to access site in case of internal jugular access

  Under ultrasound guidance, perform the Seldinger technique

  - Find target vessel and identify important adjacent structures (i.e., carotid artery if accessing internal jugular vein or common femoral artery if accessing common femoral vein)
  - Anesthetize skin with lidocaine
  - Make a shallow skin nick with #11 scalpel
    - Incision can be made prior to or after 21 g needle insertion
  - 21 g needle (with inner stylet) inserted into the vein
    - Needle tip should be always visualized
  - 0.018″ microwire advanced through needle and advanced under fluoroscopic observation
  - Microaccess sheath (with inner dilator) then advanced over microwire
  - Remove inner dilator and microwire
  - 0.035″ guidewire advanced through microaccess sheath
  - Microaccess sheath removed and desired sheath/catheter advanced over 0.035″ guidewire

- Arterial access
  - Most commonly accessed arteries are the common femoral and radial arteries
  - Indications

    Procedural access

    - Angioplasty, atherectomy, thrombolysis, stenting, and embolization

    Diagnostic arteriography
  - Pre-procedural

    Check history and review appropriate imaging

    Check labs and medications

    - Check eGFR and potential nephrotoxic medications, especially if contrast planned
    - Desired INR < 1.5 and platelets > 50,000/μL
    - Assess patient and procedural risk of bleeding; hold antiplatelets and anticoagulants per procedure/hospital protocol
    - Clopidogrel: ideally held for 5 days prior to procedure
    - Aspirin: does not need to be withheld
    - Warfarin: desired INR for most procedures is <1.5
      - FFP or vitamin K for correction if needed
    - LMWH (therapeutic dose): held morning of procedure

    NPO for at least 6 h (or per hospital policy) if sedation is planned
  - Procedural

    Patient supine on table, sterile prepped, ± analgesia/sedation

    - Wrist in hyperextension for radial access

    Under ultrasound guidance, perform the Seldinger technique

    - Find target vessel and identify important adjacent structures

- Common femoral artery access site should be over the medial 1/3rd of the femoral head; high or low puncture could lead to retroperitoneal hematoma or inadvertent superficial femoral artery access, respectively
- Radial artery access site should be ~2 cm proximal to the radial styloid process
    - Some prefer to predilate radial artery with topical nitroglycerine prior to procedure

- Anesthetize skin with lidocaine
  - Skin entry site should be ~2 cm below (for retrograde arterial access) or above (for antegrade arterial access) the arteriotomy site
- Make a shallow skin nick with #11 scalpel
  - Incision can be made prior to or after 21 g needle insertion
  - Skin nick usually not necessary for radial access
- 21 g needle (with inner stylet) inserted into the artery at 45° angle
  - Needle tip should be always visualized
- 0.018″ microwire advanced through needle and advanced under fluoroscopic observation
- Microaccess sheath (with inner dilator) then advanced over microwire
  - Specific radial artery access sheaths are available
- Remove inner dilator and microwire
  - Vasodilatory "cocktail" administered through microaccess sheath
    - Nitroglycerin (200 μg) + verapamil (2.5 mg) + heparin (3000 units)
- 0.035″ guidewire advanced through microaccess sheath
- Microaccess sheath removed and desired sheath/catheter advanced over 0.035″ guidewire

6.1.2.2 Embolization [9–18, 20–35]

- Embolization refers to the insertion of an intravascular agent to control hemorrhage or for devascularization purposes
- Indications for embolization
  - Occlude active source or potential source of hemorrhage
    - Vascular rupture, aneurysms, pseudoaneurysms, arteriovenous fistulas, and varices
  - Tumor devascularization
  - Flow redistribution to protect tissue or facilitate flow to another tissue
    - For example, gastroduodenal artery (GDA) embolization prior to chemo/radioembolization for hepatocellular carcinoma protects the tissues supplied by the GDA from receiving chemotherapy or radiotherapy
  - Treatment of congenital arteriovenous or venous malformations
  - Treatment of venous insufficiency
    - For example, saphenous vein occlusion for lower extremity venous insufficiency
- Numerous embolization agents are available and are selected based on the indication for embolization, desired duration of embolization, and specific target(s) for embolization; they can be broadly divided into temporary versus permanent embolic agents
  - For example, a permanent embolic agent would be desired in a patient with an arteriovenous fistula
  - Embolic agents can also be differentiated by size of vessel occlusion (small, medium, or large) and mechanism of action (obstructs flow, thrombosis, or sclerosis)
    - In general, smaller embolic agents will embolize more distal vessels (i.e., capillaries) while larger embolic agents will embolize more proximal vessels
    - Some embolic agents (i.e., Onyx) can conform to the vessel lumen and therefore, obstruct flow to both small and large vessels

- Temporary embolic agents
  - Gelatin sponge
    Gelfoam (Upjohn Co, Kalamazoo, MI) or Surgifoam (Ethicon, Somerville, NJ)
    - Embolic particles that temporarily obstruct flow
      - Commonly used to temporarily embolize acute arterial hemorrhage
    - Usually completely resorbs with recanalization of the treated vessel with a few weeks
    - Can be prepared as single "torpedo" or "slurry" forms depending on indication for embolization
      - A "slurry" form can be created by cutting a Gelfoam sheet into very tiny squares which can then be mixed with contrast to create a slurry
        Mixed contrast provides fluoroscopic visualization while injecting

    Relatively inexpensive and effective
  - Avitene (Davol Inc, Cranston, RI)
    Embolic particle that temporary obstructs flow
    Made of microfibrillar collagen
    Completely resorbs with recanalization of the treated vessel within 2 months
  - Autologous clot
    Delivery of patient's own thrombosed blood products
    Completely resorbs with recanalization of the treated vessel within hours (very short duration of action)
- Permanent Embolic Agents
  - Coils
    Coils are radiopaque, permanent embolic agents
    Come in various shapes and sizes and primarily work by mechanical obstruction with subsequent recruitment of the patients own clotting cascade and platelet activation for permanent vessel occlusion
    Coated with tiny fibers and/or hydrogel which initiates platelet aggregation
    To consider using coils, the catheter needs to be advanced all the way to the target vessel/embolization area
    Coils should be slightly larger than the diameter of the target vessel lumen to avoid the risk of dislodgement (approximately 10–20% larger than the vessel lumen)
    "Pushable coils": deployed through a microcatheter via a coil-pusher wire with subsequent semi-forceful injection of ~2cc saline; difficult to retrieve after deployment if malpositioned
    "Detachable coils": can be deployed either mechanically or electrically and may be retrieved if malpositioned
    - Useful for high-flow shunts or vital vessels

    Stent-assisted coil embolism
    - Use of a noncovered stent to apply coils
    - Commonly used for pseudoaneurysm or berry aneurysm treatment
      - Noncovered stent placed across pseudoaneurysm neck
      - Microcatheter maneuvered through the stent interstices
      - Coils then introduced through microcatheter
  - Particles
    Particles are essentially tiny solids that induce permanent embolism
    - Gelfoam is technically a particle that only provides temporary embolization

    Usually have good small vessel penetration (better than coils but not as good as liquid embolic agents)
    Nonspherical Embolics—Polyvinyl Alcohol (PVA)
    - PVA particles are nonspherical irregular shavings from PVA blocks that vary in size from 50 to 1200 μm
    - Embolize by clumping together after injection and mechanically occluding the vessel lumen by activating the coagulation cascade (similar to coils)

- Clumping can lead to occlusion in a wide range of vessel calibers—can occlude both small and large vessels; smaller particles (100–300 μm) penetrate more deeply and medium to large particles (300–800 μm) penetrate less deeply
  - Degree of clumping determined by concentration of PVA particles
    - A more dilute solution prevents clumping whereas a very concentrated solution will rapidly clump
  - Like glue (discussed below), PVA particles in a very concentrated solution risk occluding the proximal vessel or even the catheter during injection and therefore, should be mixed with dilute contrast prior to administration
    - Concentration of PVA to dilute contrast will vary by size of target vessel

Spherical Embolics—"Microspheres"

- Spherical embolic agents, or "microspheres," also vary in size (50–1200 μm) and tend not to clump like nonspherical PVA particles, resulting in a more predictable location of aggregation location and size of vessel occlusion
- Does not usually need to be mixed with dilute contrast prior to administration (just mix with ~3cc of contrast)
- Numerous spherical embolic agents available, including
  - Embospheres (Biosphere Medical, Rockland, MA)
    - First microspheres used in humans
  - Contour SE microspheres (Boston Scientific)
  - EmboGold Microspheres (Merit Medical, South Jordan, UT)
  - Embozene microspheres (CeloNova BioSciences, Peachtree City, GA)
- Drug Eluting Particles
  - Promising "newer" drug delivery method whereby drugs our electrically or osmotically bound to particles and gradually elute to provide its therapeutic effect
  - Currently mostly used for chemotherapy/radiation drug delivery however, many non-chemoradiation drugs are currently being researched
    - Yttrium-90—beta emitting particle used to treat hepatocellular carcinoma

- Vascular plugs
  - Expandable radiopaque nitinol mesh plug that mechanically occludes the target vessel providing permanent embolization
  - Allows for single step vessel occlusion with precise positioning
  - Should be oversized relative to the target vessel by 25–50%
  - Amplatzer Vascular Plug (St. Jude Medical, Saint Paul, MN)
    - Compact vascular plug available in four forms (AVP I, II, III, and IV)
    - Requires a guide catheter or sheath for deployment
    - Newer vascular plugs are being developed that can be deployed through a microcatheter
- Liquids
  - Liquid embolic agents usually provide excellent small vessel penetration and occlusion
    - Administration is sometimes difficult to control depending on flow dynamics and embolic agent properties
      - Greatest risk is nontarget embolization due to higher than expected vascular flow
  - Ethanol
    - Ethanol (96–98%) is a liquid embolic agent that immediately causes protein denaturing and permanent vessel thrombosis

- Can embolize an entire organ if desired
- Sometimes painful during delivery
- Not fluoroscopically visible unless mixed with Lipiodol—radiopaque substance (~4:1 mix)

Glue (N-butyl cyanoacrylate [n-BCA])

- Non-resorbable, non-radiopaque liquid embolic agent
- Most used to treat vascular malformations, particularly intracranial
- Liquid glue (cyanoacrylate) is a monomer that immediately becomes a solid polymer when contacted with ionic medium (i.e., blood or saline)
  - Glue will solidify within the catheter unless a substance is added that extends the polymerization time
  - Lipiodol (Guerbet, Paris, France)
    Lipiodol (aka ethiodized oil) is a radiopaque poppy seed oil that is typically mixed with cyanoacrylate to extend polymerization time or with ethanol for fluoroscopic visualization
    - Common to also add powdered tantalum during intracranial procedures to increase fluoroscopic visualization during injection

    Typically, ~5:1 lipiodol to cyanoacrylate ratio
    The higher the ratio, the longer the polymerization time
- Preparation and administration can therefore be a tedious and deliberate process
- The final mixture of liquid glue is injected after the catheter has been flushed with D5W
- The major disadvantage/risk of using cyanoacrylate is secondary to rapid polymerization
  - Can result in lack of nidus/small vessel penetration which can even lead to gluing the catheter in place
  - If polymerization time is too long, can pass into the venous circulation resulting in pulmonary emboli

Onyx (ev3 Endovascular Inc, Covidien, Plymouth, MN)

- Onyx is an ethylene vinyl alcohol (EVOH) copolymer mixed with dimethyl sulfoxide (DMSO) and opacified with radiopaque micronized tantalum powder (added for fluoroscopic visualization)
- When Onyx encounters blood, the DMSO rapidly diffuses away resulting in precipitation and solidification of the alcohol polymer—said to have "lava-like" flow as compared to free flowing liquid embolics, such as ethanol
- Forms an elastic "foam" that conforms to the vessel lumen
- Non-adhesive property allows for slower injection and less risk of catheter-to-vessel adhesion contrary to n-BCA glue
  - Precipitation time is mainly determined by the amount of EVOH
    More ethylene vinyl alcohol, quicker precipitation time
  - Two kinds of Onyx preparations
    Onyx 18 = 6% EVOH
    - Precipitates slower and penetrates more deeply and therefore, used for slow-flow vascular malformations/fistulas

    Onyx 34 = 8% EVOH
    - Precipitates quicker and has less penetration therefore, used for high-flow vascular malformations/fistulas

    Final solidification occurs within 5 min for both Onyx preparations

Precipitating hydrophobic embolic liquid (PHIL)

- PHIL is a newer non-adhesive liquid embolic agent made of an iodine-

bound polymer dissolved in dimethyl sulfoxide (DMSO)
  - The bound iodine provides fluoroscopic visualization
- There are four concentrations of PHIL (25%, 30%, 35% and low viscosity [LV])
- Similar to Onyx, the non-adhesive property allows for slower injection and less risk of catheter-to-vessel adhesion
- Unlike Onyx, iodine is covalently bonded to PHIL, rather than mixed with tantalum powder which leads to less glare artifact on follow-up CT scans
- Useful in embolization of neurovascular lesions (AVMs and hypervascular tumors)
- Prepared in a pre-filled sterile 1 mL syringe
- Recent studies have shown that this is a promising liquid embolic agent with very effective small vessel penetration, adequate fluoroscopic visibility, and little reflux

Thrombin
- Off-label use for treatment of arterial access complications such as pseudoaneurysm

- Sclerosants

Sclerotherapy has mostly become the first-line therapy of most venous and lymphatic malformations (low-flow vascular malformations) in the head and neck

Sclerosing agents are detergents that damage the endothelium by inducing an inflammatory reaction with eventual thrombotic vascular occlusion and sclerosis
- Liquid embolic agents are technically considered "sclerosants" however, the term is generally reserved for agents that primarily treat venous/low-flow disease

May be administered intravascularly or percutaneously
- Intravascular transcatheter balloon occlusion and/or coil/gelform embolization may be simultaneously used to prevent nontarget sclerotherapy

Numerous sclerosing agents available with differing effectiveness and side effects

Sodium tetradecyl sulfate (Sotradecol) (AngioDynamics, Latham, NR; Thrombotect, Omega, Montreal, Canada)
- Commonly used for esophageal varices, venous malformations, and varicose veins
- Liquid or foam forms

Ethanolamine oleate
- Mixture of 5% ethanolamine oleate (ethanolamine plus oleic acid) and ethiodol, ratio typically 5:1 or 5:2
- Less penetration than absolute ethanol and associated with less regional side effects (less adjacent tissue damage)
- Main side effect is nephrotoxicity as oleic acid may adhere to serum proteins and travel to the kidneys
  - Prophylactic haptoglobin (serum protein) used to reduce risk of nephrotoxicity
- Indicated for the treatment of esophageal varices that have recently bled, venous malformations, and cyst sclerosis

Bleomycin
- Effective in superficial lymphatic malformations
- Pingyangmycin is a bleomycin derivative commonly used in China

Picibanil (OK-432)
- Lyophilized mixture of group A Streptococcus pyogenes with antineoplastic activity used to treat lymphatic malformations

Doxycycline
- Inexpensive antibiotic sclerosing agent widely used for lymphatic malformations and abscesses

Ethanol

- Liquid sclerosant that immediately denatures proteins upon contact
- Effective but associated with significantly more side effects, particularly in the head and neck, such as adjacent tissue damage (nerve damage) and skin necrosis/ulceration
  - For these reasons, ethanol is not usually recommended in the head and neck

6.1.3 Section 3: Nonvascular Procedures of the Head and Neck

Discuss the distinct nonvascular procedures performed by Interventional Radiology.

1. Image-Guided Biopsies
   (a) Superficial masses may be amenable to non-image guided biopsy in the clinician's office. Deeper head and neck lesions may be percutaneously biopsied under image guidance, with CT and US being the most commonly employed imaging modalities.
   (b) After adequate head positioning, virtually all major spaces of the head and neck are amenable to image- guided biopsy. Intravenous contrast may be used to better delineate surrounding vascular structures and most procedures can be performed with local anesthetics and moderate sedation.
   (c) Biopsies of the upper cervical spine and upper aerodigestive tract may require general anesthesia.
   (d) Typically, a coaxial needle technique is used. An 18–19-gauge guiding needle is advanced near the target lesion, followed by advancement of the biopsy needle into the lesion. 20–22-gauge needles, such as a Chiba needle, are used to obtain aspirates, while a 20-gauge cutting needle can be used for acquiring core samples.
   (e) Approximately 90% of biopsies yield diagnostic samples.
   (f) Complications include pain, vasovagal reactions, bleeding, and infection. Significant blood vessel or nerve injury is rare.
2. Thermal Ablation Methods
   (a) General
      (i) Apply direct thermal therapy to a lesion with the purpose of producing significant or complete tumor ablation.
      (ii) Techniques include cryoablation, microwave ablation, and radiofrequency ablation.
      (iii) Can be used to treat benign and malignant tumors, though most commonly used for palliative treatment of unresectable malignancies or treatment of potentially resectable lesions in patients who are poor surgical candidates.
      (iv) Advantages include direct visualization of tumor response, reduced recovery time, and absence of a surgical scar.
   (b) Radiofrequency Ablation
      (i) Radiofrequency ablation is a relatively low risk procedure that utilizes electromagnetic radiation to create frictional heat and tissue necrosis. The goal is to produce a temperature between 55 and 100 °C for approximately 4–6 min. To ensure adequate tumor ablation, 0.5–1.0 cm of normal tissue surrounding the tumor must also be ablated.
      (ii) Nearby vasculature may dissipate heat and make tumor ablation harder, a concept known as heat sink. Additionally, one must be cautious of ablating tumors that are near the carotid artery, as this conveys an increased risk of stroke and carotid blowout.
      (iii) Major disadvantages include limited use with larger masses, the risk of vaporization, charring, and carbon-

ization at temperatures above 100 °C which in turn cause an insulating effect that may prevent tumor ablation, and the time to necrosis.

(iv) To treat larger masses, up to three radiofrequency probes can be placed within no more than 1 cm apart to generate a larger ablation zone.

(c) Cryoablation

(i) Cryoablation is a procedure in which there is rapid freezing of intratumoral tissue resulting in intracellular and/or extracellular ice crystal formation causing direct damage to cell structures or cell desiccation, respectively. The procedure involves several freeze and thaw cycles which can take up to 25–30 min. The goal is to produce a temperature between −35 and −20°C. Like radiofrequency ablation, a 0.5–1.0 cm margin of normal tissue ablation is recommended to ensure adequate success.

(ii) Major disadvantages include longer treatment time and the possibility of cryoreaction or cryoshock. Cryoreaction presents with tachycardia, tachypnea, fever, chills, and elevated creatinine levels. Cryoshock presents with multi-organ failure, severe coagulopathy, disseminated intravascular coagulation, and acute respiratory distress syndrome. These are thought to be the result of released cytokines from cellular debris after tumor reperfusion.

(d) Microwave Ablation

(i) Microwave ablation is a procedure that utilizes electromagnetic energy, water molecule agitation, and heat to cause coagulation necrosis. It occurs between frequencies of 900–2450 MHz, with the largest ablation zones seen at a frequency of 915 MHz.

(ii) Microwave ablation has similar results as radiofrequency ablation with the added benefits of increased speed, higher temperatures, and larger ablation zones. It is also less susceptible to electrical impedance and heat sinks.

(e) Percutaneous Sclerotherapy

(i) General

1. Involves the use of sclerosing agents administered via percutaneous catheterization to treat abnormalities of the head and neck such as low-flow vascular malformations, lymphatic malformations, plunging ranulas, sialoceles, and cysts.
2. Usually performed in the interventional suite with moderate sedation or under general anesthesia.
3. Typically, should be avoided in cystic or necrotic tumors, given the risk of producing a communication with surrounding vital structures and acutely infected lesions.

(ii) Low-flow Vascular Malformations

1. Sclerotherapy of the head and neck is most commonly performed for venous and/or lymphatic malformations. These lesions can cause symptoms ranging from pain and swelling to significant functional impairment including hemodynamic effects and airway compromise from mass effect. MRI is particularly useful for the evaluation of these lesions. The presence of phleboliths and enhancement in venous malformations helps distinguish them from lymphatic malformations.
2. The most commonly used sclerosing agents for venous malformations include ethanol, sodium tetradecyl sulfate, and polidocanol.
3. The most commonly used sclerosing agents for lymphatic malfor-

mations include picibanil (OK-432) and doxycycline.

4. Multiple sclerotherapy sessions may be needed for larger or diffuse lesions.
5. Percutaneous Sclerotherapy of Venous Malformations (Direct Stick Embolization):
   (a) A 21-gauge butterfly needle is advanced into the venous malformation under ultrasound guidance.
   (b) Venous blood is freely aspirated from the lesion, confirming the vascular nature and flow pattern of filling of the lesion.
   (c) Angiography is performed with injection of 50% contrast to evaluate the size and venous drainage pattern of the lesion, as well as to exclude arterial cannulation. Volume of the sclerosant can be estimated at this time. The lesion is then serially injected under fluoroscopic guidance with boluses of 1:1 3% sodium tetradecyl sulfate (sotradecol):ethiodized oil (ethiodol) and the amount of sclerosing agent deployed is mindfully noted. Care is taken not to allow the sclerosing agent to enter the draining veins.
   (d) The procedure is then repeated for any other venous malformation in the adjacent tissues with similar 1:1 sotradecol:ethiodol formulation, in an incremental fashion. The total sclerosing agent deployed is similar for lesions in the oral mucosa, tongue, lip, and remaining upper aerodigestive tract.
   (e) The needle is then withdrawn from the venous malformation after 5 min following completion of the injections and another 5 min of very gentle pressure are applied to the puncture site following removal of the needle. At the completion of the procedure the face, neck, and upper chest are re-cleansed with sterile saline solution. The skin of the neck and upper chest was no longer erythematous and without an urticarial reaction.
   (f) (Different case?)
   (g) A butterfly needle was then used to access the posterior pouch of the venolymphatic malformation with biplanar fluoroscopy.
   (h) Free flowing blood aspiration out of the venolymphatic pouch and a pouchogram is performed to ensure access into the venolymphatic pouch proper.
   (i) The needle is then flushed and, under biplane fluoroscopy, an injection mixture of 1:1:1 of 3% Sotradecol, Ethiodol and air (for foam) is instilled to cause sclerosis of any vascular island or pouch. Additional pools or pouches in different planes and deeper are again evaluated by pouchogram to ensure access is within the pouch and sclerosing agent is instilled in a similar fashion.
   (j) All needles are then removed and light pressure is applied for hemostasis.
   (k) Notably, intraoperative ultrasound and biplane fluoroscopy are essential in finding additional pools or pouches.

6.1.4 Section 4: Vascular Procedures of the Head and Neck

6.1.4.1 Management of Acute Hemorrhage

- Epistaxis
  - Causes
    - Idiopathic
    - Trauma with vascular injury
      - Post nasotracheal intubation
    - Tumor
      - Primary or metastatic tumors involving the nasal mucosa may present with intractable epistaxis
      - Primary tumor: classically, juvenile nasopharyngeal angiofibroma (JNA)
    - Hereditary hemorrhagic telangiectasia (HHT)
      - Osler-Weber-Rendu syndrome
      - Autosomal dominant disease that affects the nasal mucosa, abdominal viscera, and central nervous system characterized by numerous telangiectasias and AVMs
  - Treatment
    - Varies by cause
    - Majority are treated by nasal packing or cutaneous electrocauterization
    - Refractory epistaxis not responsive to anterior and posterior nasal packs associated with significant blood loss may be amenable for arterial embolization
  - Pre-procedural considerations
    - Pre-procedural imaging should be reviewed and should include a CT/CTA to exclude possible mass/tumor causing hemorrhage
    - Gather relevant past medical history and labs
      - Correct the coagulopathy if present (desired INR < 1.5)
      - Hold anticoagulation if still taking
      - CBC (desired platelets > 50,000)
  - Procedural
    - General anesthesia is typically recommended for airway protection as patient may hemorrhage while in supine position
    - Obtain arterial access
      - Most commonly right common femoral artery approach
    - Angiographic protocol for the evaluation of epistaxis includes assessment of bilateral internal/external carotids, internal maxillary (particularly sphenopalatine branches), and facial arteries
    - Vascular supply to nasal mucosa
      - Supplied by the distal internal maxillary and facial arteries (sphenopalatine branches)
      - The ophthalmic artery may supply nasal mucosa via ethmoidal branches
    - Epistaxis usually successfully treated with embolization of bilateral sphenopalatine arteries ± ipsilateral distal facial branch of internal maxillary artery
      - It is recommended that the contralateral sphenopalatine artery be angiographically evaluated even if there is unilateral bleeding as there may be contralateral collateralization
    - If epistaxis persists, then hemorrhage may be from ethmoidal branches of the ophthalmic artery which are typically not embolized due to risk of vision loss
    - Polyvinyl alcohol (PVA) or embozene particles are suitable embolic agents
  - Complications
    - Major complications include routine risks of cerebral angiography as well as ischemic stroke by inadvertent embolization of intracranial collateral vessels and skin/mucosal necrosis most commonly due to too small particle size

6.1.5 Case: Epistaxis from Traumatic Nasotracheal Intubation Requiring Embolization (Fig. 6.2)

6.1.5.1 Case: Refractory Epistaxis of Unknown Etiology

Access to the right common femoral artery was obtained with Seldinger technique. A shuttle sheath was advanced into the thoracic aorta over

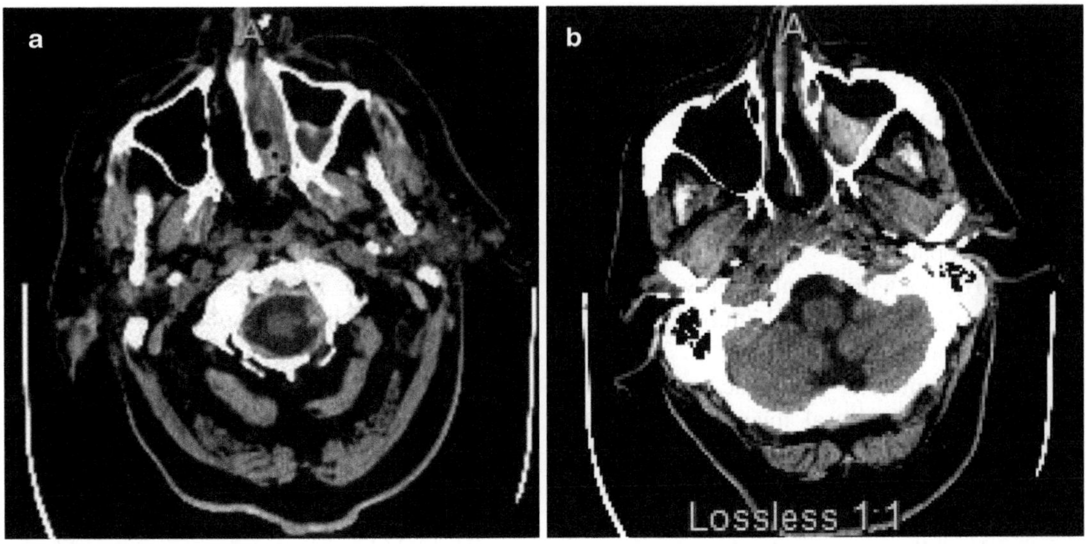

Fig. 6.2 (**a**, **b**) Non-contrast CT head demonstrating left nasal intubation with associated hemorrhage and blood products in the left maxillary antrum. Embolization was requested and performed. Patient's right groin was prepped and draped in usual sterile fashion. Right common femoral artery found to be patent by ultrasound (**c**). Ultrasound image archived. (**c**) Access was then obtained by Seldinger technique. A 5-French Berenstein catheter was advanced through the sheath into the aortic arch and the left common carotid artery was selectively catheterized. Digital subtraction arteriograms (DSA) were then obtained. (**d**) DSA of the left common carotid artery arteriogram. A microcatheter was then advanced into the left external carotid artery and eventually into the left internal maxillary artery. (**e**) DSA image demonstrating bifurcation into the left superficial temporal artery and proximal aspect of the left internal maxillary artery. (**f** and **g**) sagittal and coronal section—Microcatheter was advanced into the distal left internal maxillary artery near the bifurcation of the internal maxillary artery into the sphenopalatine artery and greater palatine artery. Digital subtraction arteriograms demonstrated hyperemia over the nasal mucosa and posterior nasal pharynx. Microcatheter could not be advanced further and the left greater palatine artery was chosen to be sacrificed. Multiple DSAs were obtained. No collateral flow to the internal carotid circulation was identified. Ophthalmic artery was not visualized. Again hyperemic flow was identified within the nasal cavity and nasal pharynx. The sphenopalatine and greater palatine arteries were then embolized with 450 μm embozene particles. A follow-up lateral DSA demonstrated obstruction of flow at the origin of the left sphenopalatine and midway through the left greater palatine artery. (**h**) Post embolization angiogram of the demonstrating lack of hyperemia or significant flow to the nasopharynx. Microcatheter was then pulled back and angiograms of bilateral maxillary, facial, and right sphenopalatine arteries were obtained which did not demonstrate hyperemia or significant flow to the nasopharynx

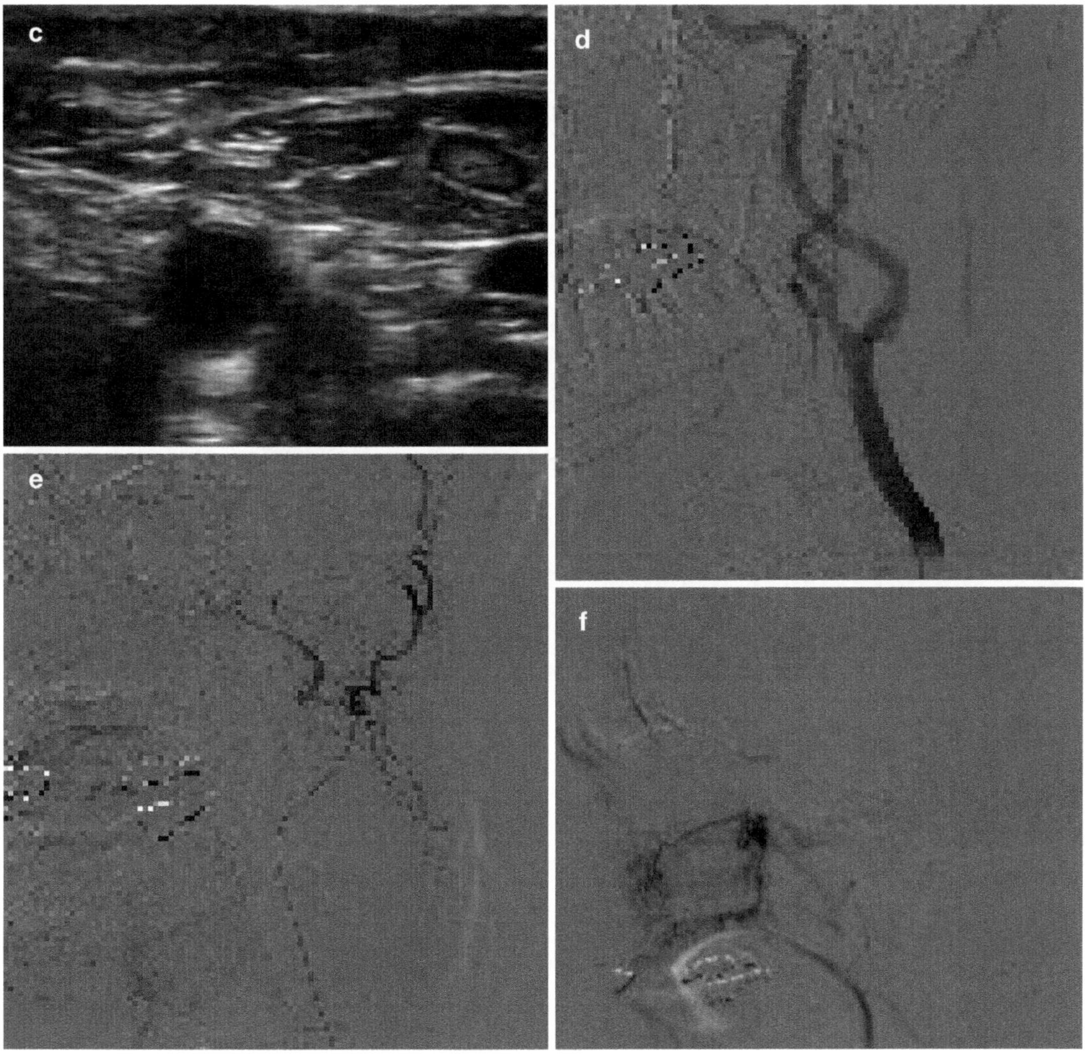

Fig. 6.2 (continued)

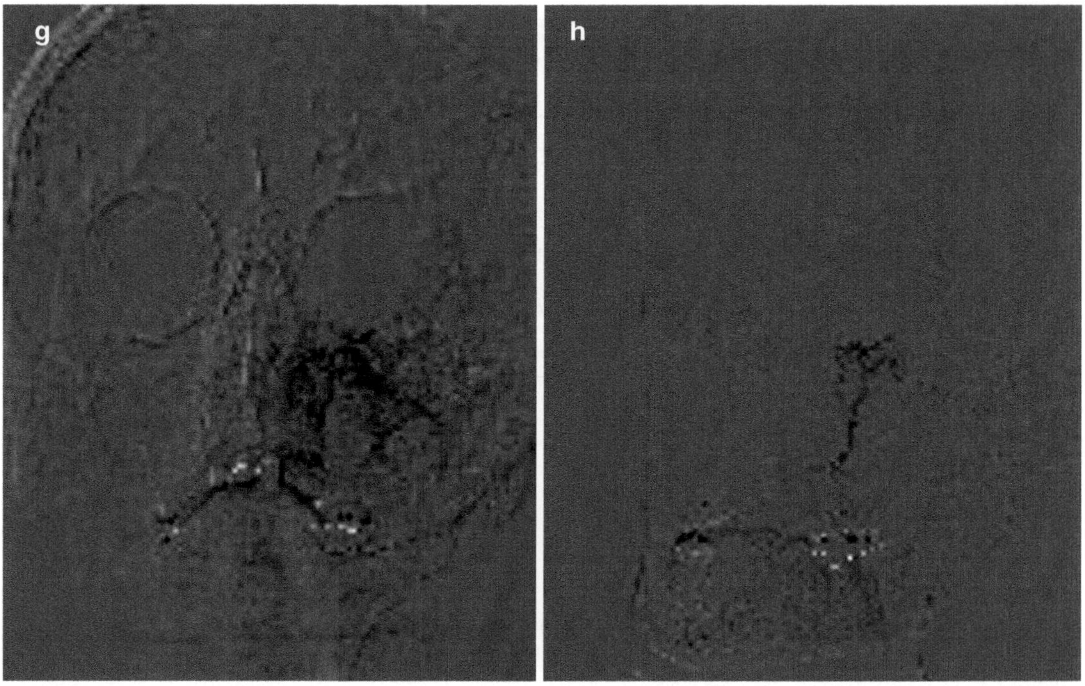

Fig. 6.2 (continued)

a Bentson guidewire. A 5-French vertebral catheter was used to navigate the great vessels of the aortic arch, and the common carotid artery was selected. Right common carotid arteriogram was performed demonstrating appropriate placement (Fig. 6.3).

6.1.5.2 Case: Large Left Glomus Vagale Paraganglioma Treated with Embolization (Fig. 6.4)

- Traumatic Vascular Injuries
  - General

    Traumatic vascular injuries of the head and neck can occur from blunt or penetrating trauma. If osseous fractures are seen adjacent to the expected location of vascular structures on CT, CTA may be necessary to further evaluate for vascular injury. In cases of penetrating injury, the injury tract can also be evaluated at time of CT. Alternatively, angiography can be performed and would also be effective at identifying vascular lacerations, occlusions, pseudoaneurysms, and/or vasospasms.

    Angiography is performed after standard heparin bolus with evaluation of the aortic arch, carotid arteries and major branches, and vertebral arteries, but the protocol may vary based on the nature of vascular injury. Routine risks of cerebral arteriography apply, including additional risk of vascular injury and stroke.

    Continuous ICU neurologic and hemodynamic monitoring may be required, particularly if there is vertebral or internal carotid artery injury or if treatment involved major vessel occlusion.
  - Oronasal bleeding from facial fractures

    Usually requires the embolization of injured ECA branches with temporary embolic agents such as PVA foam particles or gelfoam pledgets. NBCA glue or Onyx can be used for the treatment of fistulas or pseudoaneurysms.

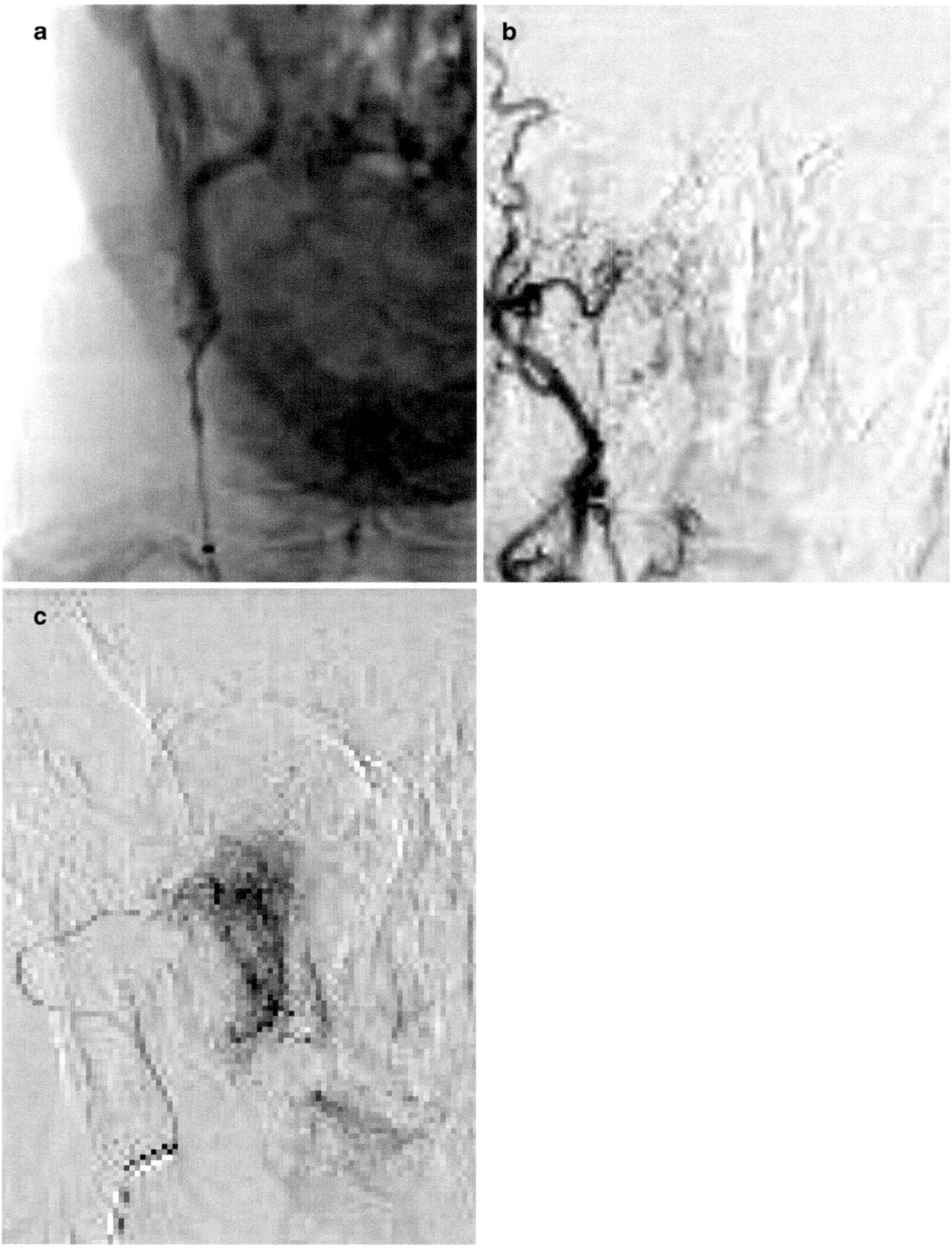

Fig. 6.3 (**a**) A right carotid arteriogram with access through the aortic arch. (**b**) Using a stiff Glidewire, the vertebral catheter was used to select the right external carotid artery. Right external carotid PA DSA was performed documenting appropriate placement of the vertebral catheter. Mild hyperemia can be seen within the sphenopalatine branch of the internal maxillary artery. (**c**) The microcatheter/microwire system was then subselectively advanced into the sphenopalatine branch of the right internal maxillary artery. Subselective DSA was performed confirming appropriate placement and demonstrating no branches supplying the orbits or other vital structures. The hyperemia is again noted. At this point, 400 μm Embozene particle embolization was performed under fluoroscopic guidance, with 1/5 of a viral used until near stasis was noted

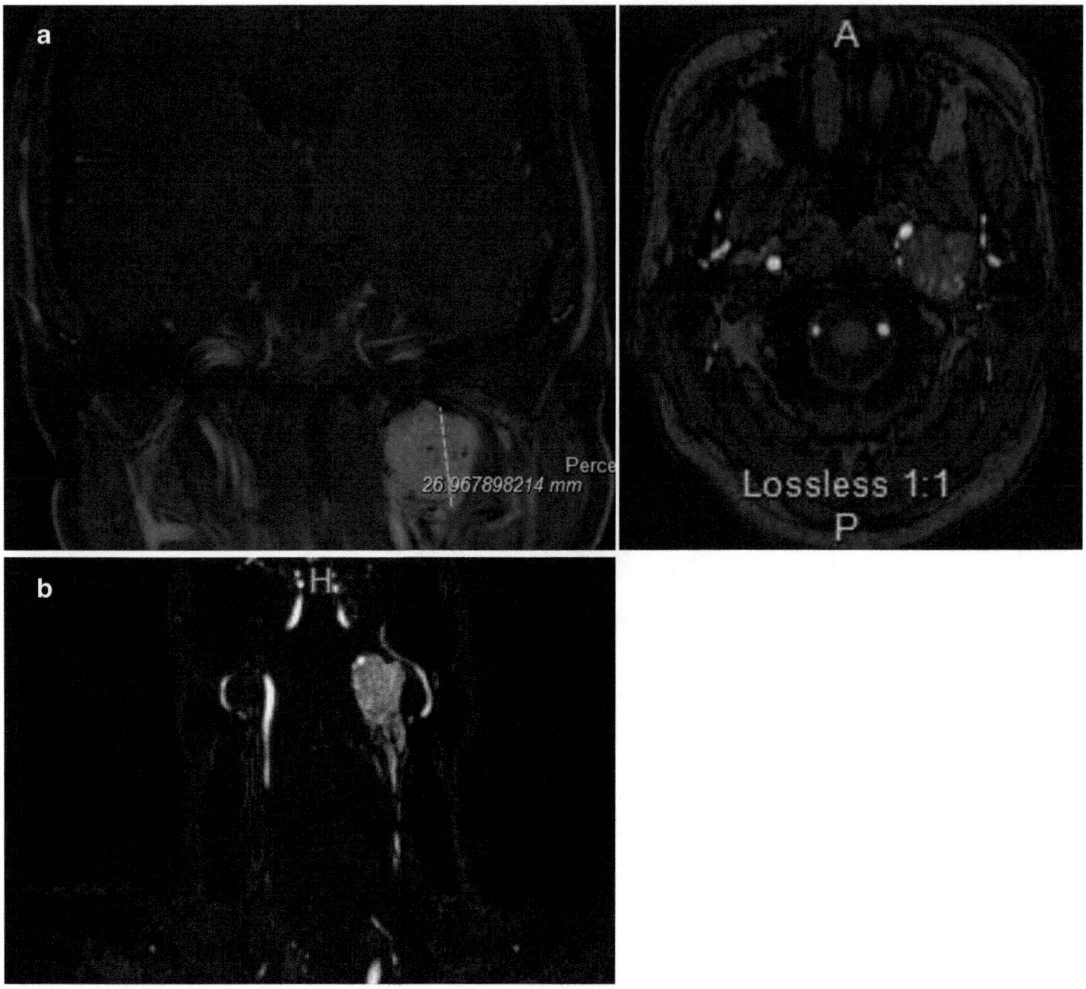

Fig. 6.4 (**a**, **b**) Post contrast coronal and axial T1, coronal time-of-flight MRA. (**c**) coronal MIP demonstrating large hypervascular mass adjacent to the left ICA near the base of the skull, characteristic of glomus vagale. Post contrast coronal T1, coronal time-of-flight MRA, and coronal MIP demonstrating large hypervascular mass adjacent to the left ICA near the base of the skull, characteristic of glomus vagale. (**c**) DSA demonstrating large hypervascular mass adjacent to the left ICA near the base of the skull, characteristic of glomus vagale. DSA demonstrating large hypervascular mass adjacent to the left ICA near the base of the skull, characteristic of glomus vagale. (**d**) DSA demonstrating feeder vessel to the glomus vagale. DSA demonstrating feeder vessel. (**e**) Subselective DSA image of hypervascular mass. (**f–h**) Subselective DSA image of hypervascular mass and Pre and Postembolization DSA demonstrating stasis of flow to the previously seen hypervascular mass. Pre and Postembolization DSA demonstrating stasis of flow to the previously seen hypervascular mass

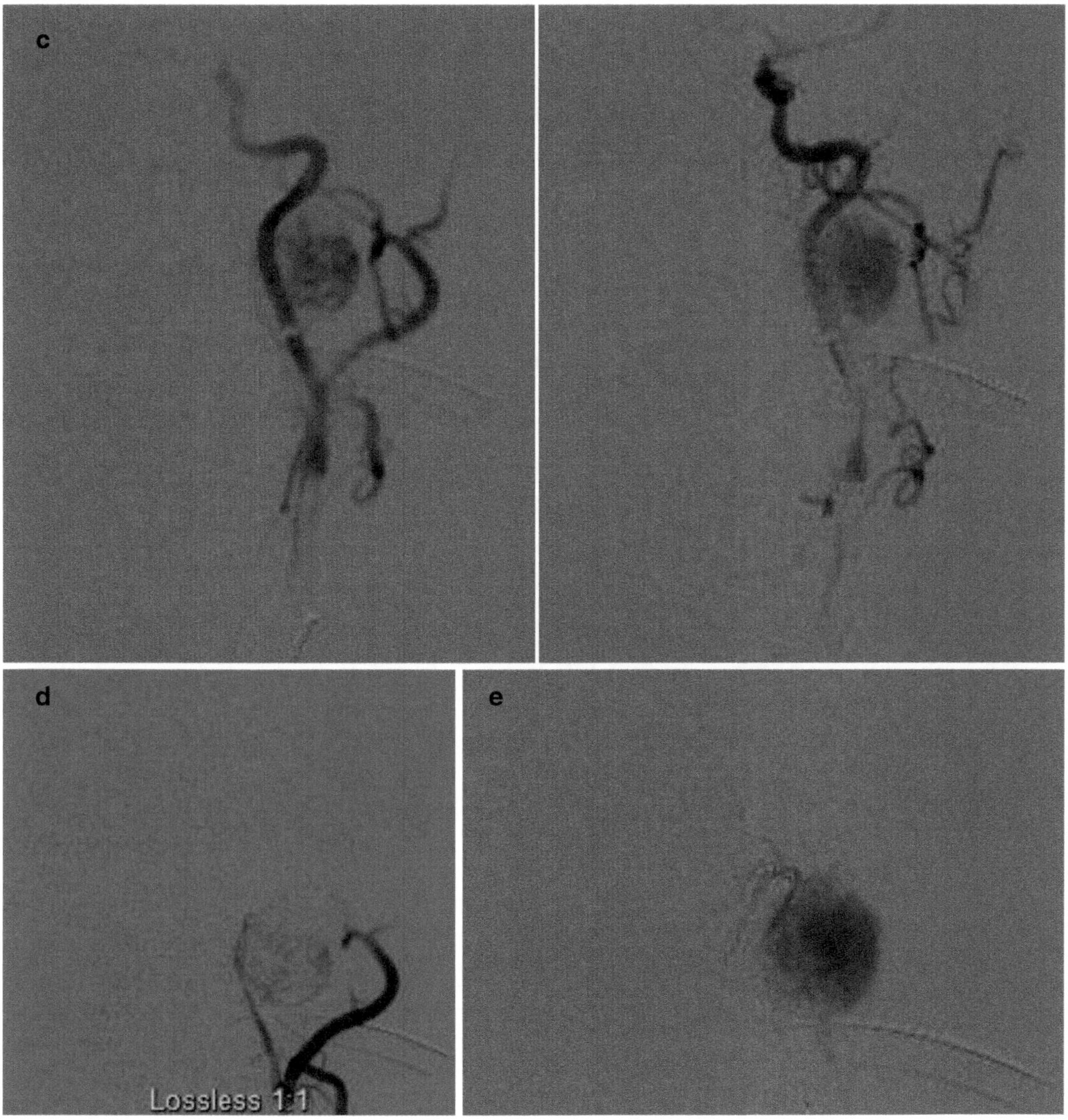

Fig. 6.4 (continued)

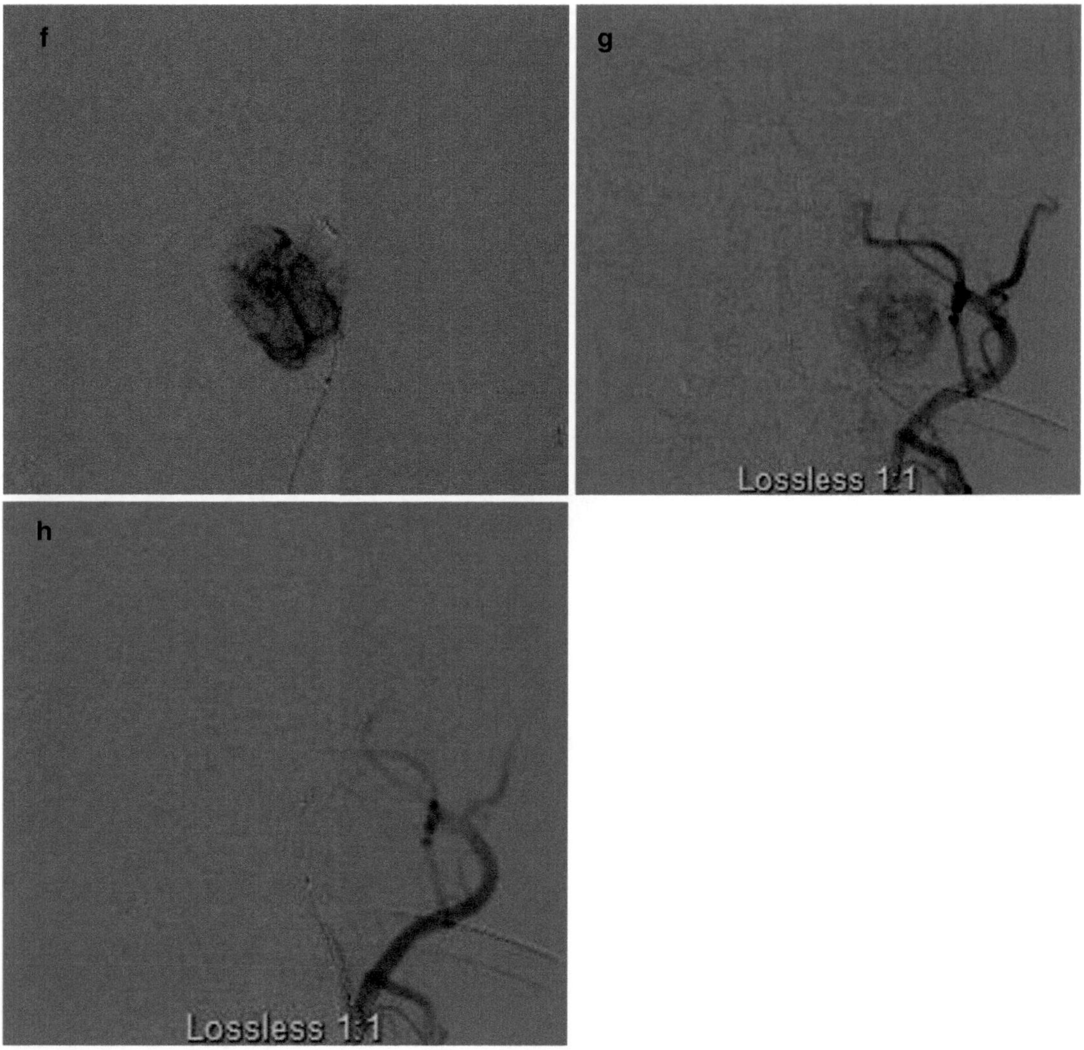

Fig. 6.4 (continued)

– Carotid/Vertebral Artery Injury

Injury in the form of laceration or rupture can occur anywhere along the course of the carotid artery and branches and special attention on imaging should be made to fixed points, such as where the internal carotid artery enters the dura or within the cavernous sinus. Ultimately, injury can lead to occlusion, pseudoaneurysm or fistula formation. Expectant management is usually employed in the event of traumatic carotid occlusion as surgical bypass is usually not possible. Pseudoaneurysms, on the other hand, may be amenable to stents ± coils deployed into the excluded pseudoaneurysm. Alternatively, surgical repair or, if adequate collateral flow is demonstrated, parent artery occlusion may be performed.

Similarly, vertebral artery injury can occur anywhere along its course and special attention on imaging should be made to fixed points, such as the entry sites into the vertebral foramen and at the craniocervical junction. As mentioned above, osseous irregularity on CT, particularly at the vertebral foramen, may prompt further evaluation with CTA to exclude underlying injury. After determination of collateral flow, vertebral artery injury may require embolization or sacrifice, which can be performed with platinum micro-coils.

- Traumatic Carotid-Cavernous/Vertebrojugular Fistulas

  Carotid-Cavernous and vetebrojugular fistulas are typically seen after penetrating trauma, however, can be seen in the setting of any severe head and neck injury, as well as iatrogenic injury. Carotid-Cavernous fistulas classically present with pulsatile exophthalmos, though symptoms largely depend on the pattern of venous drainage. Additional symptoms include chemosis, proptosis, progressive visual loss, pulsatile tinnitus, and intracranial hemorrhage, including intraparenchymal hemorrhage in the setting of cortical venous drainage. Vertebrojugular fistulas present with cerebral ischemic symptoms relating to "stolen" arterial blood from the posterior circulation or hemodynamic instability from arteriovenous shunting. Emergent treatment is usually not required unless there is risk of vision loss in the case of carotid-cavernous fistulas. For both types of fistulas, treatment usually involves the closure of the fistula using an arterial approach, but venous approach may also be employed based on fistula location or venous drainage pattern. In severe cases, parent artery occlusion or sacrifice may be necessary.

- Malignancy
  - Tumoral Hemorrhage and Carotid Blowout Syndrome [16, 22, 32]

    When assessing upper aerodigestive tract bleeding from malignant disease, it is important to also assess the extent of tumor spread in order to appropriately guide endovascular treatment. This can be done by reviewing prior imaging or performing emergent CT or MRI if the patient's condition allows.

    Bleeding can occur from increased tumor neovascularity or direct injury of adjacent vasculature. Treatment usually involves direct embolization of injured vasculature or pseudoaneurysms but may also require the occlusion or "sacrifice" of arterial branches supplying the tumor, arising either from the external, internal, or common carotid arteries. Prior to occlusion of the internal carotid artery, a Balloon Occlusion Tolerance (BOT) test can be performed to assess tolerance of carotid occlusion. It usually involves diagnostic arteriography to evaluate for collateral flow, clinical testing after temporary balloon occlusion, and HMPAO SPECT to evaluate cerebral blood flow after temporary occlusion. Endovascular occlusion is usually performed by employing detachable platinum coils with or without the use of a closure device.

    Carotid Blowout Syndrome usually refers to acute, though sometimes chronic, bleeding of the upper aerodigestive tract from direct tumor erosion of the major head and neck vasculature. It is usually treated with carotid sacrifice after performing temporary BOT testing. In some life-threatening instances, carotid sacrifice must be performed without provocative testing and the risk of stroke is significantly higher.

    Tumoral hemorrhage refers to upper aerodigestive bleeding from increased tumor vascularity or tumor injury of smaller surrounding vessels. It is usually treated with direct embolization, however, may require carotid sacrifice in more severe cases.

    Postprocedural management of carotid occlusion or sacrifice entails close neuro-intensive ICU monitoring and hemodynamic therapy (Fig. 6.5).

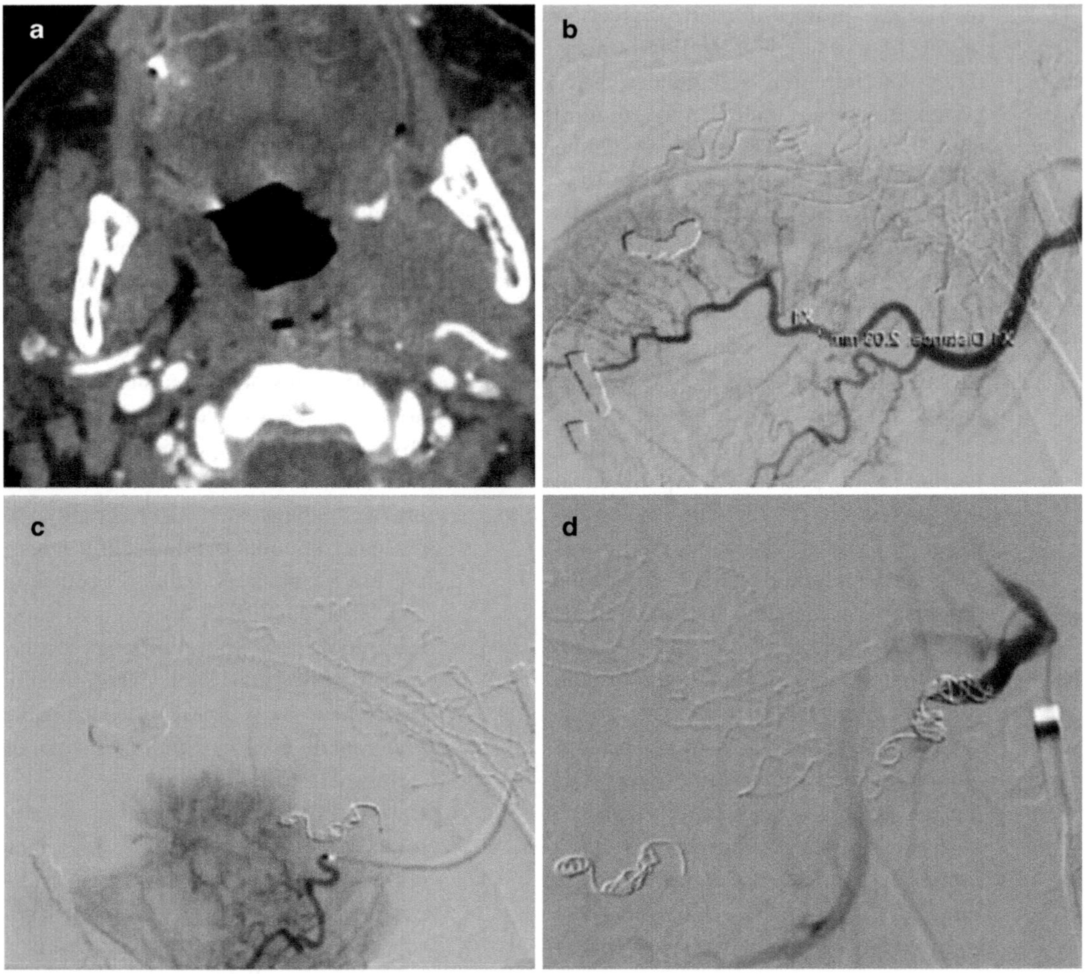

Fig. 6.5 (**a**–**d**) Case of a 73-year-old male with history of poorly-differentiated squamous cell carcinoma within the left oropharyngeal wall presenting with persistent oropharyngeal bleeding which was treated coil embolization of the left lingual artery. (**a**) Axial CTA image through the oropharynx demonstrates masslike fullness of the left oropharyngeal wall tonsillar pillar region with a small focus of contrast within the left glossotonsillar sulcus suspicious for pseudoaneurysm and hemorrhage source. (**b**) Lateral DSA image shows no clear contrast extravasation or pseudoaneurysm arising from the left lingual artery and branches. (**c, d**) Based on the location of the SCC and continued oropharyngeal bleeding, the left lingual artery was embolized. Embolization microcoils were deployed distal to the origin of the sub-lingual artery and dorsal lingual arteries to prevent backfeeding from the contralateral lingual artery. Gelfom pledgets were then injected into the sublingual artery, followed by the injection of 200 μm PVA particles at the level of the lingual artery. Finally, microcoils were deployed in the proximal portion of the lingual artery to prevent recanalization

- Management of Vascular Lesions [1, 3, 8–14]

  Intra-arterial Chemotherapy

  - Intra-arterial chemotherapy has been used to treat both intracranial and extracranial head and neck tumors. Notably in the extracranial head and neck, intra-arterial chemotherapy has been used in the treatment of carcinomas, but use has also been reported in the treatment of metastases, malignant melanoma, and neuroblastomas.
  - The radiation and platinum (RADPLAT) protocol involves the

direct tumor administration of extremely high doses of cisplatin trans-arterially, while circulating the antagonist sodium thiosulfate as to minimize systemic toxicity. The increased dose of cisplatin increases tumor cytotoxicity and increases the effectiveness of subsequent radiation therapy.

- Transfemoral carotid arteriography is performed with selective catheterization of the ECA branch supplying the tumor. Infusion of 150 mg/m^2 of cisplatin over a period of 3–5 min is performed. During this time, concomitant administration of an intravenous infusion of 9 g/m^2 of sodium thiosulfate over a period of 3–5 min is performed, followed by an administration of 12 g/m^2 over a period of 6 h. In disease extending across midline, bilateral infusions may be performed. Treatment consists of four cycles of intra-arterial chemotherapy (days 1, 8, 15, and 22) and once daily radiation therapy 5 days a week.
- Results and techniques are variable based on practitioner and institution protocol. More recent studies have shown that RADPLAT is not superior to intravenous chemoradiotherapy in the treatment of advanced head and neck cancer, however it has been suggested that further investigation is warranted.

Tumor Embolization [16–18, 20–24]

- Cerebral angiography is first performed with selective injections of the internal and external carotid arteries. The artery supplying the tumor is accessed with a microcatheter and angiography is performed with special attention to anastomoses between the carotid and vertebral arteries. Any potentially dangerous anastomoses are coil embolized prior to particulate embolization.
- The aim of tumor embolization in the head and neck is the devascularization of lesions prior to surgical excision or to stop tumoral bleeding. It is frequently performed by trans-arterial route and the goal is to selectively occlude the external carotid artery feeders that ideally supply the arteriolar capillary beds in the tumor parenchyma with embolic material, as to avoid collateralization. This minimizes blood loss during surgery, provides a clean field for the surgical resection, improves resectability, makes the lesion amenable to different surgical procedures not previously feasible, reduces morbidity, shortens hospital stay, and reduces the rate of tumor recurrence.
- Embolization is usually done 24–72 h prior to surgical resection to allow maximal thrombosis and prevent recanalization and formation of collaterals.
- Skull base tumors that are supplied by branches of the ICA can be difficult to cannulate and convey an increased risk of embolic agent reflux and nontarget embolization. In these cases, direct percutaneous embolization of the tumor can be performed with liquid embolizing agents such as NBCA glue or Onyx.
- Benign vascular lesions may be treated with embolization without the need of subsequent surgery, as is the case of some congenital hemangiomas.
- Commonly embolized tumors of the head and neck include glomus tumors, angiofibromas, and meningiomas. The most common use of embolization is seen in the management of juvenile nasal angiofibromas—highly vascular tumors originating in the pterygo-palatine fossa which can expand aggressively through the sphenopalatine foramen

to involve other surrounding regions. Other tumors amenable to preoperative tumor embolization include esthesioneuroblastomas, schwannomas, rhabdomyosarcomas, plasmacytomas, chordomas, hemangiopericytomas, diffuse neurofibromas, and metastases.

- Commonly used embolizing agents include polyvinyl alcohol (PVA) particles and embospheres, usually in the size range of 100–300 microns, as well as liquid embolic agents, Onyx, gelatin sponge, and coils. Embolization coils are typically not used if open surgical resection is to be performed, however they may be useful if endoscopic resection is planned as proximal coil embolization of the feeding artery after particulate embolization of the tumor may provide added protection from vessel injury and intraoperative bleeding.
- As mentioned previously, Onyx can be used to devascularize tumor directly with relatively low risk. It has inherent properties that allow for a more controlled injection with superior penetration than NBCA glue. It is mechanically occlusive, but does not adhere to vessel walls, allowing it to be used as a single injection administered slowly over a longer period. If unwanted filling of normal vasculature occurs, the treatment can be stopped and resumed after a short period of approximately 2 min. Solidification will continue to occur in the region of previously embolized tumor and once the injection is restarted the agent will follow the route of least resistance and continue to embolize the remaining portions of the tumor.
- Overall, tumor embolization is a safe procedure with a serious complication rate of <2%. Complications include facial numbness, mucosal necrosis, blindness, or cerebrovascular accidents which are usually related to particle reflux, poor technique, or unidentified anastomoses.

- Vascular Malformations
  - Arteriovenous Malformations/Fistulas of the Head and Neck [1–39]

    See **Percutaneous Sclerotherapy** for more information on treatment of Low-flow Vascular Malformations.

    High-flow Vascular Malformations (HFVMs) are **rare** and can involve the soft tissues and bones of the head and neck. They commonly present as cosmetic deformities, however, can also cause pain, bleeding, and high-output heart failure from arteriovenous shunting.

    HFVMs treatment can be challenging depending on the lesion characteristics and are known to **frequently recur**. **Small lesions can be treated with endovascular embolization alone, however larger lesions may require surgical resection.**

    Distinction between a **vascular nidus versus an arteriovenous fistula** proper may also be challenging. Arteriovenous fistulas are less likely to recur after treatment.

    Commonly used embolic agents include ethanol, NBCA glue, Onyx, and coils. Trans-arterial NBCA glue has been shown to be more effective and permanent when compared to other embolization particles but may require staged procedures.

    As in low-flow vascular malformations, **direct puncture embolization** or percutaneous sclerotherapy can be performed to embolize the nidus and/or draining vein with NBCA glue or Onyx. Manual digital compression of the draining vein or the application of a compression device in cases with multiple draining venous channels can be used to alter flow and facilitate complete filling of the nidus. When compared to trans-arterial embolization, direct puncture embolization is associated with decreased risk of ischemic complications and reduced procedure times.

Given the rarity of these lesions, no standard of therapy has been determined (Fig. 6.6).

6.1.6 Section 5: Complications and Post-procedure Management

Provides an overview of common complications and post-procedural management

1. Pain and Fever
   (a) Perform a brief history evaluation. The pain description will usually coincide

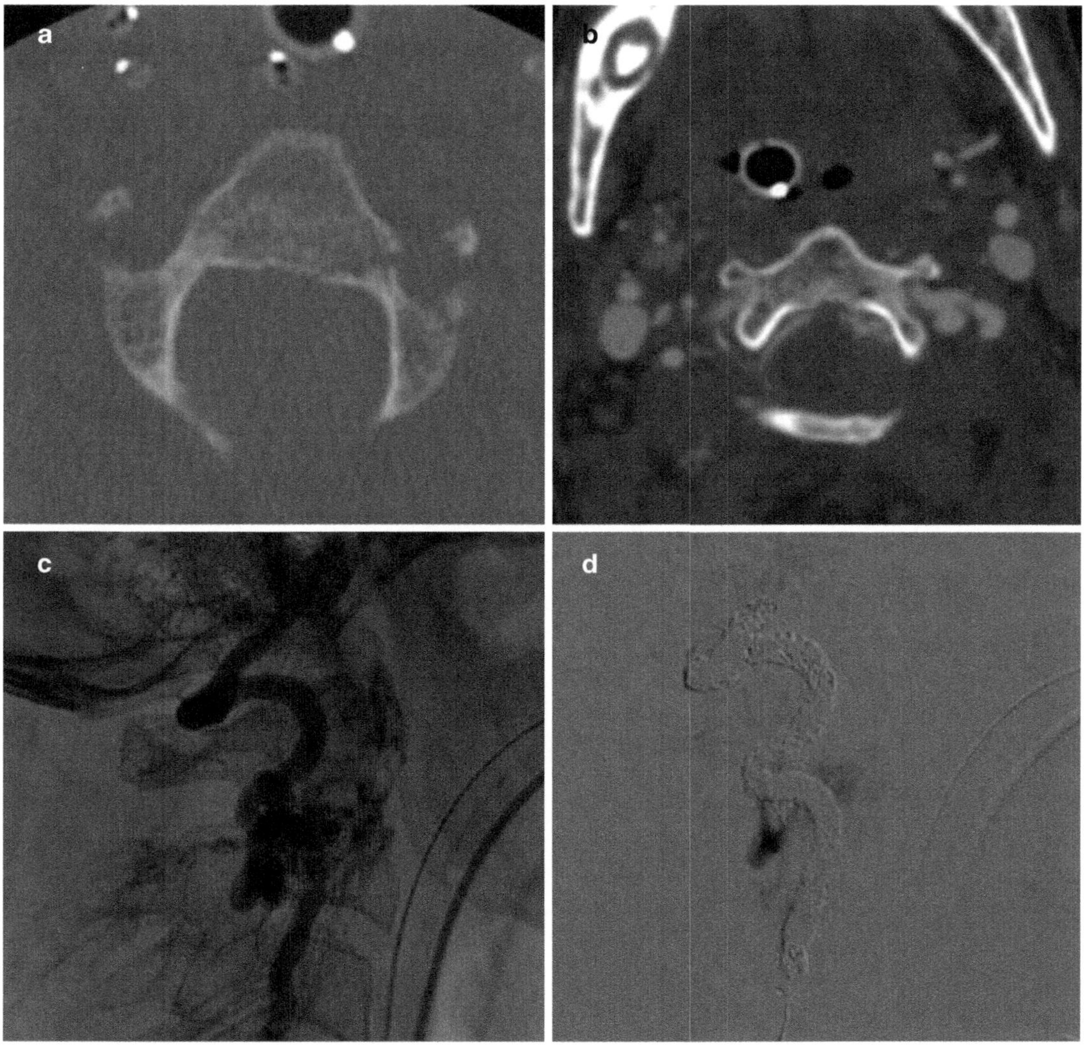

Fig. 6.6 (**a**–**d**) Case of a 72-year-old female presenting for MVC with Traumatic Vertebral Artery Pseudoaneurysm and Vertebral-Venous Fistula S/P Coil Embolization. (**a**) Axial NECT image of the cervical spine demonstrates a fracture of the dorsal C2 body with extension into the left foramen transversarium. (**b**) Axial CTA image through the level of the fracture shows a multilobulated pseudoaneurysm with suggestion of AV fistula formation. (**c**) Lateral fluoroscopic spot image during left vertebral artery angiogram confirms a large pseudoaneurysm with vertebral-venous fistula formation. (**d**) Lateral DSA image status post coil embolization

with the type of procedure performed. If the pain is greater than expected or refractory, this may prompt an investigation for an alternative cause of pain or a potential complication from the procedure.
(b) Many IR procedures will usually require minimal analgesia, if any. This can be accomplished with Acetaminophen (500–1000 mg q4 h for a maximum dose of 4 g in 24 h) or Ibuprofen (400–600 mg q4–6 h for maximum dose of 3.2 g in 24 h).
(c) Other more invasive or inherently painful procedures will require a higher level of analgesia. This can be accomplished with opioids, preferably administered PO, such as Oxycodone (PO 5–10 mg q4–6h) or Hydromorphone (PO 2–6 mg q4–6 h or IV 0.2–0.5 mg q4–6 h).
(d) Like with any other procedure, the inflammatory response may elicit a fever in the early post-operative period; however, this should prompt a brief history and physical evaluation to exclude any other underlying cause. It is important to note the type of procedure, the time since the procedure was performed, and any intraoperative complications that may have occurred. Any line, tube, or incision should be examined for signs of infection.
(e) Postembolization syndrome is a known potential complication of embolization of usually malignant soft tissue masses and is characterized by noninfectious fevers in the first 2–3 days after the procedure.
(f) Once the etiology has been identified, fever can be treated with Acetaminophen and/or Ibuprofen as clinically indicated.
(g) Deep venous thrombosis, pulmonary emboli, or drug reactions should be kept in the back of the mind for causes of fevers in the post-operative state.

2. Bleeding
   (a) Bleeding after an IR procedure can occur at the level of the puncture site, including site of vascular or percutaneous access. It is important to determine what type of procedure was performed and what kind of closure device may have been implemented.
   (b) A review of the patient's chart for any anticoagulation medication, bleeding disorders, or chronic medical condition that may lead to increased bleeding risk should be performed.
   (c) Treatment will be dictated by the patient's hemodynamic status and the characteristics of the bleed (venous vs. arterial, deep vs. superficial).
   (d) Venous or superficial bleeds may subside from holding pressure at the site of bleeding. If the patient is not on anticoagulation medication, an absorbable suture may be employed.
   (e) Arterial bleeds may also subside from holding pressure at the bleeding site, however one must be careful not to occlude the artery. A vascular surgery consult may be required if bleeding persists.
   (f) Additionally, suspicion for puncture site pseudoaneurysms can be further evaluated with US.
3. Retroperitoneal Hematoma
   (a) Arterial puncture above the inguinal ligament may lead to uncontrollable puncture site bleeding or retroperitoneal hemorrhage.
   (b) Retroperitoneal hemorrhage in turn can lead to an insidious and devastating decline in the patient's clinical condition and may be life-threatening. Hypotension and tachycardia may be the only clinical signs of ongoing retroperitoneal hemorrhage.
   (c) Depending on the patient's hemodynamic status an urgent non-contrast CT or CTA of the abdomen and pelvis may be performed as the first step in diagnostic management; however, hemorrhagic shock should prompt immediate surgical intervention.
   (d) The standard therapeutic management is immediate surgical repair, however, if surgery is unavailable or contraindicated,

a covered stent placed across the vascular injury can be employed.

4. Neurological Complications
   (a) In order to adequately assess for neurological complications during or after an IR procedure, it is important to perform a neurological exam prior to the procedure and have an idea of the patient's baseline neurological function, as subtle changes in function may indicate a possible complication.
   (b) Intracranial hemorrhage, specifically subarachnoid hemorrhage, is an uncommon complication that may result from intracranial vessel perforation when manipulating microwires or catheters in the intracranial vasculature. When small and distal branches are being canalized, fast-acting embolic agents can be immediately employed to seal the perforation site and reduce the size of hemorrhage. When perforation has occurred, the microwire or catheter may be seen outside of the vessel on imaging. Alternatively, hypotension, bradycardia, or signs of increased intracranial pressure may suggest vascular injury. Immediate neurosurgical consult may be needed if there are any signs to suggest herniation.
   (c) Small and asymptomatic ischemic infarcts can occur during head and neck IR procedures. They usually result from tiny emboli which can arise from stagnant blood in catheters to tiny air bubble from poor technique. Large or symptomatic ischemic infarcts are rare and can often be identified and treated interprocedurally with thrombectomy or thrombolysis.
   (d) Catheter-associated or mechanically induced vasospasm of the head and neck vasculature may occur when manipulating intra-arterial catheters. Not only may this prevent advancement of the catheter, but the consequent cerebral hypoperfusion may lead to thrombotic and ischemic complications. Most cases are asymptomatic and self-limiting. Patients with evidence of vasospasm during diagnostic angiography, with high levels of anxiety, or tortuous vessels are more prone to catheter-induced vasospasm. It has been suggested that a patient may be administered a tranquilizer (etizolam or brotizolam), warm compresses, and/or an intra-arterial injection of lidocaine/nicardipine either prophylactically or as a means of treatment.
   (e) Continued advancements in microcatheter design have decreased the risk of immediate and delayed complications by minimizing trauma and interruption of vascular flow. Given the continued decrease in size of microcatheters, smaller vessels can be canalized for more selective treatment, thus reducing the risk of potential complications.
   (f) https://www.ncbi.nlm.nih.gov/pmc/articles/PMC4533334/

6.1.6.1 Additional Case of Direct Stick embolization

Left hemifacial, oral and pharyngeal low-flow vascular malformation.

The case below Fig. 6.7a–d was referred to clinic for obstructive sleep apnea and vascular lesion impeding his denture wearing. He had extensive cutaneous, oromucosal lesion causing palatal, pharyngeal and nasal area petulance superiorly (Figs. 6.8 and 6.9).

21-gauge butterfly needles are easily advanced into the venous malformation of the facial areas or left cheek as illustrated (Fig. 6.7) under ultrasound guidance.

Venous blood is freely aspirated from the lesion, confirming the vascular nature and flow pattern of filling of the lesion.

Angiography is performed with injection of 50% contrast to evaluate the size and venous drainage pattern of the lesion. The lesion is then serially injected under fluoroscopic guidance with boluses of 1:1 3% sodium tetradecyl sulfate (sotradecol):ethiodized oil (ethiodol) and the amount in millileters of sclerosing agent is deployed mindfully. Care is taken not to allow the sclerosing agent to enter into the draining veins.

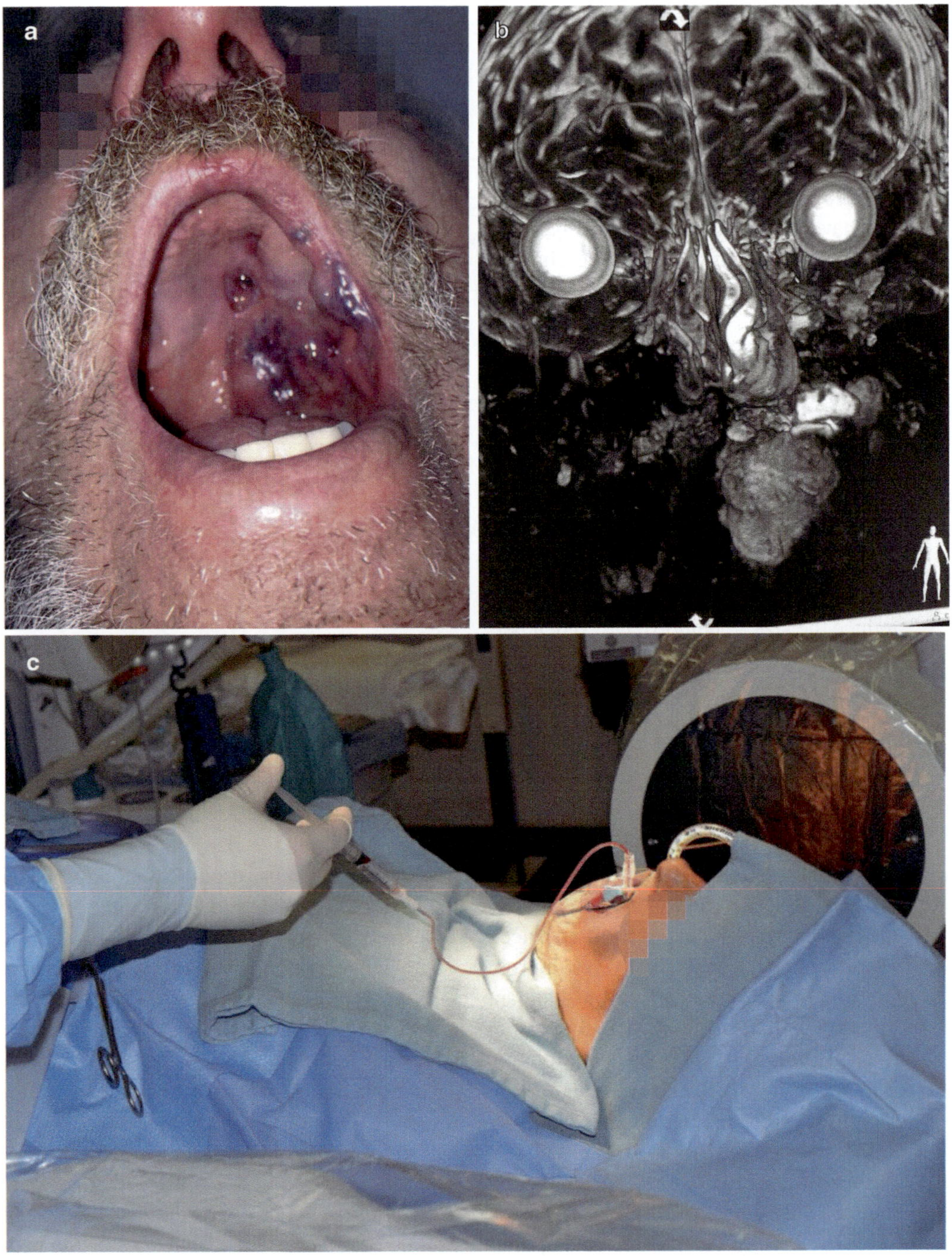

Fig. 6.7 (**a**) Has extensive lesions of low flow quality scattered on his oral, palatal, and facial areas. The center of the palate has oro-nasal fistula. (**b**) A 3D rendition of the MRI shows the extent of this lesion from the left cavernous sinus, left nasal, peri orbital, palatal, and pharyngeal flow with contrast uptake. (**c**) Venous blood is freely aspirated from the lesion, confirming the vascular nature and flow pattern of filling of the lesion. Direct stick embolization setup intraoperatively with aspiration of the lesion revealing blood in the catheter and syringe. The lesion is then serially injected under fluoroscopic guidance with boluses of 1:1 3% sodium tetradecyl sulfate (sotradecol):ethiodized oil (ethiodol) and the amount of cc of sclerosing agent deployed is mindfully noted. Care is taken not to allow the sclerosing agent to enter into the draining veins. (**d**) Post injection of sclerosant

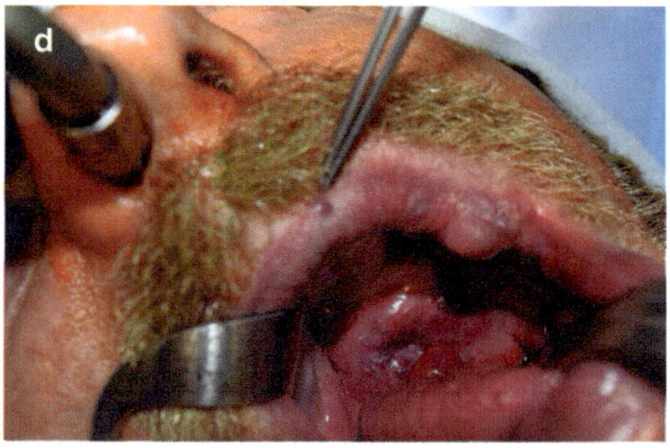

Fig. 6.7 (continued)

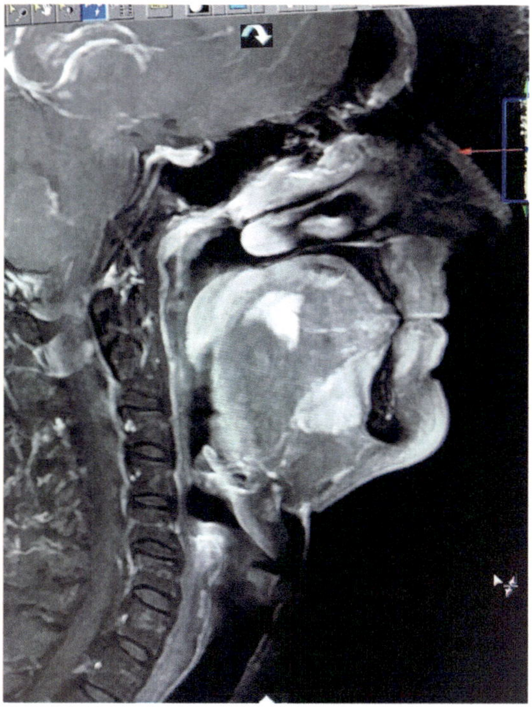

Fig. 6.8 Sagittal post contrasted MRI section reveals a blush on the tongue dorsum and floor of the mouth. Such isolated lesions are very amenable to direct stick embolization and excision

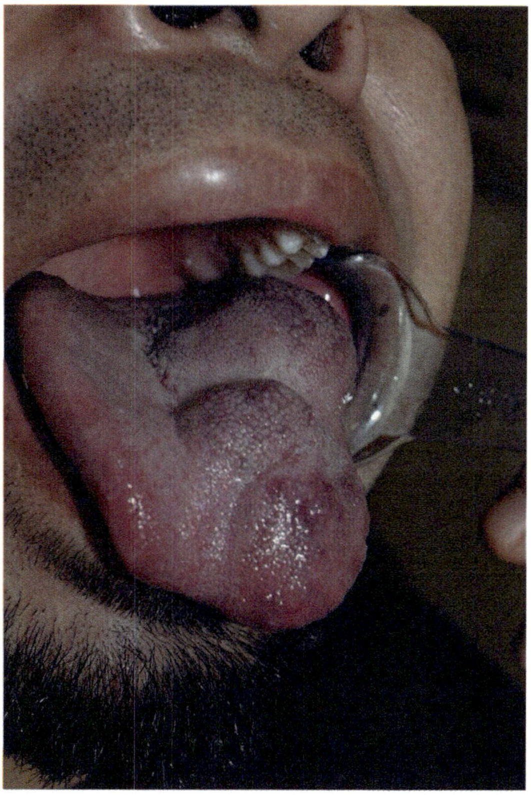

Fig. 6.9 These lingual vascular lesions are amenable to direct stick embolization with ultrasound or fluoroscopic exam. Surgically excision is amenable with proximal vascular clamp control as will be described in the surgical management section of the book with or without being sclerosed with cutaneous stick sclerotherapy

The procedure is then repeated for the venous malformation in the adjacent areas if any (idea is to do in increments) with similar 1:1 sotradecol:ethiodol total sclerosing agent deployed and similarly for the lesions in the oral mucosa, tongue, lip, upper airway, etc.

The needles were withdrawn from the venous malformations 5 min following completion of the injections and another 5 min of very gentle pressure was applied to the puncture sites following removal of the needles. At the completion of the procedure the face, neck, and upper chest were re-cleansed with sterile saline solution. The skin of the neck and upper chest was no longer erythematous and without an urticarial reaction.

The butterfly needle can be used to access the other cystic lesion or pouches of the venolymphatic malformation with biplanar fluoroscopy aids. Free flowing blood aspiration out of the venolymphatic pouch, and a pouchogram is performed to ensure that you are in the venolymphatic pouch proper.

Once this was confirmed, flush the needle, and then inject a mixture of 1:1:1 of 3% Sotradecol,

Ethiodol and air for foam solution to sclerose any vascular island or pouch. This is done under biplane fluoroscopy. Additional pools or pouches in different planes and deeper are determined again by performing a pouchogram to ensure the access is within the pouch, and then injecting a sclerosing agent in the similar dilutions.

As needles are removed, pressure application is important for hemostasis. Notably, the ultrasound is used intraoperatively and was very important in finding these pouches, as well as the biplane fluoroscopy. The authors' advice caution with risk of scatter emboli in cerebral, pulmonary draining veins, etc. Direct stick embolization can be used for bleomycin and sclerosants too.

In conclusion, majority of vascular lesions are diagnosed by presentations clinically and can be managed in a multidisciplinary team approach, there are some which will need extensive interventional diagnostic and therapeutic techniques. These can help surgical approach, morbidity reduction, and optimal outcomes.

The multidisciplinary team of authors as reflected in a vascular anomaly clinic team have taken the liberty to tackle the other vascular cases and emergencies encountered in head and neck practice.

References

1. Gandhi D, Gemmete JJ, Ansari SA, Gujar SK, Mukherji SK. Interventional neuroradiology of the head and neck. Am J Neuroradiol. 2008;29(10):1806–15. https://doi.org/10.3174/ajnr.A1211.
2. Broomfield S, Bruce I, Birzgalis A, Herwadkar A. The expanding role of interventional radiology in head and neck surgery. J R Soc Med. 2009;102(6):228–34. https://doi.org/10.1258/jrsm.2009.080240.
3. Tulunay-Ugur OE, Kocdor P, Rutledge JW, Akdol MS, Erdem E, Vural E. The role of interventional radiology in head and neck cancer. Otolaryngol Head Neck Surg. 2013;149(2_suppl):P192. https://doi.org/10.1177/0194599813496044a150.
4. Kulkarni SS, Shetty NS, Dharia TP, Polnaya AM. Pictorial essay: vascular interventions in extra cranial head and neck. Indian J Radiol Imaging. 2012;22(4):350–7. https://doi.org/10.4103/0971-3026.111490.
5. Storck K, Kreiser K, Hauber J, et al. Management and prevention of acute bleedings in the head and neck area with interventional radiology. Head Face Med. 2016;12:6. https://doi.org/10.1186/s13005-016-0103-3.
6. Cooke D, Ghodke B, Natarajan SK, Hallam D. Embolization in the head and neck. Semin Intervent Radiol. 2008;25(3):293–309. https://doi.org/10.1055/s-0028-1085929.
7. Manzoor NF, Rezaee RP, Ray A, Wick CC, Blackham K, Stepnick D, Lavertu P, Zender CA. Contemporary management of carotid blowout syndrome utilizing endovascular techniques. Laryngoscope. 2017;127:383–90. https://doi.org/10.1002/lary.26144.
8. Kovács AF, Turowski B. Chemoembolization of oral and oropharyngeal cancer using a high-dose cisplatin crystal suspension and degradable starch microspheres. Oral Oncol. 2002;38(1):87–95. https://doi.org/10.1016/s1368-8375(01)00088-4.
9. Cullen MM, Tami TA. Comparison of internal maxillary artery ligation versus embolization for refractory posterior epistaxis. Otolaryngol Head Neck Surg. 1998;118(5):636–42. https://doi.org/10.1177/019459989811800512.
10. Elden L, Montanera W, Terbrugge K, Willinsky R, Lasjaunias P, Charles D. Angiographic embolization for the treatment of epistaxis: a review of 108 cases. Otolaryngol Head Neck Surg. 1994;111(1):44–50. https://doi.org/10.1177/019459989411100110.
11. Moreau S, De Rugy MG, Babin E, Courtheoux P, Valdazo A. Supraselective embolization in intractable epistaxis: review of 45 cases. Laryngoscope. 1998;108:887–8. https://doi.org/10.1097/00005537-199806000-00018.
12. Levy EI, Horowitz MB, Cahill AM. Lingual artery embolization for severe and uncontrollable postoperative tonsillar bleeding. Ear Nose Throat J. 2001;80:208–11.
13. Siniluoto TM, Luotonen JP, Tikkakoski TA, Leinonen AS, Jokinen KE. Value of pre-operative embolization in surgery for nasopharyngeal angiofibroma. J Laryngol Otol. 1993;107:514–21. https://doi.org/10.1017/S002221510012359X.
14. Tikkakoski T, Luotonen J, Leinonen S, Siniluoto T, Heikkilä O, Päivänsälo M, et al. Preoperative embolization in the management of neck paragangliomas. Laryngoscope. 1997;107:821–6. https://doi.org/10.1097/00005537-199706000-00018.
15. Pletcher JD, Newton TH, Dedo HH, Norman D. Preoperative embolization of juvenile angiofibromas of the nasopharynx. Ann Otol Rhinol Laryngol. 1975;84:740–6. https://doi.org/10.1177/000348947508400603.
16. Tang IP, Shashinder S, Gopala Krishnan G, Narayanan P. Juvenile nasopharyngeal angiofibroma in a tertiary centre: ten-year experience. Singap Med J. 2009;50:261–4.
17. Persky MS, Berenstein A, Cohen NL. Combined treatment of head and neck vascular masses with preoperative embolization. Laryngoscope. 1984;94:20–7. https://doi.org/10.1002/lary.5540940105.

18. Valavanis A. Preoperative embolization of the head and neck: indications, patient selection, goals, and precautions. AJNR Am J Neuroradiol. 1986;7:943–52.
19. Gemmete JJ, Ansari SA, McHugh J, Gandhi D. Embolization of vascular tumors of the head and neck. Neuroimaging Clin N Am. 2009;19(2):181–98.
20. Wittekind C. Prognostic factors in patients with squamous epithelium carcinoma of the head and neck area and their evaluation. Laryngorhinootologie. 1999;78:588–9. https://doi.org/10.1055/s-1999-12971.
21. Greve J, Bas M, Schuler P, Turowski B, Scheckenbach K, Budach W, et al. Acute arterial hemorrhage following radiotherapy of oropharyngeal squamous cell carcinoma. Strahlenther Onkol. 2010;186:269–73. https://doi.org/10.1007/s00066-010-2114-5.
22. Lowe LH, Marchant TC, Rivard DC, Scherbel AJ. Vascular malformation: Classifications and terminology the radiologist needs to know. Semin Rotengenol. 2012;47:106–17.
23. Armstrong DC, ter Brugge K. Selected interventional procedures for pediatric head and neck vascular lesions. Neuroimaging Clin N Am. 2000;10:271–92.
24. Erdmann MW, Jackson JE, Davies DM, Allison DJ. Multidisciplinary approach to the management of head and neck arteriovenous malformations. Ann R Coll Surg Engl. 1995;77:53–9.
25. Arat A, Cil BE, Vargel I, Turkbey B, Canyigit M, Peynircioglu B, et al. Embolization of high-flow craniofacial vascular malformations with onyx. AJNR Am J Neuroradiol. 2007;28:1409–14.
26. Berenguer B, Burrows PE, Zurakowski D, Mulliken JB. Sclerotherapy of craniofacial venous malformations: Complications and results. Plast Reconstr Surg. 1999;104:1–11.
27. Cabrera J, Cabrera J Jr, Garcia-Olmedo MA, Redondo P. Treatment of venous malformations with sclerosant in microfoam form. Arch Dermatol. 2003;139:1409–16.
28. Ryu CW, Whang SM, Suh DC, Kim SM, Jang YJ, Kim HJ, et al. Percutaneous direct puncture glue embolization of high-flow craniofacial arteriovenous lesions: a new circular ring compression device with a beveled edge. AJNR Am J Neuroradiol. 2007;28:528–30.
29. Wakhloo AK, Juengling FD, Van Velthoven V, Schumacher M, Hennig J, Schwechheimer K. Extended preoperative polyvinyl alcohol microembolization of intracranial meningiomas: assessment of two embolization techniques. AJNR Am J Neuroradiol. 1993;14:571–82.
30. Pérez Higueras A, Saura Lorente P, García Alonso J, de las Heras García JA. Diagnosis and treatment of head and neck paragangliomas. Uses of angiography and interventional radiology. Acta Otorrinolaringol Esp. 2009;60:53–67.
31. Gruber A, Bavinzski G, Killer M, Richling B. Preoperative embolization of hypervascular skull base tumors. Minim Invasive Neurosurg. 2000;43:62–71.
32. Chaloupka JC, Putman CM, Citardi MJ, Ross DA, Sasaki CT. Endovascular therapy for the carotid blowout syndrome in head and neck surgical patients: diagnostic and managerial considerations. AJNR Am J Neuroradiol. 1996;17:843–52.
33. Goodman DN, Hoh BL, Rabinov JD, Pryor JC. CT angiography before embolization for hemorrhage in head and neck cancer. AJNR Am J Neuroradiol. 2003;24:140–2.
34. Morrissey DD, Andersen PE, Nesbit GM, Barnwell SL, Everts EC, Cohen JI. Endovascular management of hemorrhage in patients with head and neck cancer. Arch Otolaryngol Head Neck Surg. 1997;123:15–9.
35. Sittel C, Gossmann A, Jungehülsing M, Zähringer M. Superselective embolization as palliative treatment of recurrent hemorrhage in advanced carcinoma of the head and neck. Ann Otol Rhinol Laryngol. 2001;110:1126–8.
36. Chang FC, Lirng JF, Luo CB, Guo WY, Teng MM, Tai SK, et al. Carotid blowout syndrome in patients with head-and-neck cancers: Reconstructive management by self-expandable stent-grafts. AJNR Am J Neuroradiol. 2007;28:181–8.
37. Dubose J, Recinos G, Teixeira PG, Inaba K, Demetriades D. Endovascular stenting for the treatment of traumatic internal carotid injuries: expanding experience. J Trauma. 2008;65:1561–6.
38. Santhosh J, Rao VR, Ravimandalam K, Gupta AK, Unni NM, Rao AS. Endovascular management of carotid cavernous fistulae: observation on angiographic and clinical results. Acta Neurol Scand. 1993;88:320–6.
39. Gobin YP, Garcia de la Fuente JA, Herbreteau D, Houdart E, Merland JJ. Endovascular treatment of external carotid-jugular fistulae in the parotid region. Neurosurgery. 1993;33:812–6.

7 General, Surgical, and Functional Anatomy for Vascular Lesions of Head and Neck

Srinivasa R. Chandra, Sunil Shroff, Steven Curry, Amelia Christabel Rajasekaran, and Sanjiv C. Nair

An understanding of the complex nature and involvement of various structures in vascular lesions of the head and neck is essential. Thorough knowledge of the primary cross-sectional anatomy of this region is invaluable. Most of these lesions are composite and involve more than a single layer in various proportions.

Nair et al.'s anatomical classification and its various modifications help understand these lesions' real involvement. Hence, the familiarity of different structures with a three-dimensional mental picture makes their treatment planning and subsequent management comprehensive.

Command over the vascular anatomy, identifying potential flow dynamics of the head and neck vasculature would assist in decision-making toward surgery alone or in combination with embolization.

We will review the surgical anatomy of different layers of the face, scalp, and neck. Also, the network of arteries, veins, and lymphatics is discussed. This is useful in approaching and surgically debulking these vascular lesions, which we have discussed as various approaches.

7.1 Layers of Scalp, Face, and Neck (Superficial to Deep)

Skin and subcutaneous tissue are common throughout the scalp, face, and neck, with their thickness varying in different areas. The skin over the scalp is thickest, followed by mid and lower face, thin in the anterior neck, and most delicate in the eyelids. It has a superficial epidermis and deeper dermis, which are the two identifiable skin layers to the naked eye. Vascular lesions involving the thin skin are more expansile due to its elasticity.

The thickness of the subcutaneous tissue usually corresponds to the skin above it due to varying subdermal fat. The subcutaneous and dermal appendages can get thin due to expansile and pressure atrophy, further getting missed or altered in Type-I and Type-II lesions.

The original version of this chapter was revised. The correction to this chapter can be found at https://doi.org/10.1007/978-981-15-2321-2_11

S. R. Chandra (✉)
Oral & Maxillofacial- Head & Neck Oncology Reconstructive Surgery, Oregon Health & Science University Portland, Portland, OR, USA
e-mail: chandrsr@ohsu.edu

S. Shroff
Department of Oral and Maxillofacial Surgery, Bhagwan Mahaveer Jain Hospital, Bengaluru, India

S. Curry
Department of Otolaryngology, University of Nebraska Medical Center, Omaha, NE, USA
e-mail: Steven.Curry@unmc.edu

A. Christabel Rajasekaran
UIH Chicago, Chicago, IL, USA

S. C. Nair
Department of Maxillofacial Surgery, B.M. Jain Hospital, Bangalore Institute of Dental Science, Bangalore, Karnataka, India

S. C. Nair, S. R. Chandra (eds.), *Management of Head and Neck Vascular Lesions*,
https://doi.org/10.1007/978-981-15-2321-2_7

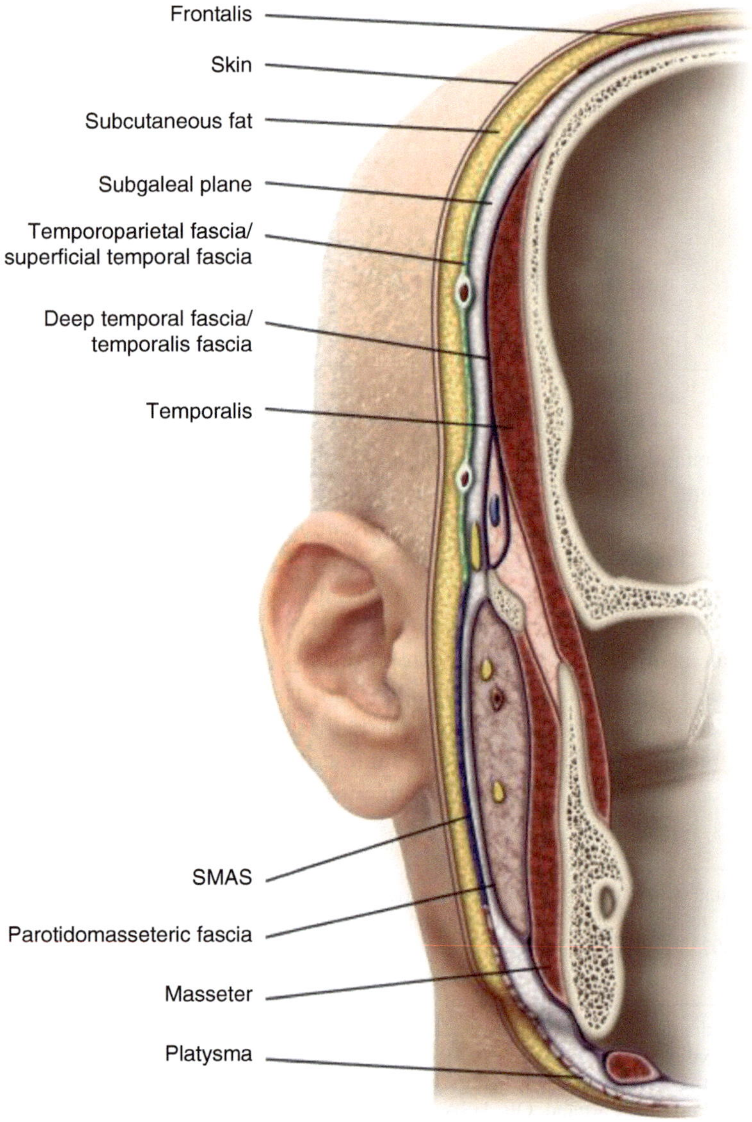

Fig. 7.1 Layers of the face from skin to deep. The SMAS layer and its continuation over the scalp and neck is seen

The layers below the skin and subcutaneous tissue can vary depending on the head and neck area. Scalp has the *musculoaponeurotic layer* (Fig. 7.1) with a strip of muscular component (frontalis anteriorly and occipital group posteriorly) and a deeper avascular aponeurotic layer (subgaleal plane). There is an excellent dissecting plane beneath the aponeurosis and is used to raise a flap or excise lesions above it.

Laterally, the aponeurosis forms the *temporoparietal layer* over the temporal area, splits into superficial, and deep temporalis fascia incorporating the superficial temporal fat pad in between and temporalis muscle underneath it (Fig. 7.2). The superficial temporalis fascia is in communication with the zygomatic arch and its superior border—the superficial temporalis fascia then continues over the face as the *SMAS (superficial musculoaponeurotic system)*.

The SMAS is thickened over the parotid gland and masseter muscle (parotido-masseteric fascia) and is easily identifiable in these areas. This layer further continues around the face but becomes

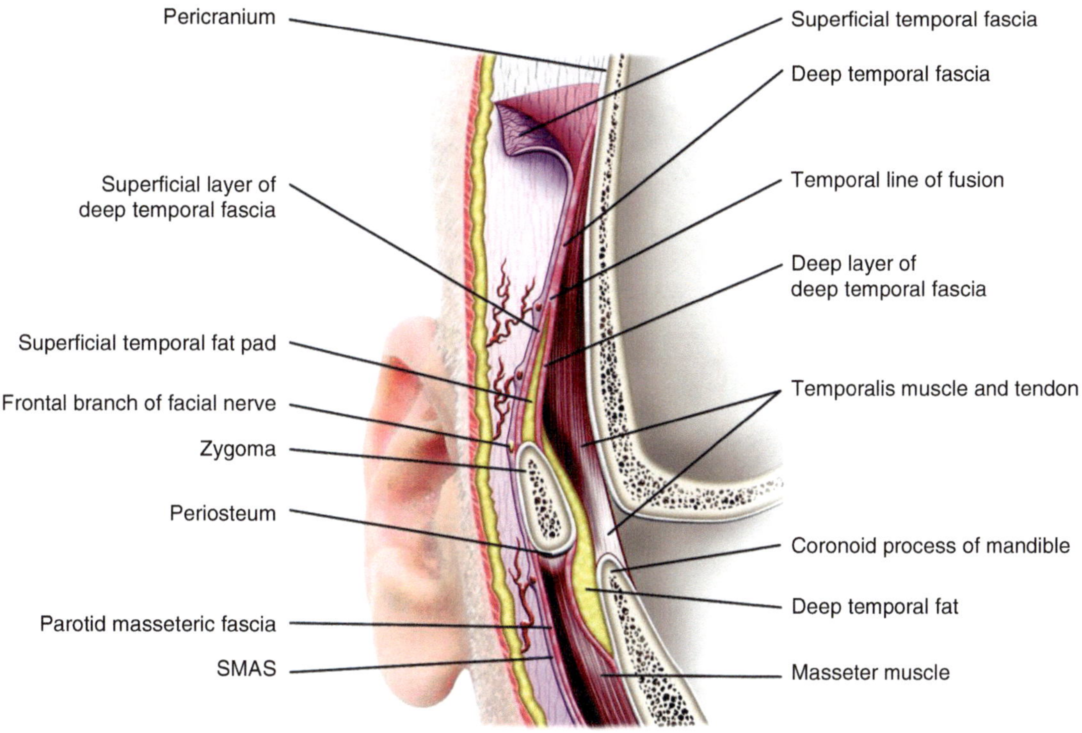

Fig. 7.2 Layers of temporal scalp and preauricular region

less conspicuous around the lips, nose, and eyes. Inferior to the mandible, SMAS continues as the platysma all around the anterior and lateral neck except slightly deficient in the midline.

The aponeurosis, SMAS, and platysma establish the skin tension's continuity over the face and neck (Fig. 7.1). This anatomical continuity aids in the reapproximation of expanded facial and neck skin after the excision of large vascular lesions to prevent sagging deformities and keep the incision lines cosmetic.

The *muscles* of the face and neck lay deep to the SMAS. Facial expressions amplify over the skin due to the SMAS interconnecting the facial muscles to the skin's dermis. Resuspend the SMAS to the dermis and facial muscles during surgery, whenever possible.

The *neck's deep cervical fascia* (Fig. 7.3) lies beneath the platysma and is divided into—investing layer, pre-tracheal fascia, prevertebral fascia, and carotid sheath.

The investing layer encloses the parotid gland, submandibular gland, sternomastoid, and trapezius muscles. This layer also forms a capsule over the parotid and submandibular glands.

The pre-tracheal layer lies in the midline and has muscular and visceral parts. The muscular layer encloses the midline neck's strap muscles, and the visceral layer surrounds the esophagus and trachea in the neck.

The prevertebral fascia encloses the vertebral column and prevertebral group of muscles.

The *carotid sheath* (Fig. 7.3) encloses the common carotid artery (CCA), internal carotid artery (ICA), internal jugular vein (IJV), and vagus nerve. The sympathetic trunk lies in the posterior sheath, and the ansa cervicalis lies in the anterior sheath.

Periosteum and bone are the next deep layers to the salivary glands and facial muscles in the region. The scalp has pericranium and is bone-deep to the aponeurosis.

The neck has the *major vessels* enclosed by the deep cervical fascia laterally and hyoid bone, thyroid, and cricoid cartilage medially. The lar-

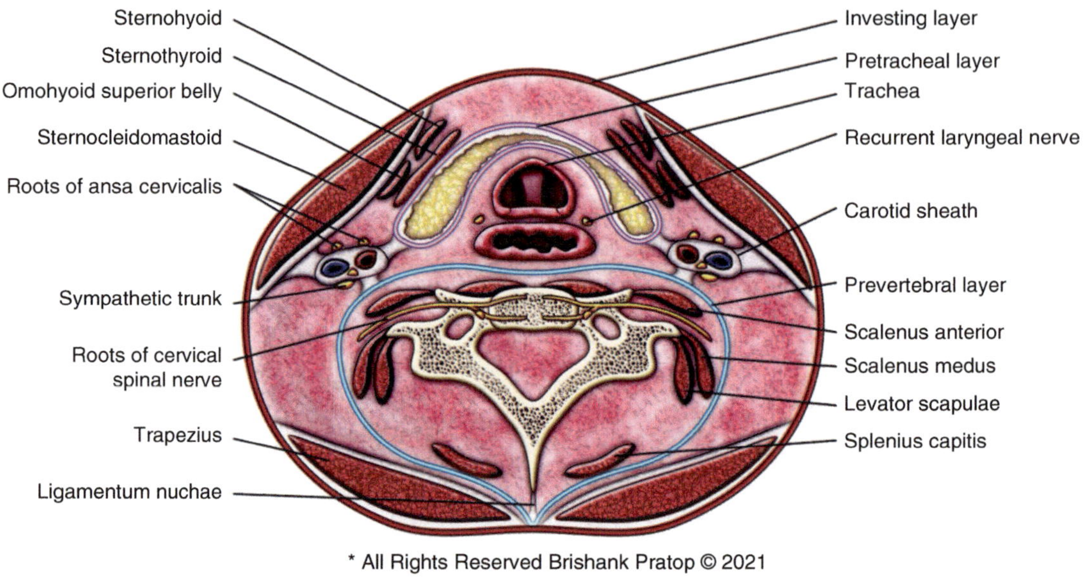

Fig. 7.3 Deep cervical fascia of the neck and its associations

ynx lies deep to it and extends until the lower end of the cricoid, where the trachea starts. The esophagus is present behind the trachea and in front of the prevertebral fascia (Fig. 7.4).

A *planned surgical airway* is many times necessary for large vascular lesions of the neck and is usually done around 1 cm below the cricoid cartilage in the area of the 2nd or 3rd tracheal ring. An *emergency airway* is usually established through the cricothyroid membrane. These should be in the surgeon's armamentarium of skills as large vascular lesions, especially long-standing venous and lymphatic malformations, can cause pressure symptoms over the trachea and esophagus, causing dyspnea and dysphagia.

The thyroid gland is located just below the thyroid cartilage's prominence, with its two lobes on either side of the trachea.

Intraorally, the tongue and floor mouth are present medial to the mandible and the pharyngeal space posterior to it.

Zygomatic body projection forms the face's malar prominence with the maxilla anteromedially and orbits superomedially, forming the "zygomaticomaxillary complex" and "orbito-zygomatic complex." The frontal bone lies superior to the orbits, with nasal and ethmoid bones medial to it, forming the "fronto-orbito-naso-ethmoid" complex in the midline. The complex has the frontal sinus, dura mater, and brain deep to it.

Intrabony vascular lesions are generally high flow in nature and occasionally demand extracorporeal curettage and fixation in uncontrollable bleeding cases.

7.2 Important Nerves of Head and Neck

The facial nerve (7th cranial nerve) is a motor nerve exiting the stylomastoid foramen in the skull base after having originated from the pons and having a long, tortuous course intracranially (Fig. 7.5). After its exit, it stems out—the posterior auricular nerve, nerve to stylohyoid, and nerve to the posterior belly of digastric. It then proceeds forward to the posteromedial surface of the parotid gland, where it divides into temporofacial and cervicofacial branches just behind the retromandibular vein and before entering the gland. Within the gland, it lies in close proximity to the ECA, forms a plexus of nerves superficial to the ECA and retromandibular vein. It then gives its terminal branches over the face, namely temporal, zygomatic, buccal (upper and lower),

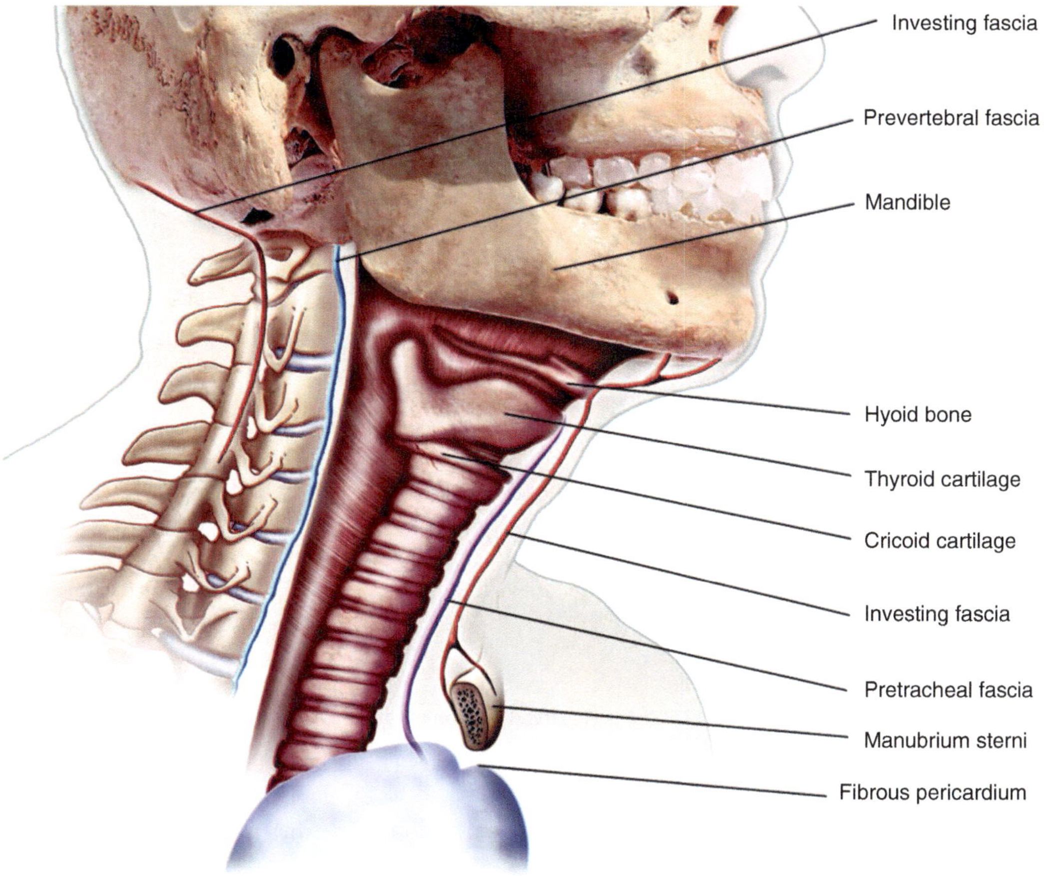

Fig. 7.4 Saggital view of midline structures in the neck

marginal mandibular, and cervical. All these branches supply the facial musculature and are solely responsible for their animation. They usually anastomose with the terminal branches from the opposite side.

The facial nerve is the most common nerve at risk of being damaged during the management of vascular lesions of the face. Every effort is made to preserve these branches by the operating surgeon. Raising large flaps using the rhytidectomy approach is one of the recommended ways while surgically treating lesions of the cheek to avoid risk to the zygomatic, buccal, and marginal mandibular branches. Sometimes the plane of dissection is determined by the lesion, which may be involving the SMAS plane, in which case sacrifice of the facial nerve is inevitable (Fig. 7.6).

Various facial animation procedures can be done to compensate for this partially. Corset suturing is recommended by Nair et al., to prevent long-term damage to the facial nerve in treating large low flow vascular lesions of the face and neck. The marginal mandibular nerve runs in the fascia over the facial vessels curving anteriorly to supply the lower lip. This can be protected when possible by ligating the facial vessels about 1–1.5 cm below the lower border of the mandible and swinging the upper part superiorly (Fig. 7.7).

The *hypoglossal* (12th cranial nerve) nerve is identified below the posterior belly of digastric muscle in the neck, and every effort is made to preserve it. Care is taken not to damage the nerve in this level during dissection around the deep

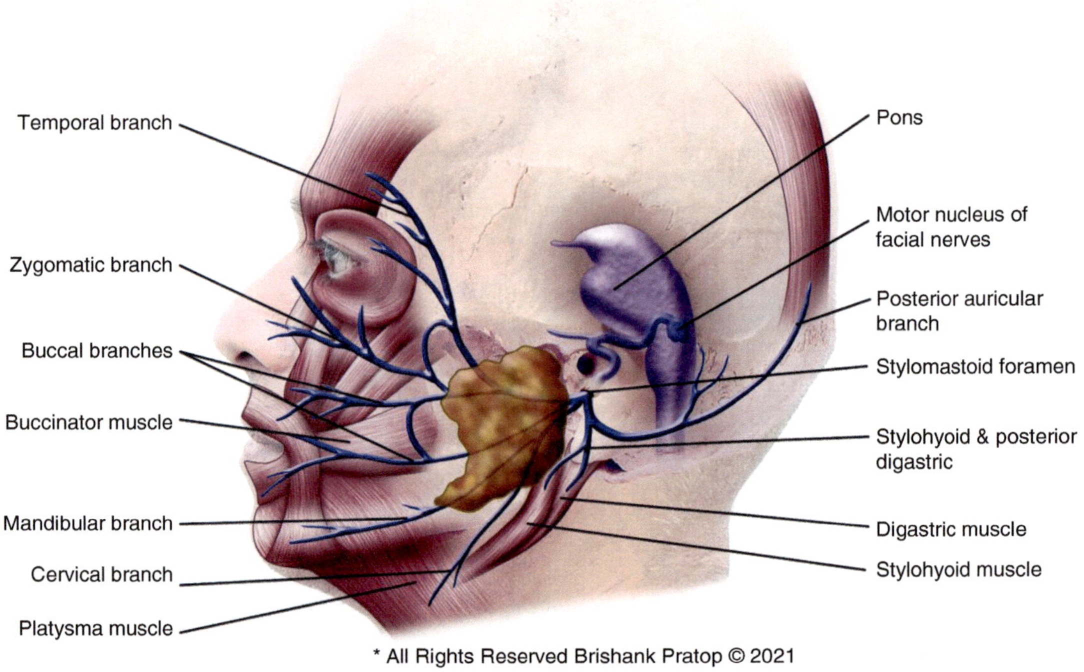

Fig. 7.5 Facial nerve origin, exit from skull and extracranial branches

Fig. 7.6 Relationship of facial nerve and its overlying structures over midface and upper neck

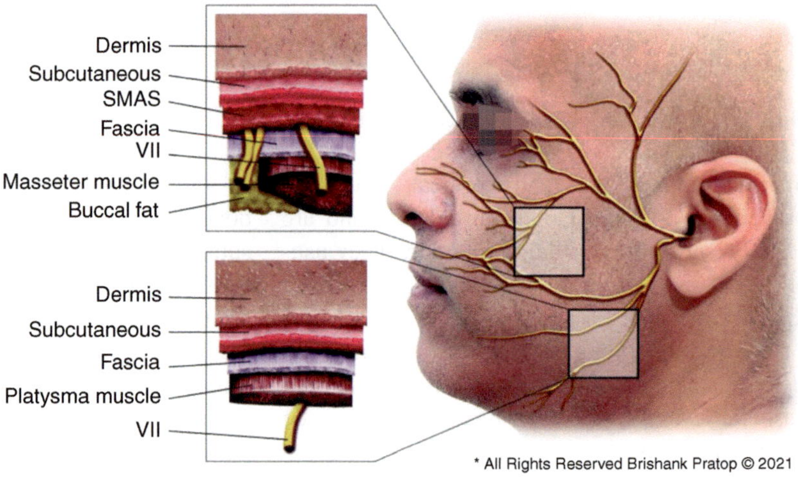

part of the submandibular gland and identification of the deep part of the facial artery.

This nerve can be located by following the ansa cervicalis cranially over the carotid sheath.

The *spinal accessory nerve* is located in the upper part of the posterior triangle beneath and behind the sternomastoid, over the scalene muscles. The great auricular nerve is a good landmark to preserve. The spinal accessory nerve is located about 1–1.5 cm below and behind the great auricular nerve (Fig. 7.8).

The terminal branches of the *trigeminal nerve (5th cranial nerve)* namely infraorbital nerve, inferior alveolar and mental nerves,

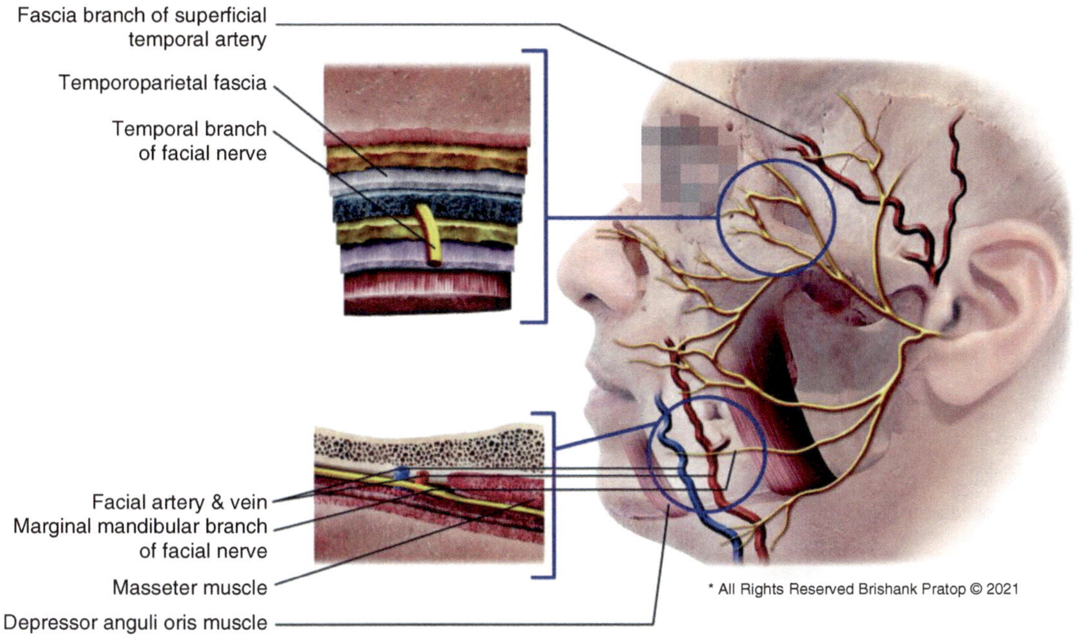

Fig. 7.7 Facial nerve in relation to facial artery and superficial temporal artery

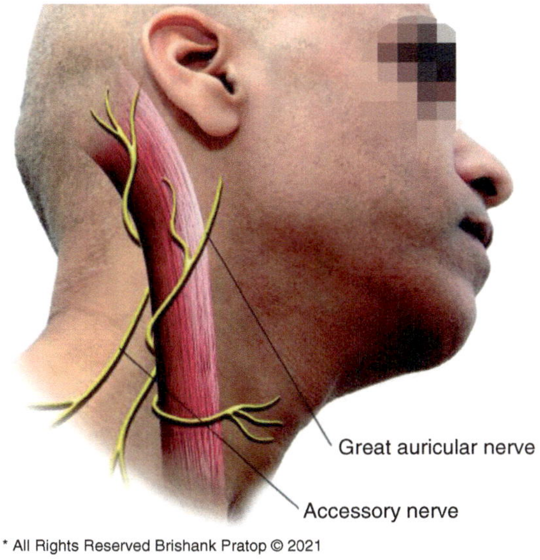

Fig. 7.8 Relation of Spinal accessory nerve to Great auricular nerve

greater palatine and nasopalatine nerves, posterior superior alveolar nerves are also encountered during surgical management of these lesions which if sacrificed or disturbed should be well consented for with the patient to avoid postoperative mishaps.

7.3 Arterial Supply of Head and Neck (Figs. 7.9, 7.10, and 7.11)

The arteries majorly of interest in the treatment of extracranial vascular lesions are *the external carotid artery and its branches*. Of all the branches of ECA, the facial, lingual/faciolingual trunk, maxillary and superficial temporal arteries supplying areas in front of the auricle and posterior auricular, occipital arteries supplying areas posterior to the auricle, are commonly encountered during treatment of these lesions.

The *ophthalmic artery*, the first major branch of the internal carotid artery intracranially, has terminal branches over the face via the supraorbital, supratrochlear, and lacrimal, dorsal nasal, and external nasal arteries supplying the central forehead, eyelids, and upper part of the nose.

The ECA is identified at its bifurcation from the CCA at the level of the upper border of the thyroid cartilage. The superior thyroid artery is sometimes seen at its origin and runs medially into the thyroid gland.

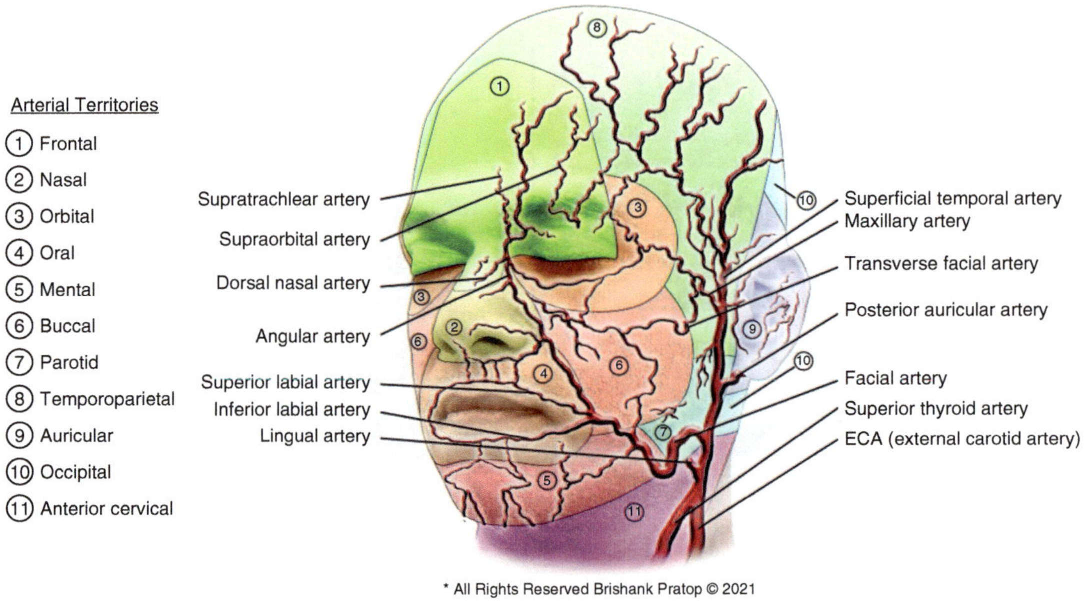

Fig. 7.9 Superficial arteries of face

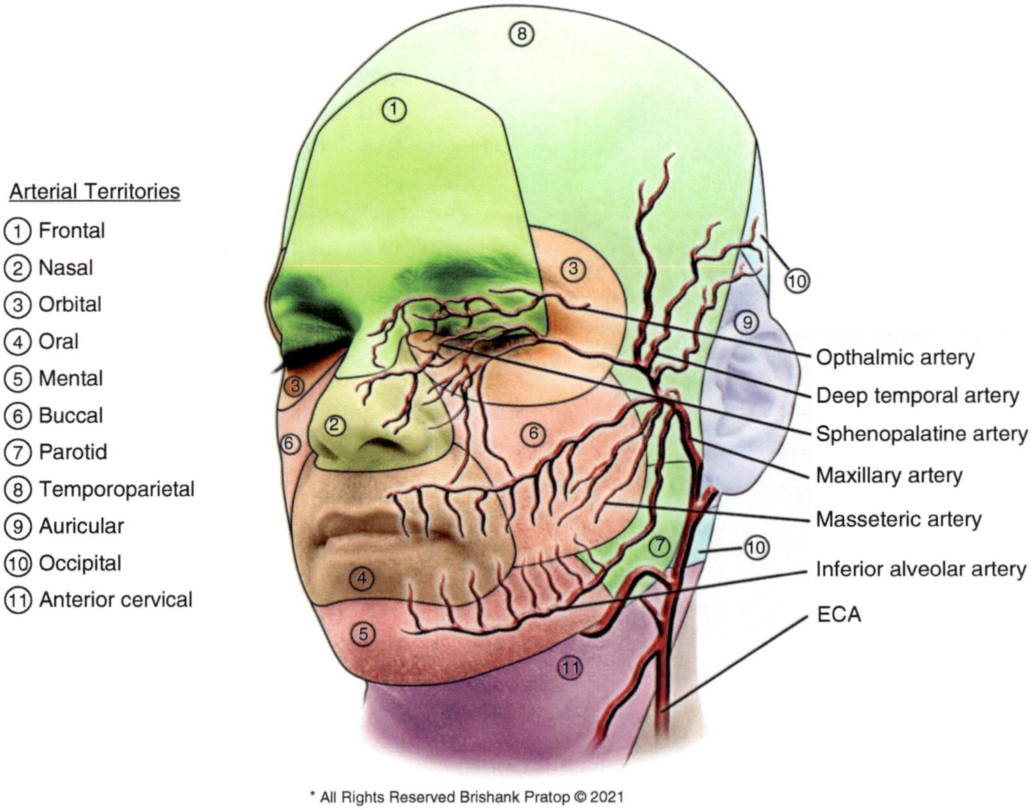

Fig. 7.10 Deep arteries of face

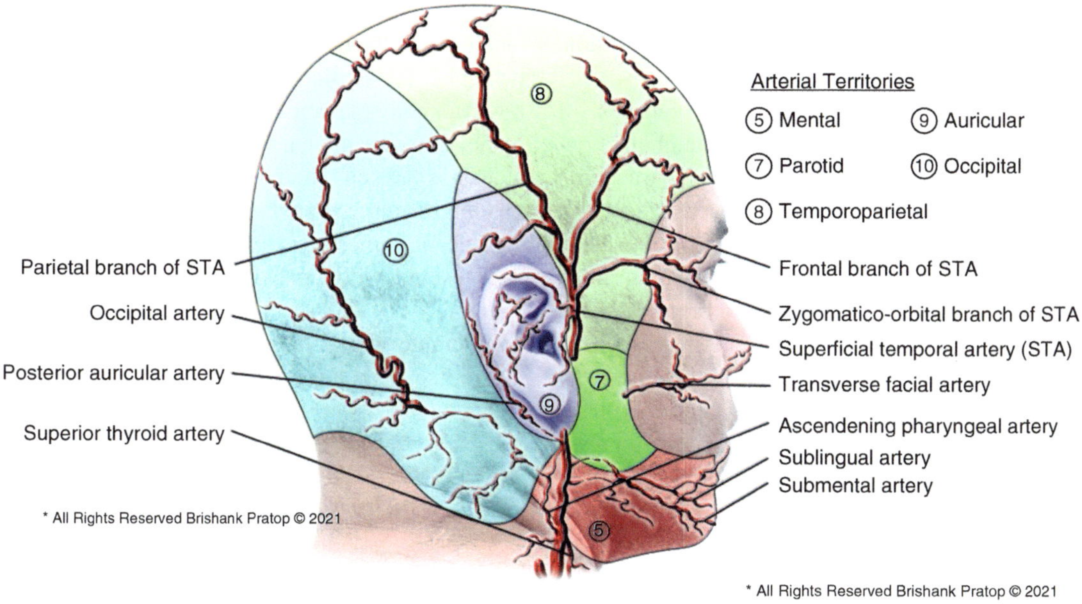

Fig. 7.11 Posterolateral arteries of face

The *lingual artery* can originate at the same level or slightly above the origin of the ECA, at the level of the greater cornu of hyoid bone and runs medially below the hyoglossus muscle, gives a sublingual branch to the anterior floor of the mouth, and continues further behind as the deep lingual artery to supply the lateral and posterior tongue. Care is taken to try and preserve the lingual artery to prevent avascularity of the lateral tongue, especially if the lingual artery on the opposite side is compromised, which usually has collateral branches to take over the blood supply.

The *facial artery*, the 4th branch of the ECA, is given off anteromedially above the bifurcation. It sometimes is the conglomerate of facio-lingual trunk. The facial artery then courses deep through the posterior belly of the digastric muscle. Commonly it then lodges in a groove at the posterior end of submandibular gland. It then runs a tortuous course between the submandibular gland and mandible, winding around the mandible at the anteroinferior angle of masseter to enter the face. It is easily identified and ligated here if necessary. Over the face, the facial artery gives ascending palatine, inferior and superior labial, tonsillar, glandular, lateral nasal, submental, muscular, and angular arteries. Angular artery is the terminal branch of the facial artery, which gives anastomotic branches to the infraorbital artery (terminal branch of maxillary artery). It also anastomoses with the inferior palpebral and dorsal nasal branch of the ophthalmic artery forming a communication with the ICA.

The *submental artery* is encountered in the submental triangle during dissection of the anterior neck, hyoglossus, and mylohyoid muscle.

The superior and inferior labial arteries are commonly compressed digitally to achieve a reduction in blood flow in vascular lesions involving the upper and lower lips, until they are excised and then released or ligated if necessary. It is a simple maneuver that is helpful during surgery and emergencies.

The maxillary and the superficial temporal arteries are the terminal branches of the ECA in the head and neck. In the facial region, the *maxillary artery* branches out of the ECA at the neck of condyle and travels around the mandibular neck, through the pterygoid musculature and pterygopalatine fossa further giving terminal branches in the nasal cavity, palate, and infraorbital region. The maxillary artery through its course gives various branches and sub-branches, supply the bones of face, calvarium, dura mater, floor of middle cranial fossa, external ear, middle ear, and tympanic membrane.

The *superficial temporal artery* branches off the ECA again at the neck of the mandibular condyle and enters the parotid gland, travelling upward toward the temporal area and scalp. It gives off a parotid branch and transverse facial artery within the parotid gland, zygomatic-orbital, middle temporal, anterior auricular branches at the level of zygomatic arch and anterior frontal, posterior parietal as terminal branches higher above.

The *posterior auricular artery* branches from the ECA just above the bifurcation travels upward between the parotid gland and styloid process to reach behind the auricle, runs between the auricular cartilage and mastoid process, thereafter anastomosing with the occipital artery. During its course, it supplies the sternomastoid, stylohyoid, digastric, posterior belly of occipitofrontalis, tympanic membrane, skin over medial surface of auricle, and provides oxygenated blood to the facial nerve.

One of many branches can be enormous and significantly increased in size, especially high-flow lesions, with a palpable bruit being the most characteristic feature. The bruit is palpable or dopplerable with a hand-held device throughout the course of the lesion.

7.3.1 Vessel and Luminal Dimensions

Internal carotid artery (ICA)		
Orbital and extracranial branches	Outer diameter (mm)	Inner diameter (mm)
Ophthalmic artery [1]		1.35–1.37 ± 0.16–0.18
Orbital group		
Anterior ethmoidal artery [2]	0.88–0.92 ± 0.15–0.20	
Posterior ethmoidal artery [2]	0.63–0.66 ± 0.19–0.21	
Dorsal nasal artery [3, 4]	0.74–0.88 ± 0.12–0.26	
Supratrochlear artery [3, 4]	0.74–0.91 ± 0.17–0.20	
Supraorbital artery [4]	0.84 ± 0.16	
Superior and inferior medial palpebral arteries [4]	0.43 ± 0.13	
Lacrimal artery [5]	1.02–1.03 ± 0.16–0.17	
Superior and inferior lateral palpebral arteries, zygomaticofacial artery, zygomaticotemporal artery [6, 7]		
Ocular group		
Ciliary arteries		
Central retinal artery		
Muscular branches		

External carotid artery (ECA)		
Arteries and branches	Outer diameter (mm)	Inner diameter (mm)
Superior thyroid artery [8–11]	2.1–3.53 ± 1.17–1.4	1.4–1.9 ± 0.3–0.7
Infrahyoid branch, superior laryngeal branch, sternomastoid branch, cricothyroid branch, glandular branches [12]		
Ascending pharyngeal artery [13, 14]	1.4–1.54 ± 0.25–0.3	
Posterior meningeal artery, pharyngeal branches, inferior tympanic artery		
Lingual artery [8–11]	2.2–3.06 ± 0.65–1.1	1.6–1.8 ± 0.4
Deep lingual artery, sublingual artery, dorsal lingual branches, suprahyoid branch		
Facial artery [8–11]	2.7–3.35 ± 0.68–1.6	1.9–2.2 ± 0.4–0.5
Cervical branches: ascending palatine artery, tonsillar branch, submental artery, glandular branches*Facial branches*: inferior labial, superior labial, inferior alar artery, lateral nasal artery, angular artery, forehead branch [15, 16]		

External carotid artery (ECA)		
Arteries and branches	Outer diameter (mm)	Inner diameter (mm)
Occipital artery [17, 18]	1.9–2.6	
SCM branches, meningeal branch, occipital branches, auricular branch, descending branch [19]		
Posterior auricular artery [20, 21]	0.7–1.2	
Stylomastoid artery, stapedial artery, auricular branch, occipital branch, parotid branch		
Maxillary artery [10, 22–24]	3.2–3.67 ± 0.07	2.1–2.3 ± 0.3–0.7
See table		
Superficial temporal artery [9, 10, 25]	2–2.73 ± 0.51–1.4	1.7 ± 0.4–0.5
Transverse facial artery, zygomatico-orbital artery, middle temporal artery, anterior auricular branch, frontal branches, parietal branch		

7.3.2 Maxillary Artery Branches

Maxillary artery			
Divisions and branches	Foramina	Outer diameter (mm)	Inner diameter (mm)
Mandibular segment [23, 24]		3.67 ± 0.07	2.1 ± 0.7
Deep auricular artery [23]	Squamotympanic fissure	1.0 ± 0.09	
Anterior tympanic artery [23]	Petrotympanic fissure	0.7 ± 0.002	
Middle meningeal artery [23, 24]	Foramen spinosum	2.53 ± 0.38	1.2 ± 0.2
Accessory meningeal artery [23]	Foramen ovale	1.9 ± 0.22	
Inferior alveolar artery [23, 24]	Mandibular foramen	1.3 ± 0.07	0.6 ± 0.1
Mylohyoid artery[a]			
Mental artery	Mental foramen		
Pterygoid segment [23]		3.24 ± 0.2	
Anterior deep temporal artery [23, 24]		1.45 ± 0.10	0.7 ± 0.2
Posterior deep temporal artery [23, 24]		1.48 ± 0.01	0.7 ± 0.1
Masseteric artery [23]		1.03 ± 0.02	
Buccal artery [23, 24]		1.05 ± 0.07	0.6 ± 0.2
Pterygoid branches [23]		0.7 ± 0.003	
Pterygopalatine segment [23]		2.75 ± 0.04	
Descending palatine artery	Greater palatine canal		
Greater palatine artery [23]	Greater palatine foramen	0.71	
Lesser palatine artery	Lesser palatine foramina		
Posterior superior alveolar artery [23, 24]	Pterygomaxillary fissure	1.31 ± 0.07	1.0 ± 0.2
Infraorbital artery [23, 24]	Infraorbital foramen	1.3 ± 0.08	1.0 ± 0.3
Anterior and middle superior alveolar arteries[b]			
Sphenopalatine artery [23, 24]	Sphenopalatine foramen	1.76 ± 0.48	1.2 ± 0.2
Lateral posterior nasal branches			
Posterior septal branches			
Pharyngeal artery	Pharyngeal (palatovaginal) canal		
Artery of the pterygoid canal (Vidian artery) [23]	Pterygoid canal	0.7 ± 0.005	

[a]The mylohyoid artery branches proximal to the mandibular foramen

[b]The anterior and middle superior alveolar arteries branch from the infraorbital artery proximal to the infraorbital foramen

7.3.3 Arterial Supply of the Neck

Subclavian artery
Arteries and extracranial branches
Vertebral artery
Thyrocervical trunk
Inferior thyroid artery
Inferior laryngeal artery, tracheal branches, esophageal branches, pharyngeal branches, glandular branches
Transverse cervical artery
Superficial branch, dorsal scapular artery
Suprascapular artery
Acromial branch
Ascending cervical artery
Costocervical trunk
Deep cervical artery, superior intercostal artery

7.4 Venous Drainage of Head and Neck (Fig. 7.12)

Veins of the head and neck drain into external and internal jugular veins. Most extracranial veins are named according to the accompanying arteries and areas they drain. The *external jugular vein* along with the vertebral vein drains into the subclavian vein. The *internal jugular vein (IJV)* and *subclavian vein* drain into the *brachiocephalic vein*, which then drains into the *superior vena cava* and *right atrium* of the heart.

Venous blood from the intracranial cavity is picked up by multiple sinuses, which drain ultimately into the sigmoid sinus, which further

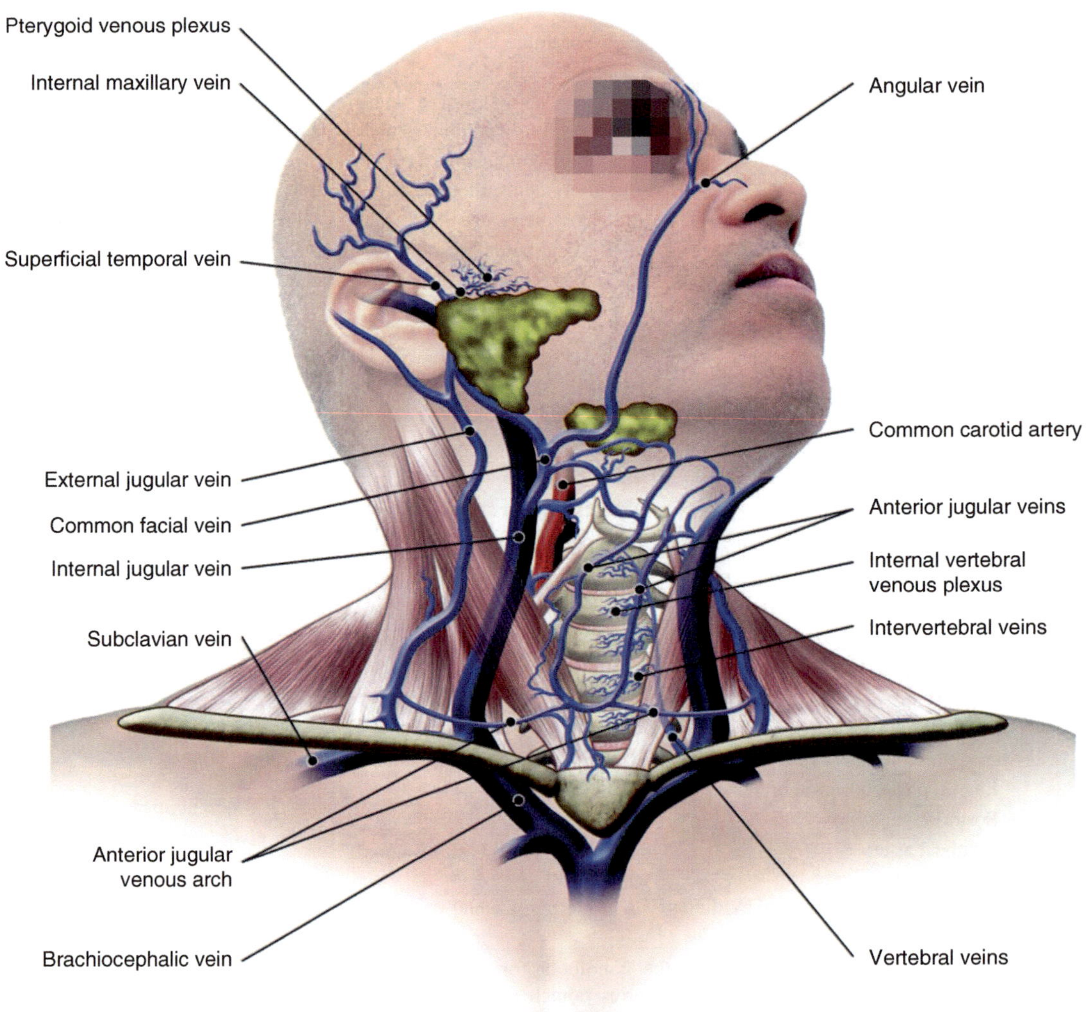

Fig. 7.12 Venous drainage of head and neck

drains into the IJV before leaving the jugular foramen. The ophthalmic vein and facial vein give communications to the cavernous sinus, which then drains into the IJV via the sigmoid and petrosal sinuses. The superficial temporal vein also drains into the internal jugular vein.

The superior and middle thyroid veins drain into the IJV in the neck.

The *facial vein* and its communications are commonly in a plexus in most venous malformations and AVM of the face. The vein lies posterior to the facial artery over the face and then joins the anterior branch of the retromandibular vein at the lower pole of the parotid gland to become the common facial vein, which drains into the IJV.

The *retromandibular vein* is another important vein formed by the merger of superficial temporal and maxillary veins. This runs through the parotid gland, posterior to the ramus of mandible, gives anterior branch as described above and a posterior branch which meets the external jugular vein. The occipital and posterior auricular veins also drain into the external jugular vein from behind the ear.

Since veins are thin-walled, low in blood flow, and so many in number over the face, they have a potential to expand easily on head-down posture, which is usually the first sight of these lesions in most small-sized venous malformations.

7.5 Lymphatic Drainage of Head and Neck (Fig. 7.13)

Lymphatic malformations of the head and neck are commonly seen in children and young adults. They are sometimes disfiguring and cause skeletal deformations over the long term due to its pressure effects. The lymphatics of the head and neck are divided into superficial and deep systems.

The *superficial system* drains the scalp, face, and neck into occipital, mastoid, pre-auricular, parotid, facial, submandibular, submental, and superficial cervical nodes.

The *deeper system* collects lymph from the entire head and neck and drains within a vertical chain into the carotid sheath. The superior and inferior deep cervical nodes are primarily laryngeal, pre-tracheal, retropharyngeal, jugulodigastric, jugular-omohyoid, and supraclavicular nodes. Efferent vessels from the above converge to form the jugular lymphatic trunks. The left jugular lymphatic trunk joins the thoracic duct at

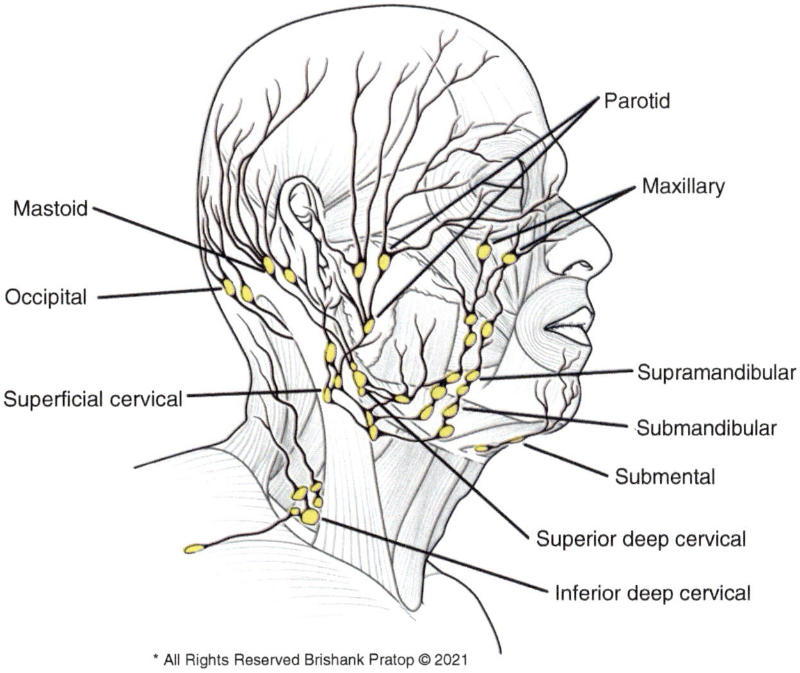

Fig. 7.13 Common lymphatics of face and neck

the root of the neck to drain into the left subclavian vein. The right jugular lymphatic trunk forms the right lymphatic duct at the root of the neck, which drains into the right subclavian vein.

Most lymphatic malformations are diffuse due to their widespread network in the head and neck. They are most times easily excised but quite incompletely. These lesions pose a challenge in areas close to the orbit, and alternate options to facilitate lymph drainage is sought recently. Good knowledge of the way our lymphatic system works helps in treatment of these lesions.

7.5.1 Approaches to the Face for Vascular Tumors and Malformations

Surgery of the face is different from surgery in the rest of the body due to the prime reason of aesthetics; hence, the placement of an incision should be inconspicuous and involve scar management postoperatively. The muscles of facial expression lay below the skin and if the incision traumatize their nerve supply, it can have disastrous functional and cosmetic outcomes. Of importance are the sphincter muscles—orbicularis occuli and orbicularis oris, as reconstruction of their dynamic function may be difficult. The surgeon must also be cognizant of the nerves exiting various foramina of the skull while planning their incisions and dissections so as to not disrupt sensory information to the skin. The coronal approach is an excellent example of a hidden scar while providing almost entire visibility of the upper facial skeleton. Incisions are placed parallel to the direction of the hair so as not to transect the hair follicles. To prevent stretching of sensitive tissue due to traction, the incisions are made long enough. Closure of incision should be considered while planning incisions to avoid marginal necrosis or overlapping, hence designing of incision plays a vital role in the success of a surgery. Aging skin provides us with the resting skin tension lines which occur due to the skin's adaptation to repetitive function and the elastic nature of the underlying dermis (Fig. 7.14).

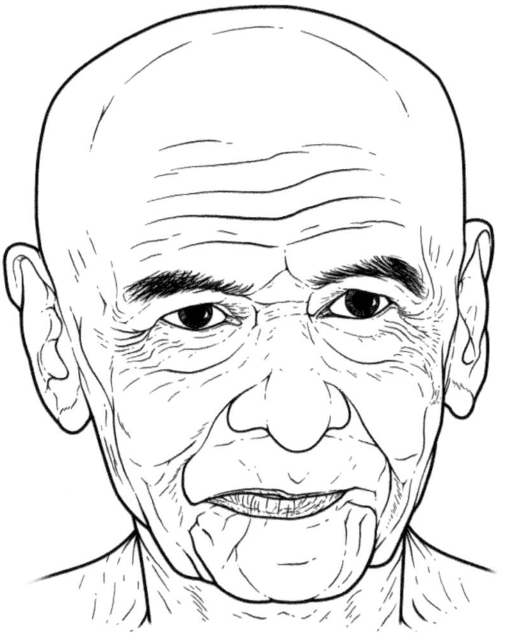

Fig. 7.14 Resting skin tension lines conspicuous in the aged face and are good choices for incision

Incisional wound closures are under the influence of elastin whereas excision wounds depend on collagen, this knowledge would minimize scarring [26]. These relaxed skin tension lines should never be crossed as they would leave behind a conspicuous scar which is unacceptable on the face. However, if an incision cannot be placed in the lines of minimal tension, it can be kept within an orifice such as nasal cavity, mouth, eyelid, or hair-bearing area to keep it inconspicuous. The same purpose is served by placing incision at the junction of two anatomic landmarks such as aesthetic subunit of the face, e.g., nasolabial crease (Fig. 7.15) [27].

The face can be divided into specific "aesthetic units," within which the skin has similar characteristics like color, thickness, subcutaneous fat, and texture. These units are separated by "aesthetic borders" which are hairline, eyebrows, philtrum, labiomental fold, nasolabial fold, and the vermillion (Fig. 7.15) [28]. These can also be further divided into smaller "aesthetic subunits" (Fig. 7.16) [28].

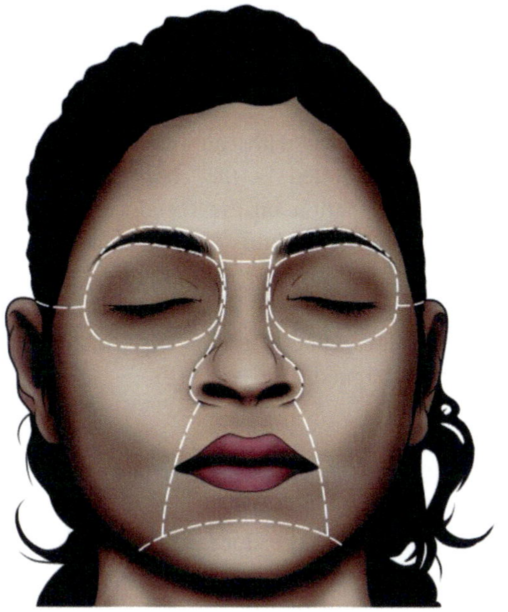

Fig. 7.15 Aesthetic borders

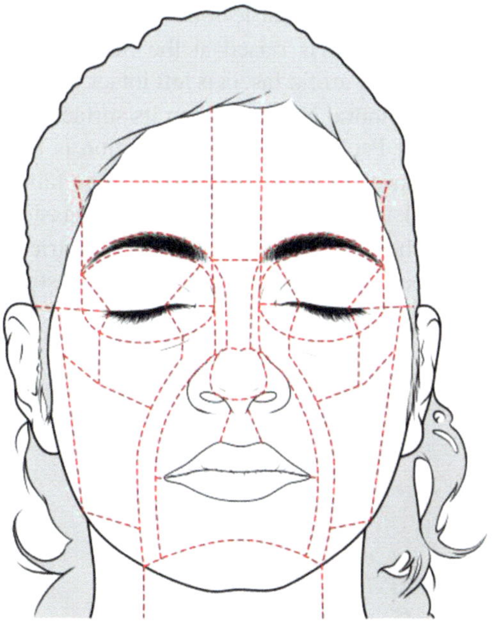

Fig. 7.16 Aesthetic subunits

The various incisions over the face are given keeping in mind these aesthetic units as described above (Fig. 7.17).

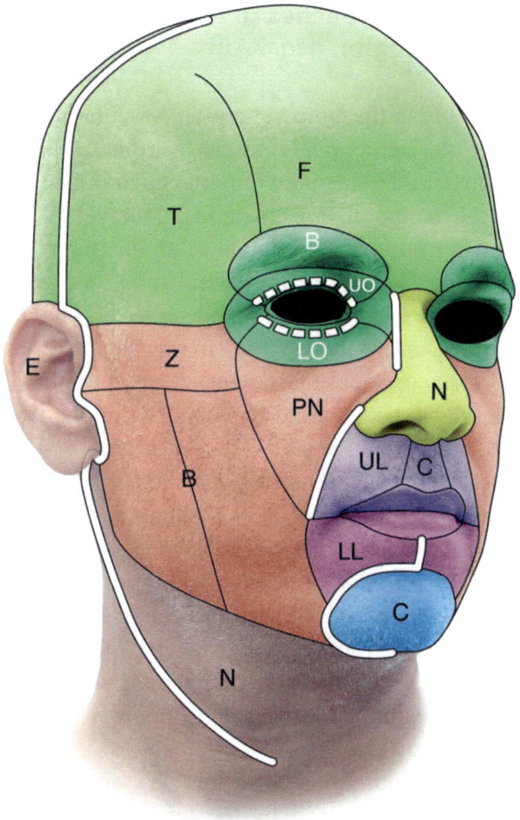

Fig. 7.17 Facial incisions based on aesthetic subunits

7.6 Approaches to Upper Face and Temporal Region

The forehead is limited by the hairline superiorly and the supraorbital margin, brow, and glabella inferiorly. The hairline, however, is an important but highly variable boundary between the scalp and the forehead [29].

The muscles in the forehead are the frontalis, the corrugator supercilii oblique and transverse, depressor supercilia, the procerus, and parts of orbicularis oculi. The movement of these muscles as in frequent frowning or as a person ages provides transverse lines on the forehead, while forming oblique and vertical lines between medial eyebrows. These lines are used to place incisions in a less conspicuous manner.

7.6.1 Approaches to the Temporal Region (Fig. 7.18)

Laterally in the temporal region, vascular lesions over the temporalis muscle warrant a lateral approach. Of anatomic importance in this region is the temporal branch of facial nerve. A line drawn from a point 5 mm beneath the tragus to a point 15 mm above the lateral brow charts the course of this branch [30] and serves as an aid to the surgeon while operating in this area.

The superior attachment of the temporalis muscle is the temporal line which is on the frontal and parietal bones. The superficial and the deep temporal fascia fuse with the periosteum of the central forehead at the temporal line. The frontal branch of the facial nerve travels within the temporoparietal fascia after its exit from the parotid gland [31]. Sharp dissection is done to transition the subperiosteal layer of the central forehead [30]. The superficial musculoaponeurotic system (SMAS) layer in this region is the temporal fascia.

The deep temporal fascia is separated to superficial and deep by the temporalis muscle which attaches to the zygoma and infratemporal fossa (Fig. 7.2). Hence, lesions deep to the temporalis muscle can be approached from the infratemporal fossa. Larger lesions superficial to the temporalis can be approached by a preauricular with Al-Kayat and Bramley extension [32], which is very versatile and provides access to a larger area while contributing to a cosmetic scar (Fig. 7.19). Since this incision is proximal to the facial nerve branches, the surgeon should approach this zone with caution. The approach has been elaborated in the chapter, including detailed information on the facial nerve in the area. The advantage of this incision is the aesthetics and the visibility for the surgeon. This provides access to temporal region, malar area, and the temporomandibular region for which it was primarily designed.

7.6.2 Approaches to Parotid

Approach to the TMJ is done through a Blair [33] incision (later modified by Bailey) [34]. The superficial lobe of the parotid gland, enclosed in the parotid masseteric fascia overlaps the capsule of the TMJ in front of the external auditory meatus, hence the modified incision is used to access the intraglandular lesions (Type III) [35].

The facial flap is raised at the SMAS layer (Fig. 7.1). The Parotid fascia is left intact with the Auriculo temporal Nerve seen on its surface. For exposure of Facial Nerve, the dissection is kept on the surface of the tragal cartilage. The tail of the parotid is freed off the sternocleidomastoid muscle. The posterior belly of the digastric is traced superiorly to its insertion on the mastoid,

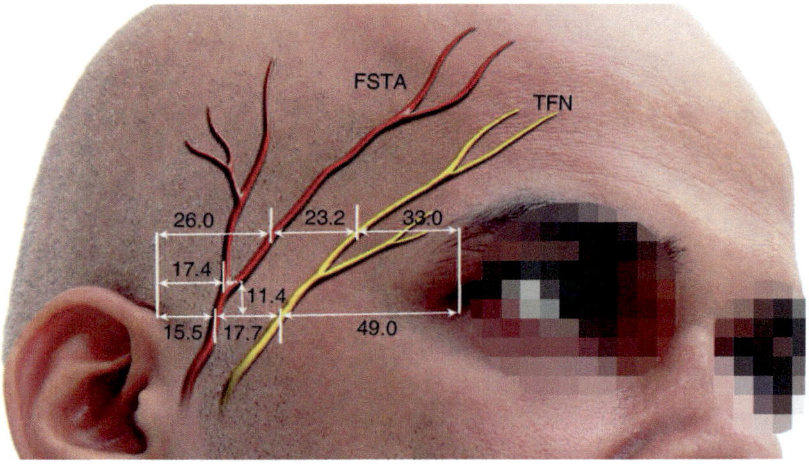

Fig. 7.18 Relations of facial nerve in temporal region (in mm)

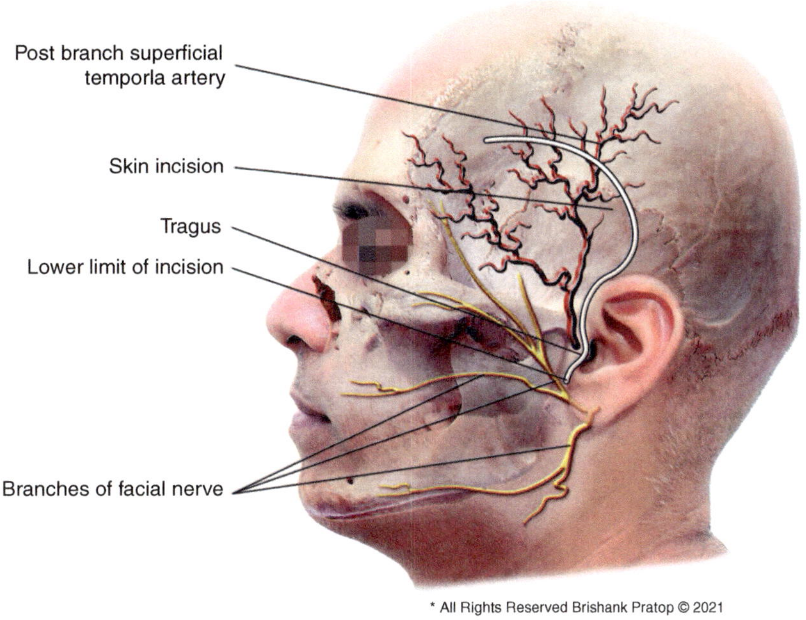

Fig. 7.19 Preauricular with Al-Kayat and Bramley extension

beneath the SCLDM. The facial nerve is identified at this point approximately 1 cm deep and anterior to the tragal pointer. Brisk bleeding is encountered from small vessels overlying the main trunk of the facial nerve. Further dissection is carried out bluntly on the surface of the nerve keeping it in sight at all times.

The deep portion of the gland is found in areas beneath the nerve and over the masseter muscle. It also has a retromandibular portion [36]. Dissection here is complicated by the presence of the auriculotemporal nerve, superficial temporal vessels, and facial nerve. The superficial temporal artery is a terminal branch of the external carotid, bifurcating within the gland and is accompanied by the superficial temporal vein, the artery also is posteriorly accompanied by the auriculotemporal nerve. The other terminal branch of the external carotid is the maxillary artery, and both superficial temporal and maxillary artery - the terminal arteries could be potential bleeders. Placing an incision close to cartilaginous part of the external acoustic meatus will reduce injury to the auriculotemporal nerve. Also, since temporal branch of the facial nerve is seen 8–35 mm anterior to the external auditory meatus, incisions in this zone are placed less than 8 mm away. Since some surgeons use the nerve stimulator to identify branches of the facial nerve, vasoconstrictor injection should be subcutaneous and not deep. The incision is carried out through skin, subcutaneous tissue, and temporal fascia which is hypovascular. When bleeders are coagulated, this flap along with the superficial temporal vessels and auriculotemporal nerve are retracted anteriorly to reach the parotid. The modified facelift approach is also used, and it has incisions in three regions including preaural, postaural, and hairline [37] (Fig. 7.20).

Post-auricular approach has better cosmetic outcomes and prevents injury to the auriculotemporal nerve. The incision is arc shaped and transects the external auditory canal, then the ear is reflected anteriorly, however, it presents a smaller access. Parotidectomy has been performed through a 4–5 cm incision in the postaural sulcus. However, this approach is for most small (Fig. 7.21) to medium size parotid tumors located in the mid and lower pole regions of the parotid gland [38]. VM within the parotid or preauricular region is tough to deal with this approach.

Deep lobe of the parotid if involved in the vascular lesion would require a trans-parotid approach, trans-parotid approach with mandibu-

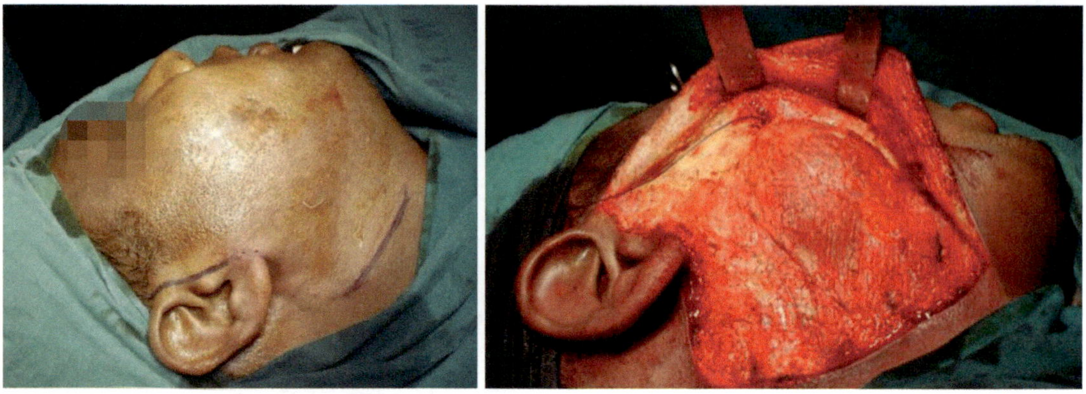

Fig. 7.20 Modified facelift incision (SMAS layer) for parotid and lesions of pre-auricular region

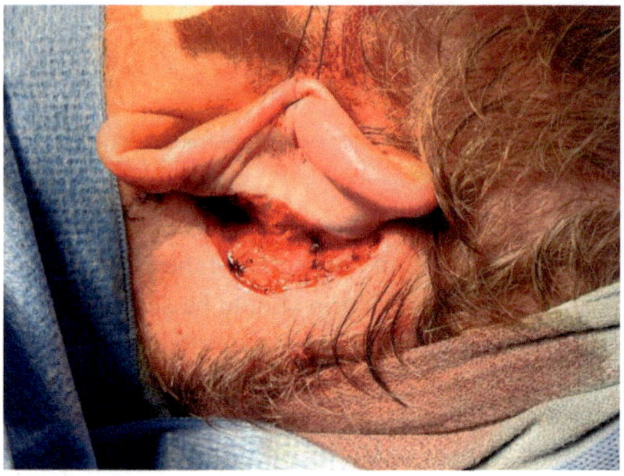

Fig. 7.21 Post-auricular approach

lotomy, trans-cervical approach, or a combined trans-parotid and trans-cervical approach [39]. The trans-cervical approach is for lesions with para-pharyngeal extension of the tumor. Frey's syndrome is caused by damage to auriculotemporal nerve, which innervates the skin of the tragus and the temple and it, gives secretomotor branches to the parotid gland. Damage to this nerve produces functional morbidity and should be prevented, discussion of which is beyond the scope of this chapter.

Bicoronal Approaches to the Cranium, cranial cavity, frontal, and orbital regions can be through the Bicoronal incision with elevation of the scalp. The bicoronal incision begins inferiorly in the preauricular crease bilaterally and is restricted to the inferior limit of the tragus. The incision in the preauricular skin crease is curved posteriorly onto the scalp. It is concealed within the hairline superiorly. The scalp flap is raised at the relatively avascular loose areolar level easily and bluntly, modified depending on the location of the VM. Lesions on the bone may need a pericranial elevation. The exposure is obtained inferiorly from the Zygomatic root on either side, temporal region and parietal areas. Anteriorly the Frontal zone, Nasal bridge, and Superior Orbital rims can be exposed conveniently. The supraorbital foramen and its contents can be protected by staying subperiosteal . An osteotome can be used to free the Supra orbital Nerve from the foramen.

Lateral elevation of the flap is deep to the superficial layer of the deep temporal fascia, this protects the zygomatic and temporal branches of the facial nerve (Fig. 7.22).

7.6.3 Supra Orbital Approach

A commonly used approach in the upper face is the supraorbital approach, which provides access to the frontozygomatic area. The scar resulting from this incision is not conspicuous. The incision is placed within the eyebrow hair (Fig. 7.23) and made through the skin and subcutaneous tissue till periosteum. There are no important neurovascular structures in this region. If extended exposure is desired, incision can be extended into the crow's feet line, lateral to the lateral canthus. It is vital to stay in the subperiosteal zone of dissection to avoid injury to the eyeball. Periosteum integrity should be maintained so as to avoid herniation of the lacrimal gland.

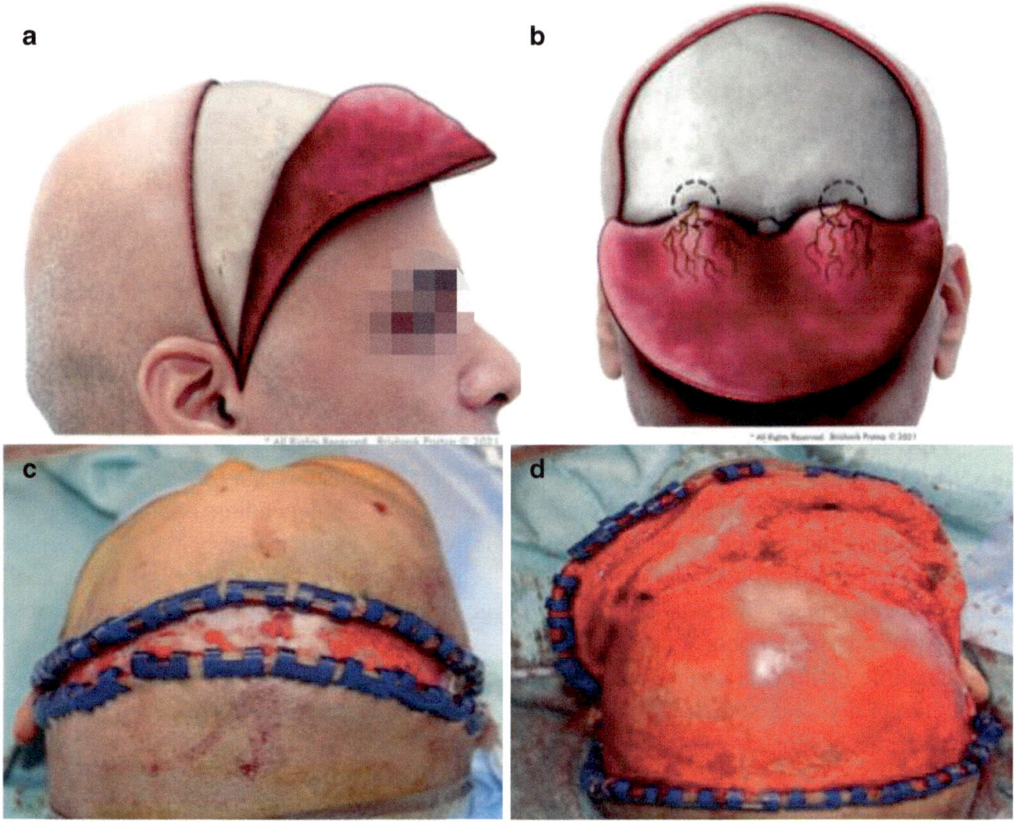

Fig. 7.22 Bicoronal approach. (**a**) Schematic lateral view (**b**) Schematic frontal view (**c**) Bicoronal skin incision, and (**d**) Bicoronal flap elevated to expose LM in right fronto-orbital region

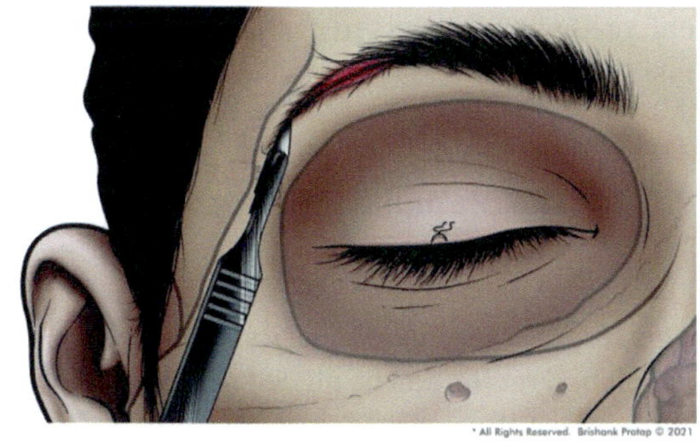

Fig. 7.23 Supraorbital approach with incision in the hairline

7.6.4 Upper Eyelid Approach

Another approach that gained popularity due to its aesthetic outcome is the upper eyelid approach also known as the supra-tarsal fold approach. The incision follows the natural crease of the upper eyelid, which is present in most individuals (Fig. 7.24). Lateral extension of this incision into a crows feet skin crease allows good exposure. About 1 cm above the eyelid margin slanting downward and 6 mm above the lateral canthus laterally. Once the incision is placed, a skin muscle flap is raised and the incision can be undermined until the periosteum to provide enhanced visualization. This approach provides access to the upper bony orbit and can be used to excise tumors of soft tissue around the upper eye (Fig. 7.24b) while producing almost an invisible scar.

7.7 Approaches to the Midface

Midface is one of the regions of the face that has shown to have the most congenital problems [40]. The midface encompasses the cheek and nose aesthetic subunits. The most important fac-

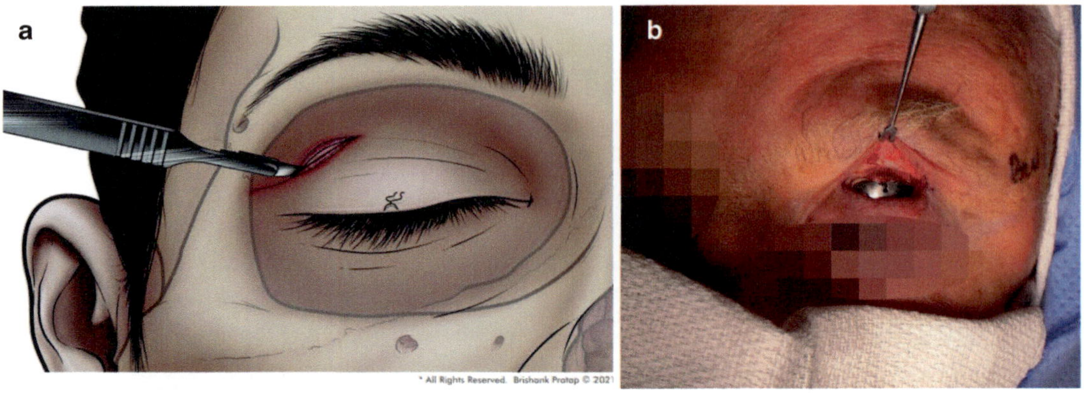

Fig. 7.24 (a) Upper eyelid crease approach. (b) Excision of lesion in mid upper eyelid

tor to consider is the position of the lesion. If they can be approached and excised completely via an intraoral approach that should be the first choice for a surgeon. What aids in making that decision usually is whether the lesion can be accessed below or above a muscle or bone. Lesions involving the mandible or maxilla can most times be accessed intraorally and sometimes combined with other approaches for extended access.

7.7.1 Subciliary Incision

Subciliary incision with dissection exposes areas in the infraorbital and supra zygomatic zone (Fig. 7.25a–d). Vascular sacs present in this area are mostly VM. They are seen in the subcutaneous plane. Adhering to the infraorbital periosteum protects the Infraorbital neurovascular bundle. The vascular sac can be identified and dissected out.

7.7.2 Lateral Rhinotomy Incision

The first lateral rhinotomy incision was introduced by Moure in 1902 [28]. The rhinotomy incision (Fig. 7.26) provides access to the nasal cavity, ethmoidal sinuses, maxillary sinuses, and nasopharynx. It has the advantage of creating a minimal cosmetic or functional disability. Intraoral extensions can be performed on a case-by-case basis, depending on the extent of the lesion. The incision line below the medial eyebrow, along the deepest part of nasomaxillary groove and curves below the ala of the nose. If extension is desired the philtral ridge down the upper lip and intraorally. Once intraoral, a buccal sulcus incision till the first molar with dissection provides a wide exposure. The anterior and posterior ethmoid arteries can be identified in or above the fronto-ethmoid suture. Lesions arising from these vessels can be identified here and the vessels may be ligated. The maxillary antrum can be accessed via this approach as well through the anterior maxillary wall and the antrostomy can be enlarged with ronguers to maximize visualization inside the antrum [41].

7.7.3 Nasolabial with Subciliary Extension

The surgical approach to lesions presents in the nasolabial region can be placed in the Nasolabial skin crease. Lesions beneath the skin and subcutaneous plane, either superficial to or in between the paranasal muscles such as levator labii superioris, Zygomaticus major and minor can be exposed and excised. The scar is concealed within the nasolabial skin crease (Fig. 7.27).

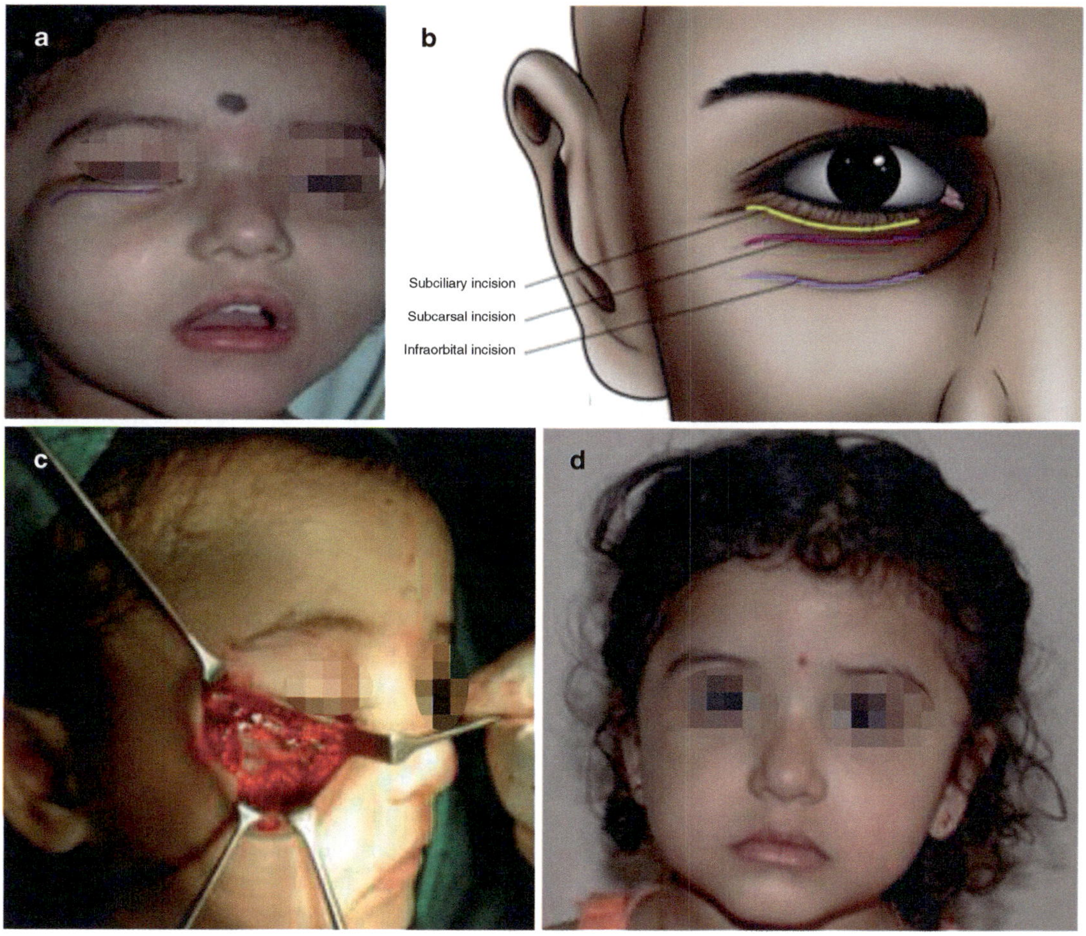

Fig. 7.25 (**a–d**) Subciliary incision for exposure of VM in infraorbital and zygomatic region (**a**, **b**) incision marking (**c**) excision of lesion (**d**) Postoperative healing without obvious scar)

7.7.4 Weber–Fergusson Approach

The Webber–Fergusson's incision and its modifications are used for approach to the anterior maxilla [42] another approach is the Midface degloving incision [43]. The former incision remains a controversy. Gensoul (1893) was believed to have first described it and later popularized by Weber and Fergusson. Another theory exists about it being first described Weber in German literature and later modified by Fergusson in English literature [44]. This standard technique, which follows the facial subunits, underwent various modifications depending on the extent of the tumor [45]. The various modifications of the weber-ferguson insicion for accessing the maxillofacial and skull base are [46]:

The Weber–Fergusson incision is suitable for superficial lesions which cannot be approached intraorally or when wide excision of the maxilla is required for type IV intraosseous lesions [35]. Due to the various modifications available, the incision has diverse utilities producing a less conspicuous scar.

The incision line is drawn through the vermillion border, along the philtrum of the lip, extending around the base of the nose and along the facial nasal groove (Fig. 7.28). It then extends infraor-

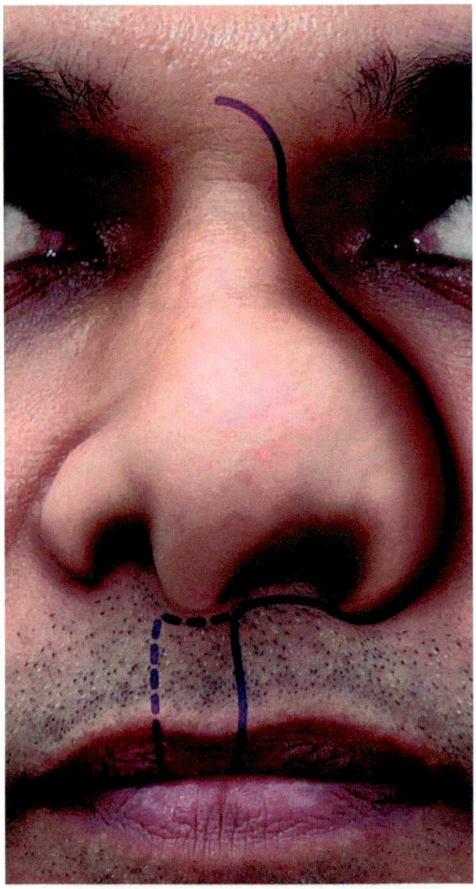

Fig. 7.26 Lateral rhinotomy incision

bitally 3–4 mm below the cilium to the lateral canthus. The intraoral part of the incision continues along the inner mucosal part of the upper lip proceeding laterally along the Gigivo buccal sulcus unto desired posterior extension. The soft tissue of the cheek is raised from the anterior surface of the maxilla, transecting the infraorbital nerves and vessels should the superior and lateral walls of the maxilla need to be approached.

The Lynch modification is used to approach tumors involving the frontal sinus. lateral extension up to the level of the lateral canthus, or inferiorly to be included in a lateral rhinotomy incision. The incision may be along the lower border of the eyebrow or in a skin crease along the upper eyelid. The incision is extended down, 0.5 cm medial to the medial canthus.

The Dieffenbach modification is used for lesions occurring at the infraorbital margin, anterior floor of orbit, and the zygomatic bone.

7.7.5 Intraoral Approach to Maxilla

Location of the lesion, access to the lesion, and need for reconstruction are usually three reasons to decide if an intraoral or extraoral approach is warranted. For example, lesions medial to the buccinator, can be accessed intraorally while if

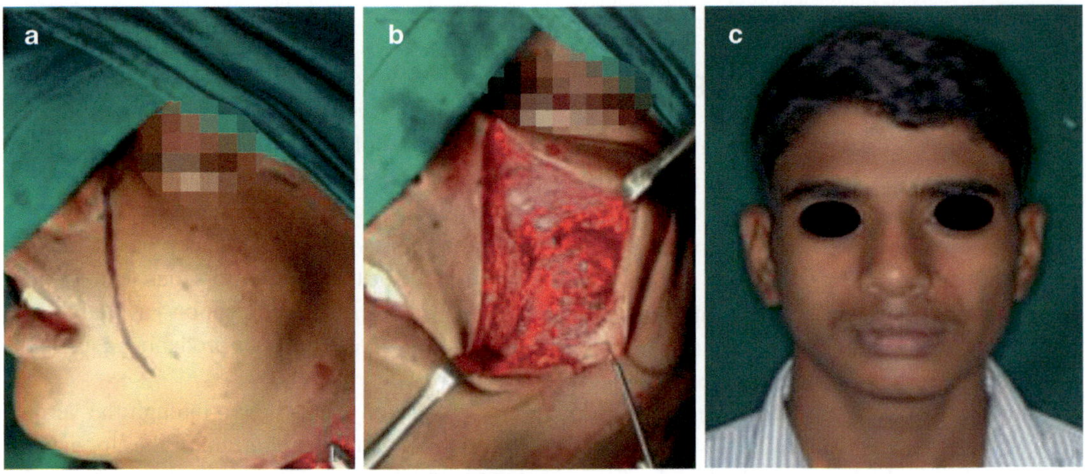

Fig. 7.27 (**a**–**c**) Nasolabial incision to expose the VM in the Sub Zygomatic area. Subciliary extension may be required for better access. (**a**) Incision (**b**) Exposure, (**c**) Post-operative

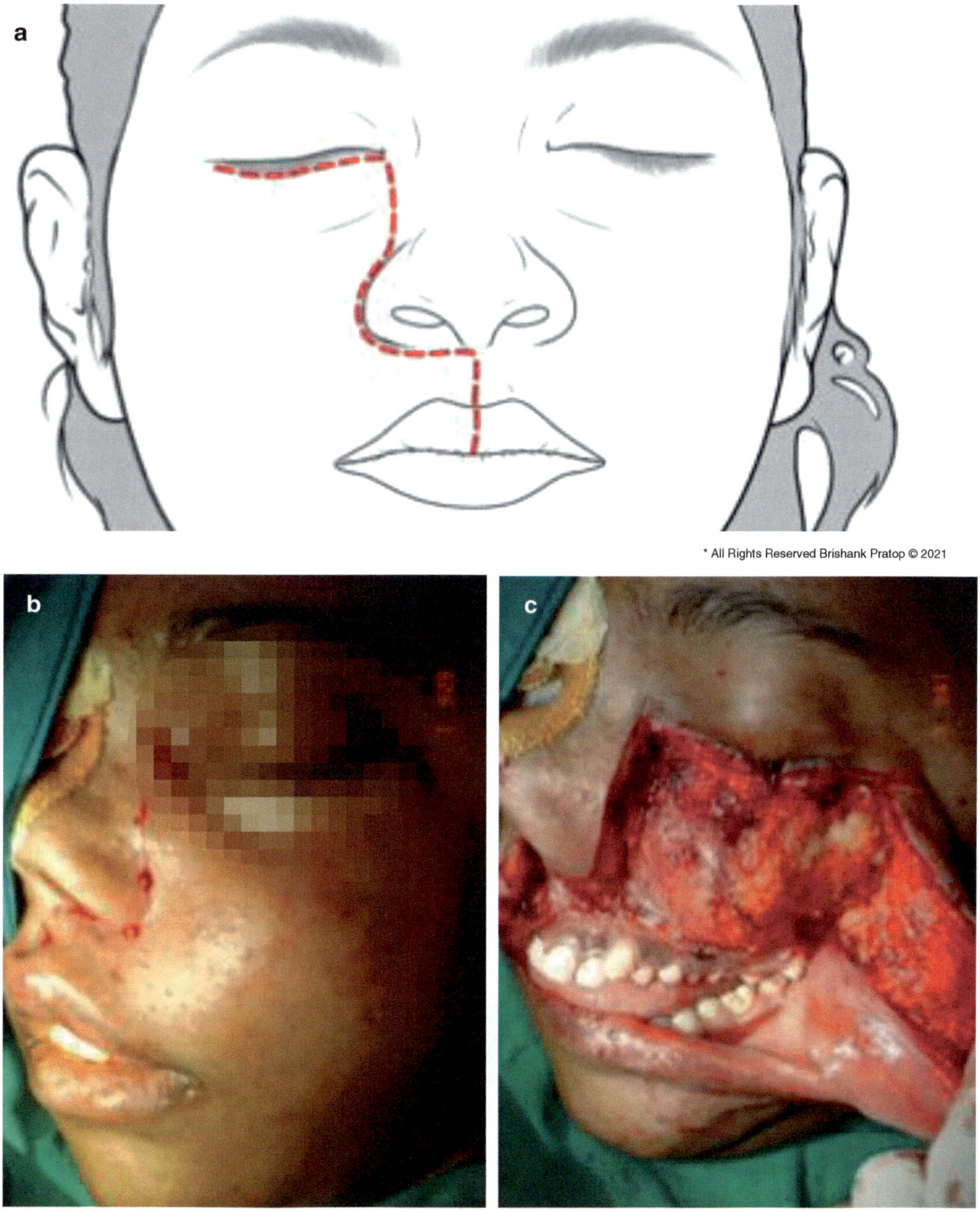

Fig. 7.28 (**a–c**) Dieffenbach's modification of Weber–Fergusson's approach. (**a**) Incision outline (**b**, **c**) Intraoperative incision and exposure

lateral to the buccinator an extraoral approach would provide better access.

Relevant anatomy for the surgeon while performing a maxillary intraoral approach is the infraorbital nerves and the buccal fat pad posteriorly. The infraorbital nerve supplies sensation to the ipsilateral upper lip, side and ala of the nose, and lower eyelid. This nerve must be preserved while dissection from the maxilla to the orbital bone, as it exits the infra-orbital foramen less than a centimeter inferior to the orbital rim. The buccal fat pad will be discussed in the intraoral mandibular approach in detail, the surgeon needs to be cautious while incising around the maxillary second molar. This approach can be used for intraosseous maxillary tumors.

Before infiltration, the upper lip midline is marked on the mucogingival junction to aid proper closure. Vestibular/sublabial incision is made as far as the first molar tooth in the sulcus with adequate attached gingiva for closure. The incision is made till the periosteum and then the bone is exposed subperiosteally (Fig. 7.29). Subperiosteal dissection is carried out till piriform aperture and strip its attachments to perinasal musculature, while posterior extend is till the pterygomaxillary fissure. While dissecting the nasal region injury to nasal mucosa should be prevented, bleeding can be expected in this zone which is easily controlled with packing. The dissection is extended superiorly till the orbital rim with caution around the infraorbital nerve. Even with cautious dissection, some amount of temporary paraesthesia can be expected. This approach exposes the entire maxilla for intraosseous lesions or even lesions of the nasal cavity and maxillary sinus. This gives access to lesions in the anterior nasal area and maxillary sinus. A Lefort 1 osteotomy with down fracture of the maxilla allows access to vascular tumors such as Nasopharyngeal Angiofibroma in the posterior maxillary space.

7.7.6 Midface Degloving Approach

This is an all-inclusive approach with no extraoral scar and hence an excellent choice for large tumors of the midface region (Fig. 7.30). Due to the nature of the incisions, it is performed under oro-endotracheal intubation. It begins with an intranasal incision which is made circumferentially on the mucosa followed by a transfixion incision that spans the membranous septum, between the lower end of the cartilaginous septum and the medial crura of the lower lateral cartilages. Now an inter-cartilaginous incision is made to release the soft tissue from the upper lateral nasal cartilage and bone, this is done in a subperiosteal plane. Now, an incision is placed intraorally along the buccal sulcus till the molars (as in trauma or orthognathic surgery) and the entire midface can be raised till the infraorbital rim and glabella Access can be made via various osteotomies to the central cranial base as well if needed, from the frontal base down to the upper cervical spine [47]. The exposure obtained using the degloving approach is excellent and the absence of the resultant facial scar or deformity makes this a popular approach in the midface. Nasal obstruction and infraorbital paresthesia can result from this approach.

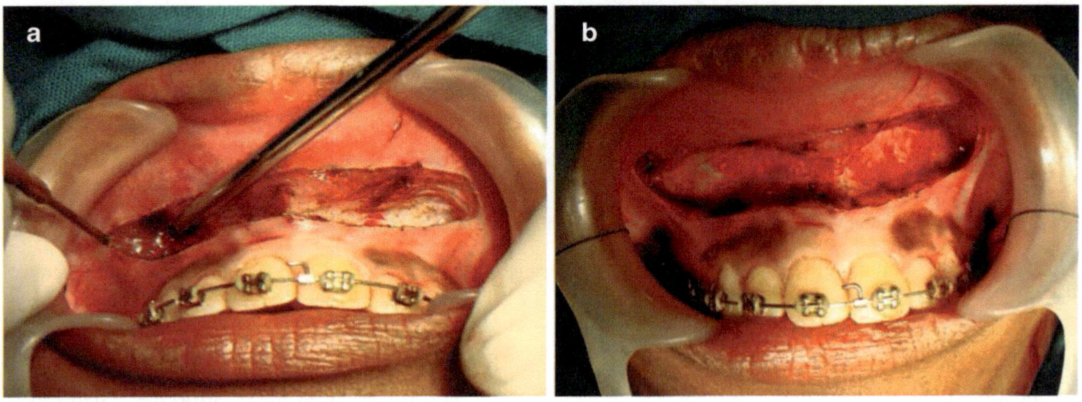

Fig. 7.29 (**a**, **b**) Intraoral approach: Maxillary Vestibular approach

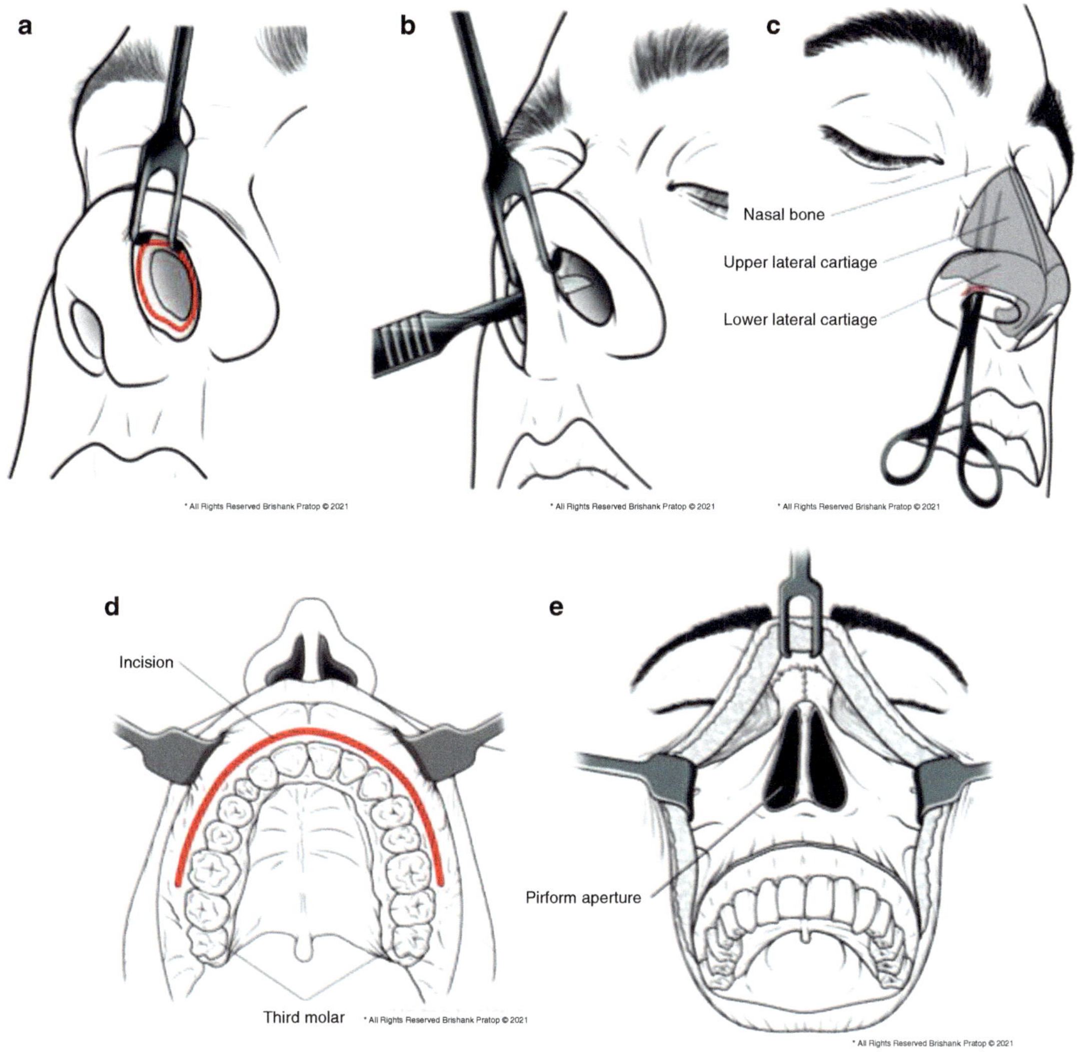

Fig. 7.30 Midface degloving approach (steps **a**–**e**)

7.8 Approaches to the Lower Face

7.8.1 Mandibular Vestibular Approach

Intraoral vascular lesions within the substance of the vestibule and deep to the SMAS/buccinator, it is wise to approach this intraorally via a vestibular approach. The anatomy to be aware of the mandibular vestibular approach are mental vessels, facial vessels, mentalis muscle, and buccal fat pad. The mental nerve is of significance when accessing the soft tissue or bone anterior to the molar region. Mucosal incisions are made anterior and posterior to this region, pass through submucosa and periosteum (Fig. 7.31). The nerve needs to be isolated while accessing this region. The facial vessels can be encountered in the inferior border of the mandible and in this region, the only structure separating them from bone is the periosteum. Since the facial artery arises from the

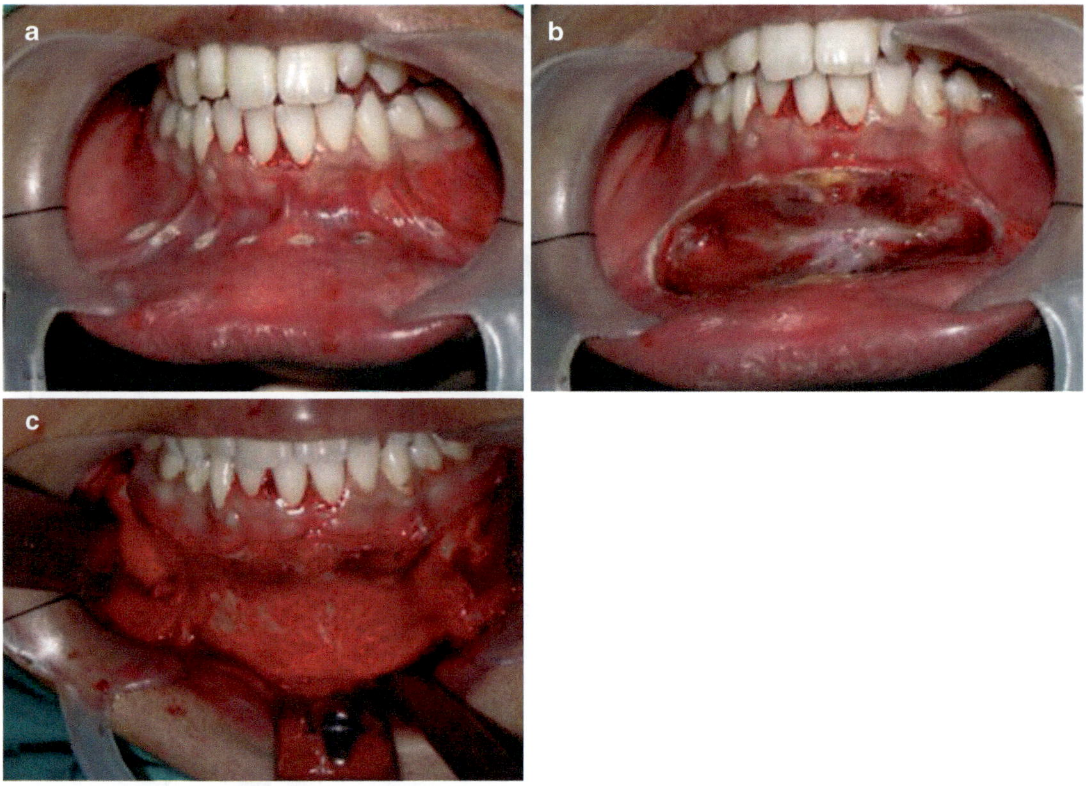

Fig. 7.31 (**a**–**c**) Mandibular vestibular approach

external carotid, vascular lesions arising from this vessel must be ligated prior to accessing this lesion. The mentalis muscle is the elevator of the lower lip and chin and without proper approximation will cause the chin to droop and expose the lower anterior teeth. This muscle is innervated by the marginal branch of the facial nerve and passes from the bony chin to the skin of the chin, hence can be transected in subperiosteal dissections of this zone. The buccal fat pad is a unique structure, which has four extensions: buccal, temporal, pterygoid, and pterygomandibular. The buccal extension is superficial and imparts fullness to the cheek while the rest are deeply seated. The parotid duct travels superficial to the fat pad and penetrates the oral mucosa through the fat pad and buccinator muscle to enter the oral cavity opposite the second molar. Intraoral incision should not be placed, if possible, higher than the occlusal plane of mandibular teeth, to prevent herniation of the buccal fat pad. The incision is placed with these structures in mind, on the sulcular mucosa extending all the way to the external oblique ridge. Exposure is achieved till the lateral border of the ramus of the mandible and even to the condylar neck and coronoid. It is to be noted that in edentulous mandible that incisions should be made on the alveolus, in older patients the resorption causes the mental nerve move closer to the superficial surface.

7.8.2 Visor Incision

Submandibular, submental, and cervical parts of the head and neck are accessible through the cervical visor incision (Fig. 7.32). The flap is raised in a sub-platysmal plane all the way to the lower border of the mandible. The EJV can be identified and ligated at the level of the incision or raised off the flap. Investing layer of the deep cervical fascia is exposed. Supra-platysmal dissec-

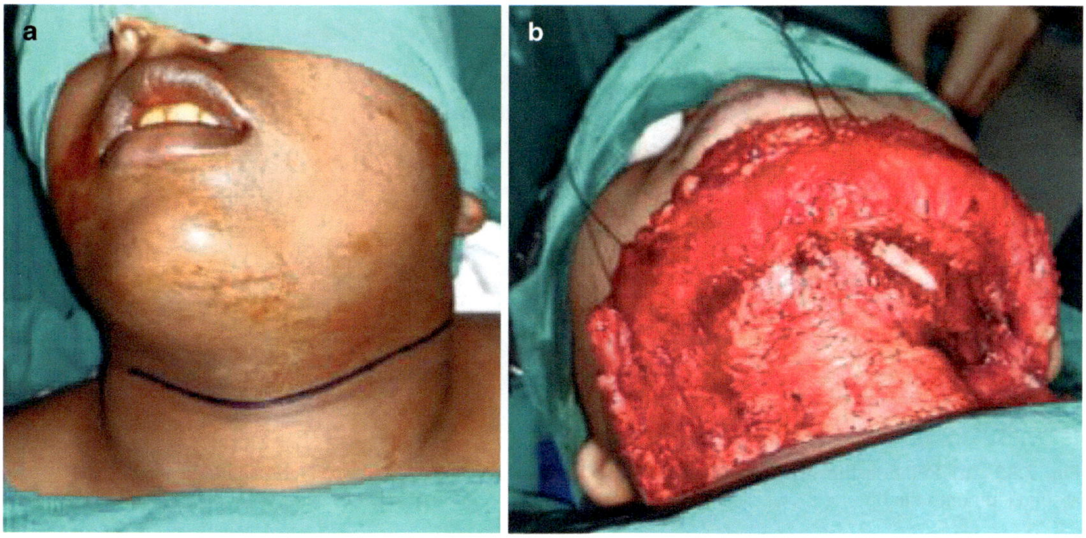

Fig. 7.32 The visor incision is an ample access to the neck, mandible, skull base and parotid areas. (**a**) skin incision (**b**) elevation of the skin and platysma flap elevation to the inferior border of the mandible

tion is required for lesions present in the subcutaneous plane. Care taken not to perforate the flap.

The marginal mandibular and cervical branch of the facial nerve can be identified deep to the investing layer of cervical fascia and is identified at the lower mandibular border emerging below the cervical fascia to cross the facial artery (Fig. 7.7). From here on the nerve is traced posteriorly into the lobe of the parotid gland.

Vascular lesions present in the subcutaneous plane (Type II), Submandibular Gland (Type III), Deep to Mylohyoid, and sternocleidomastoid (SCM), and supraclavicular region can be accessed. The posterior retraction of the SCM exposes the contents of the Carotid sheath (common Carotid Artery, IJV, and vagus nerve). Control of External Carotid can be achieved as well through this approach.

7.8.3 Submandibular Approach

These approaches are for lesions usually deep to the SMAS layer but superficial to the mylohyoid and facial muscles and cannot be accessed intraorally. The relevant anatomy to this region is the facial artery, facial vein, and the marginal branch of facial nerve (Figs. 7.7 and 7.33a). The facial artery, a tortuous branch of the external carotid, arises medial to the mandible, passes the submandibular salivary gland and circles around the lower border of the mandible, anterior to the masseter, and is anterior to the facial vein. The facial vein is formed as a direct continuation of the angular vein which joins the retromandibular vein to form the common facial vein and drains into the internal jugular vein. The facial vein is not as tortuous as the artery. The marginal mandibular branch arises from the facial nerve when it divides in the parotid, extend inferiorly, and supply motor fibers to the facial muscles of the lower lip and corner of the mouth. Injury to this nerve results in facial asymmetry, deviation of the contralateral angle of the mouth, drooling of saliva, and difficulty of speech and chewing. Multiple variations have been mentioned in literature of this nerve. In a study by P.G. Balagopal et al. [48], 161 of the 202 patients (79.7%) the nerve was a single division, formed of two branches in 26 (12.9%) patients, three branches in 14 (6.9%) patients, and four branches in one patient. In patients with a single branch, the nerve crossed the facial artery below the lower border of the mandible in 97/161 (60%) patients, at the lower border of the mandible in 42/161 (26%) patients and above the lower border in 22/161 (14%) patients. The furthest distance the nerve

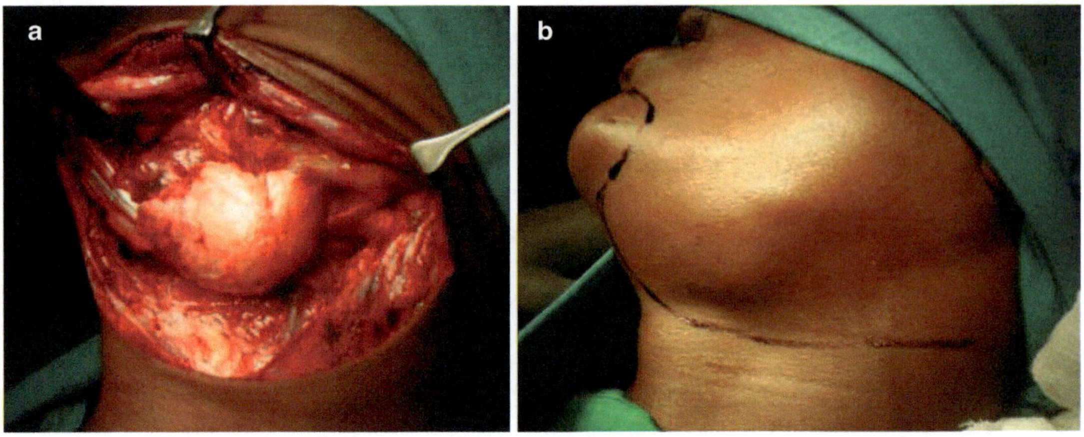

Fig. 7.33 (**a**) Relationship of marginal mandibular nerve and facial vessels (**b**) Submandibular incision extended around chin unto the lip

has been reported from the lower border of the mandible is 1.5 cm and hence incisions for submandibular approach are always placed 1.5–2 cm away from the inferior border. Incisions to ligate the facial artery or vein at this location should follow a low cervical approach.

The layers encountered in this region are skin, subcutaneous tissue, platysma muscle which extends from subcutaneous tissue of periclavicular region to insert into symphysis menti and merge with orbicularis oris. Elevating a subplatysmas flap will expose the superficial layer of deep cervical fascia and in this region, we can encounter the facial vessels and/or the marginal mandibular branch of the facial nerve. The facial vessels can be ligated if necessary or retracted anteriorly depending on the location of the lesion. The capsule of the submandibular gland and the submandibular node can also be encountered here. Further dissection leads to the mandibular periosteum at the lower border of the mandible and the pterygomasseteric sling, This avascular zone is sharply incised in the inferior border of the mandible.

7.9 Mandibular Access Osteotomy [35]

The incision is placed in the submandibular skin crease as described previously and extended anteriorly in a wavy curve toward the mid part of the chin, follows the submental skin crease laterally and continuing around the bulbous part of the chin onto the lower part of the face (Fig. 7.34a). The lip split may be done either medial to the corner of the mouth or carried closer to the midline of the lip with a stagger. Across the vermilion onto the labial mucosa and continued upward to the gingival mucoperiosteum anterior to the desired osteotomy line. Lingual mucosal incision may be placed along the floor of the mouth, at its junction with the attached lingual muco periosteum or a lingual crevicular gingival incision is placed. The lingual mucoperiosteal incision at the junction of the floor and mucoperosteum has the risk of damaging the submandibular duct, sublingual gland, and more importantly the lingual nerve. The lingual incision is extended to the retromolar region around the last erupted tooth and continued buccally at 45°. The mandible is split anterior to the mental foramina between two teeth (usually canine and premolar).

Prior to the osteotomy, a 4-holed plate is adapted on the desired split site, the osteotomy is initiated with a saw preferably to allow good osteosynthesis (Fig. 7.34b). The lingual mucosa or the mucoperiosteum is elevated with the lingual nerve in sight. Posteriorly the medial pterygoid is stripped off the mandible. Lateral traction to the mandible gives good visibility and eases dissection. Medial side of the ramus is visualized and the inferior alveolar neurovascular bundle can be seen before it enters the canal (Fig. 7.34d) Temporalis

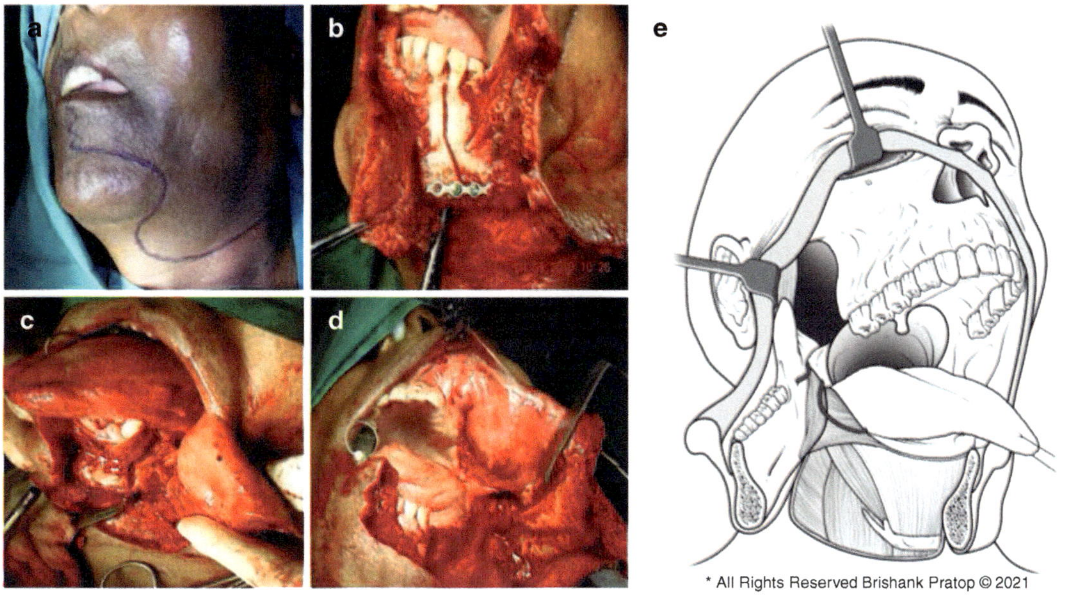

Fig. 7.34 Mandibular access osteotomy. (**a**) Skin marking of the incision (**b**) Mini-plate adapted prior to osteotomy (**c**) Osteotomy completed (**d**) Mandible swung laterally after stripping muscles (**e**) Diagrammatic illustration of the procedure

fibers from the anterior margin of the ramus are elevated using a monopolar cautery. This allows a good lateral and upward swing of the mandible.

The mandibulotomy allows access to lesions in the deep lobe of parotid, parapharynx, and infra-temporal fossa. Following access and excision of the lesion, after obtaining homeostasis the mandible is swung back and plated. Two 4-holed plates are used for fixation in this region. In case of intraoral defect caused by mucosal excision, a temporoparietal flap or radial forearm vascularized flap is used. The rest of the surgical wound is closed in layers with a vacuum drain in situ.

Incisions placed in the head and neck regions are objectively done bearing in mind good access is obtained for excision of the lesion and the scars are well concealed in skin creases or at junctions of aesthetic facial subunits. All wounds are closed in layers with underlying muscles restored to restore function. Skin sutures are placed with 4/0 monofilament non absorbable sutures. Subcuticular sutures are preferred in straight-line wounds. The sutures are removed on the 7th post-operative day.

References

Section A

1. Zhang T, Fan S, He W, Zhang T, Wang Y. Ophthalmic artery visualization and morphometry by computed tomography angiography. Graefes Arch Clin Exp Ophthalmol. 2015;253(4):627–31.
2. Erdogmus S, Govsa F. The anatomic landmarks of ethmoidal arteries for the surgical approaches. J Craniofac Surg. 2006;17(2):280–5.
3. Erdogmus S, Govsa F. Arterial features of inner canthus region: confirming the safety for the flap design. J Craniofac Surg. 2006;17(2):280–5.
4. Tansatit T, Apinuntrum P, Phetudom T. An anatomic basis for treatment of retinal artery occlusions caused by hyaluronic acid injections: a cadaveric study. Aesthet Plast Surg. 2014;38(6):1131–7.
5. Erdogmus S, Govsa F. Importance of the anatomic features of the lacrimal artery for orbital approaches. J Craniofac Surg. 2005;16(6):957–64.
6. Bozikov K, Shaw-dunn J, Soutar DS, Arnez ZM. Arterial anatomy of the lateral orbital and cheek region and arterial supply to the "peri-zygomatic perforator arteries flap". Surg Radiol Anat. 2008;30(1):17–22.
7. Choi DH, Eom JR, Lee JW, et al. Zygomatico-orbital artery: the largest artery in the temporal area. J Plast Reconstr Aesthet Surg. 2018;71(4):484–9.

8. Ozgur Z, Govsa F, Ozgur T. Assessment of origin characteristics of the front branches of the external carotid artery. J Craniofac Surg. 2008;19(4):1159–66.
9. Bettoni J, Pagé G, Salsac AV, et al. 3T non-injected phase-contrast MRI sequences for the mapping of the external carotid branches: in vivo radio-anatomical pilot study for feasibility analysis. J Craniomaxillofac Surg. 2018;46(1):98–106.
10. Shintani S, Terakado N, Alcalde RE, Tomizawa K, Nakayama S, Ueyama Y, Ichikawa H, Sugimoto T, Matsumura T. An anatomical study of the arteries for intraarterial chemotherapy of head and neck cancer. Int J Clin Oncol. 1999;4(6):327–30.
11. Shima H, von Luedinghausen M, Ohno K, Michi K. Anatomy of microvascular anastomosis in the neck. Plast Reconstr Surg. 1998;101(1):33–41.
12. Ozgur Z, Govsa F, Celik S, Ozgur T. Clinically relevant variations of the superior thyroid artery: an anatomic guide for surgical neck dissection. Surg Radiol Anat. 2009;31(3):151–9.
13. Cavalcanti DD, Reis CV, Hanel R, et al. The ascending pharyngeal artery and its relevance for neurosurgical and endovascular procedures. Neurosurgery. 2009;65(6 Suppl):114–20. discussion 120
14. Wang C, Kundaria S, Fernandez-Miranda J, Duvvuri U. A description of arterial variants in the transoral approach to the parapharyngeal space. Clin Anat. 2014;27(7):1016–22.
15. Pinar YA, Bilge O, Govsa F. Anatomic study of the blood supply of perioral region. Clin Anat. 2005;18(5):330–9.
16. Al-Hoqail RA, Meguid EM. Anatomic dissection of the arterial supply of the lips: an anatomical and analytical approach. J Craniofac Surg. 2008;19(3):785–94.
17. Ateş O, Ahmed AS, Niemann D, Başkaya MK. The occipital artery for posterior circulation bypass: microsurgical anatomy. Neurosurg Focus. 2008;24(2):E9.
18. Keser N, Avci E, Soylemez B, Karatas D, Baskaya MK. Occipital artery and its segments in vertebral artery revascularization surgery: a microsurgical anatomic study. World Neurosurg. 2018;112:e534–9.
19. Alvernia JE, Fraser K, Lanzino G. The occipital artery: a microanatomical study. Neurosurgery. 2006;58(1 Suppl):ONS114-22. discussion ONS114-22
20. Kobayashi S, Nagase T, Ohmori K. Colour Doppler flow imaging of postauricular arteries and veins. Br J Plast Surg. 1997;50(3):172–5.
21. Gómez Díaz OJ, Cruz Sánchez MD. Anatomical and clinical study of the posterior auricular artery angiosome: in search of a rescue tool for ear reconstruction. Plast Reconstr Surg Glob Open. 2016;4(12):e1165.
22. Akiyama O, Güngör A, Middlebrooks EH, Kondo A, Arai H. Microsurgical anatomy of the maxillary artery for extracranial-intracranial bypass in the pterygopalatine segment of the maxillary artery. Clin Anat. 2018;31(5):724–33.
23. Alvernia JE, Hidalgo J, Sindou MP, et al. The maxillary artery and its variants: an anatomical study with neurosurgical applications. Acta Neurochir. 2017;159(4):655–64.
24. Otake I, Kageyama I, Mataga I. Clinical anatomy of the maxillary artery. Okajimas Folia Anat Jpn. 2011;87(4):155–64.
25. Pinar YA, Govsa F. Anatomy of the superficial temporal artery and its branches: its importance for surgery. Surg Radiol Anat. 2006;28(3):248–53.

Section B

26. Rajmohan S, Tauro D, Bagulkar B, Vyas A. Coronal/hemicoronal approach—a gateway to craniomaxillofacial region. J Clin Diagn Res. 2015;9(8):PC01.
27. Paul SP. Are incisional and excisional skin tension lines biomechanically different? Understanding the interplay between elastin and collagen during surgical procedures. Int J Biomed. 2017;7(2):111–4.
28. Paluch J, Markowski J, Pilch J, Piotrowska-Seweryn A, Kwiatkowski R, Lewin-Kowalik J, Zralek C, Gorzkowska A. Interdisciplinary surgical management of orbital and maxillo-ethmoidal complex disorders. In: Clinical management and evolving novel therapeutic strategies for patients with brain tumors. Intech; 2013.
29. Ilankovan V, Ethunandan M, Seah TE. Local flaps in facial reconstruction: a defect based approach. Cham: Springer; 2015.
30. Garritano FG, Quatela VC. Surgical anatomy of the upper face and forehead. Facial Plast Surg. 2018;34(02):109–13.
31. Babakurban ST, Cakmak O, Kendir S, Elhan A, Quatela VC. Temporal branch of the facial nerve and its relationship to fascial layers. Arch Facial Plast Surg. 2010;12(1):16–23.
32. Al-Kayat A, Bramley P. A modified pre-auricular approach to the temporomandibular joint and malar arch. Br J Oral Surg. 1979;17(2):91–103.
33. Blair VP. Surgery and diseases of the mouth and jaws: a practical treatise on the surgery and diseases of the mouth and allied structures. St. Louis: Mosby; 1917. p. 492–523.
34. Bailey H. The treatment of tumours of the parotid gland with special reference to total parotidectomy. Br J Surg. 1941;28(111):337–46.
35. Nair S, Sridhar KR, Shah A, Kumar B, Shetty P. Maxillectomy through mandibulotomy—a retrospective clinical review. J Oral Maxillofac Surg. 2011;68:2040–7.
36. Olsen KD, Quer M, de Bree R, et al. Deep lobe parotidectomy—why, when, and how? Eur Arch Otorhinolaryngol. 2017;274:4073–8. https://doi.org/10.1007/s00405-017-4767-5.
37. Appiani E, Delfino MC. Plastic incisions for facial and neck tumors. Ann Plast Surg. 1984;13(4):335–52.
38. Yuen AP. Small access postaural parotidectomy: an analysis of techniques, feasibility and safety. Eur Arch Otorhinolaryngol. 2016;273(7):1879–83.
39. Casani AP, Cerchiai N, Dallan I, Seccia V, Franceschini SS. Benign tumours affecting the deep

lobe of the parotid gland: how to select the optimal surgical approach. Acta Otorhinolaryngol Ital. 2015;35(2):80.
40. Baxter DJ, Shroff M. Congenital midface abnormalities. Neuroimaging. Clinics. 2011;21(3):563–84.
41. Schramm VL, Myers EN. Lateral rhinotomy. Laryngoscope. 1978;88(6):1042–5.
42. Chiodo AA, Strumas N, Gilbert RW, Birt BD. Management of odontogenic myxoma of the maxilla. Otolaryngol Head Neck Surg. 1997;117(6):S73–6.
43. Zaghloul AS, Nouh MA, Fatah HA. Midfacial degloving approach for malignant maxillary tumors. J Egypt Natl Canc Inst. 2004;16(2):69–75.
44. Fernandes R, Ord R. Access surgery for oral cancer. Oral Maxillofac Surg Clin North Am. 2006;18(4):565–71. https://doi.org/10.1016/j.coms.2006.06.008.
45. Rajasekhar G, Vura NG, Sudhir R, Dhanala S, Alwala AM. Versatility of Dieffenbach's modification of Weber Fergusson's approach for treatment of maxillary pathologies. J Maxillofac Oral Surg. 2012;11(4):416–9.
46. Stell PM, Maran AG, Gaze M, Wilson JA. In: Maran AGD, Gaze M, Wilson JA, editors. Stell and Maran's head and neck surgery. Oxford: Butterworth-Heinemann; 1993. p. 381–9.
47. Torrens M, Al-Mefty O, Kobayashi S. Operative skull base surgery. New York: Churchill Livingstone; 1997. p. 107–15. [33]
48. Balagopal PG, George NA, Sebastian P. Anatomic variations of the marginal mandibular nerve. Indian J Surg Oncol. 2012;3(1):8–11.

8 Surgical Management

Sanjiv C. Nair, Sunil Shroff,
and Srinivasa R. Chandra

8.1 Introduction

Vascular lesions are a diverse group of anomalies, presenting in different areas of the head and neck predominantly. These can be seen in children and adults involving different layers of the face, oral cavity and deep visceral spaces. Management of this group of lesions is complex and governed by the age of presentation and anatomical structures involved. Their treatment should be tailored as per the nature and extent of lesion as, '***one size does not fit all***'.

Neonates, infants and children up to the age of 3 years are best managed with pharmacotherapy unless involving critical areas like airway, vital structures like eyes causing severe functional problems. Most other patients benefit from surgery alone or surgery in combination with pharmacotherapy, sclerotherapy or embolisation.

The role of various drugs and embolisation with their mechanism of action has been discussed elsewhere in the text, and surgical management alone will be dealt with in the rest of this chapter.

Unlike in the past, most low and high-flow vascular anomalies can be managed with surgery by either excision or debulking. Smaller-sized lesions are almost always excised completely. On the contrary, larger-sized lesions are mostly debulked and may require multiple procedures. External carotid artery (ECA) control and/or Endovascular embolisation is used to aid in primary haemostasis during surgical debulking of high-flow lesions [1].

8.2 Decision-Making

As in any surgical treatment, is the most important aspect in the management of vascular lesions. This commences at the time of their presentation. In head and neck anomalies, surgery is chosen in the following situations:

1. Presence of Functional problems such as breathing, speech or bleeding episodes.
2. The Lesions present significant cosmetic challenge.
3. Failure of all other treatment modalities which are less intrusive. Flow dynamics of the lesion dictate the surgical therapy. The Small low flow vascular malformations (venous/lymphatic/lympho venous) are treated either with sclerotherapy followed by surgery or surgery alone. Larger low flow lesions are subjected to

S. C. Nair (✉)
Department of Maxillofacial Surgery, B.M. Jain Hospital, Bangalore Institute of Dental Science, Bangalore, Karnataka, India

S. Shroff
Department of Oral and Maxillofacial Surgery, Bhagwan Mahaveer Jain Hospital, Bengaluru, India

S. R. Chandra
Oral & Maxillofacial- Head & Neck Oncology Reconstructive Surgery, Oregon Health & Science University Portland, Portland, OR, USA
e-mail: chandrsr@ohsu.edu

S. C. Nair, S. R. Chandra (eds.), *Management of Head and Neck Vascular Lesions*,
https://doi.org/10.1007/978-981-15-2321-2_8

debulking or corseting [2] with or without sclerotherapy.

High-flow vascular lesions are subjected to either surgical debulking or excision assisted with intra-operative ECA control/pre-operative embolisation/both. These lesions can demand primary reconstruction if involving the aesthetic subunits of the face and oral cavity.

An algorithm has been designed as a guide for surgical intervention (Fig. 8.1a, b).

For simplicity, the author's own anatomical classification [1] (Table 8.1) is followed as it makes the understanding of various surgical

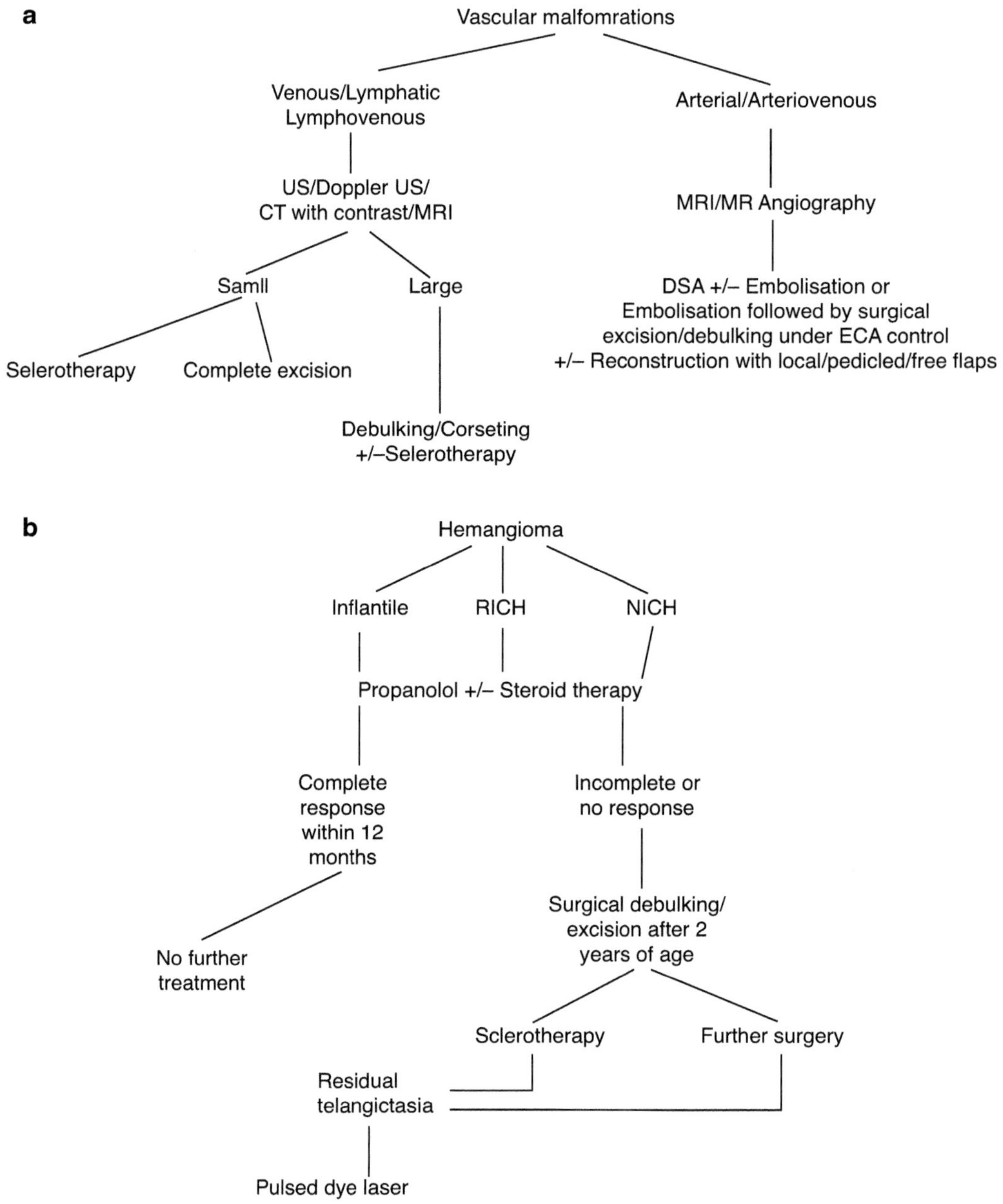

Fig. 8.1 (**a**) Algorithm for management of vascular malformations. (**b**) Algorithm for management of vascular malformations

Table 8.1 Anatomical classification of Vascular malformations (Figs. 8.2, 8.3, 8.4, 8.5, and 8.6)

Type I	Mucosal/cutaneous
Type II	Submucosal/subcutaneous
Type III	Glandular
Type IV	Intraosseous
Type V	Deep visceral

approaches and the rationale behind them more lucid and comprehensible. Also, the concept of '*corset suturing*' [2] will be explained with its specific indications.

The surgical anatomy has been explained elsewhere in this book. It is very important to be familiar with the various anatomical subunits of the face to define the extent and involvement of these lesions. Surgical approaches to these units are almost always kept along the skin tension lines leaving the final results aesthetically acceptable.

An understanding of the different layers and planes of dissection in the head and neck is important to approach and treat these vascular anomalies. Layers of the face (Fig. 8.2) from superficial to deep are skin, subcutaneous tissue, SMAS layer, parotid fascia (preauricular)/deep cervical fascia (submandibular), salivary gland (parotid and submandibular regions), muscle, periosteum and bone. The scalp has a loose areolar plane and all other tissues attached. The neck has vital structures like the carotid artery, jugular vein, spinal accessory nerve, cervical plexus and other muscles superficial and deep to them. The surgical anatomy is discussed in detail in Chap. 7.

A knowledge of origin, insertion and course of these structures is indispensable for adequate understanding and surgical management of these lesions.

The key to successful excision is obtaining vascular control at the time of excision. There are different modalities a surgeon can use to achieve this.

(a) Intra lesional embolisation is employed in low flow venous malformations using agents such as *N*-butyl cyanoacrylate [3]. This helps solidify the lesion within the venous pool (Fig. 8.13).
(b) Endovascular embolisation is the use of absorbable/nonabsorbable agents (PVA particles, Silicone beads , Ti coils) injected into the nidus of the lesion through feeder vessels. More of this technique is discussed in detail in Chap. 6.
(c) Feeder vessel ligation/control. The main feeder vessel to the maxillofacial region is the External Carotid Artery and its branches, control of blood flow would significantly reduce intra-operative haemorrhage.

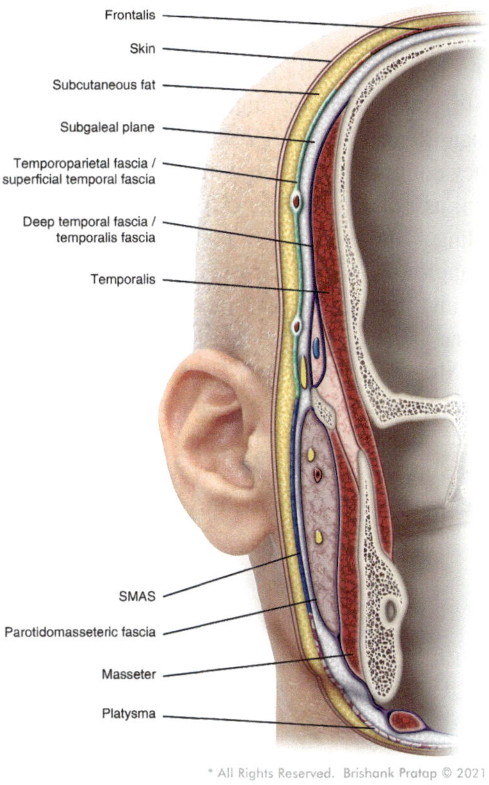

Fig. 8.2 Facial layers (Superficial to deep)

8.3 Case Series

According to the author's classification [1] (Table 8.1), vascular malformations are categorised into five types depending on their anatomy and depth of location in the head and neck region. This is a good guide for selecting the type of surgical management and reconstruction.

Type I These are superficial lesions involving the various layers of skin (epidermis/dermis) and/or mucosa of the oral cavity. They arise from the papillary dermis. They could be either Vascular malformations, mostly low flow type that extends up to the skin or mucosa or superficial Hemangiomas. These lesions are easy to diagnose as they commonly present with a bluish discolouration, associated with a well defined or diffuse swelling. The swelling in the case of involuted Hemangiomas is fibrofatty tissue. Such lesions, when involving critical structures like eyes, pharynx and larynx, are challenging to examine and treat. Most of these lesions can be excised with the skin or mucosa to remove in toto. Care is taken to place incisions along the skin tension lines of the face and neck to avoid unaesthetic results. It is challenging to select these lines in young individuals, and every attempt is made to lay the incision on prominent skin creases like nasolabial, mentolabial, preauricular, lower skin crease of the neck. Tongue lesions, if well circumscribed are mostly excised in toto or debulked in a V-shaped fashion to achieve primary closure. Defect reconstruction can be managed with:

1. Primary Closure
2. Local advancement Flaps
3. Regional pedicle Flaps
4. Microvascular composite flaps.

Cases Selection

Case 1 (Fig. 8.3): Twenty-three-year-old female with an involuted lesion across the left cheek.

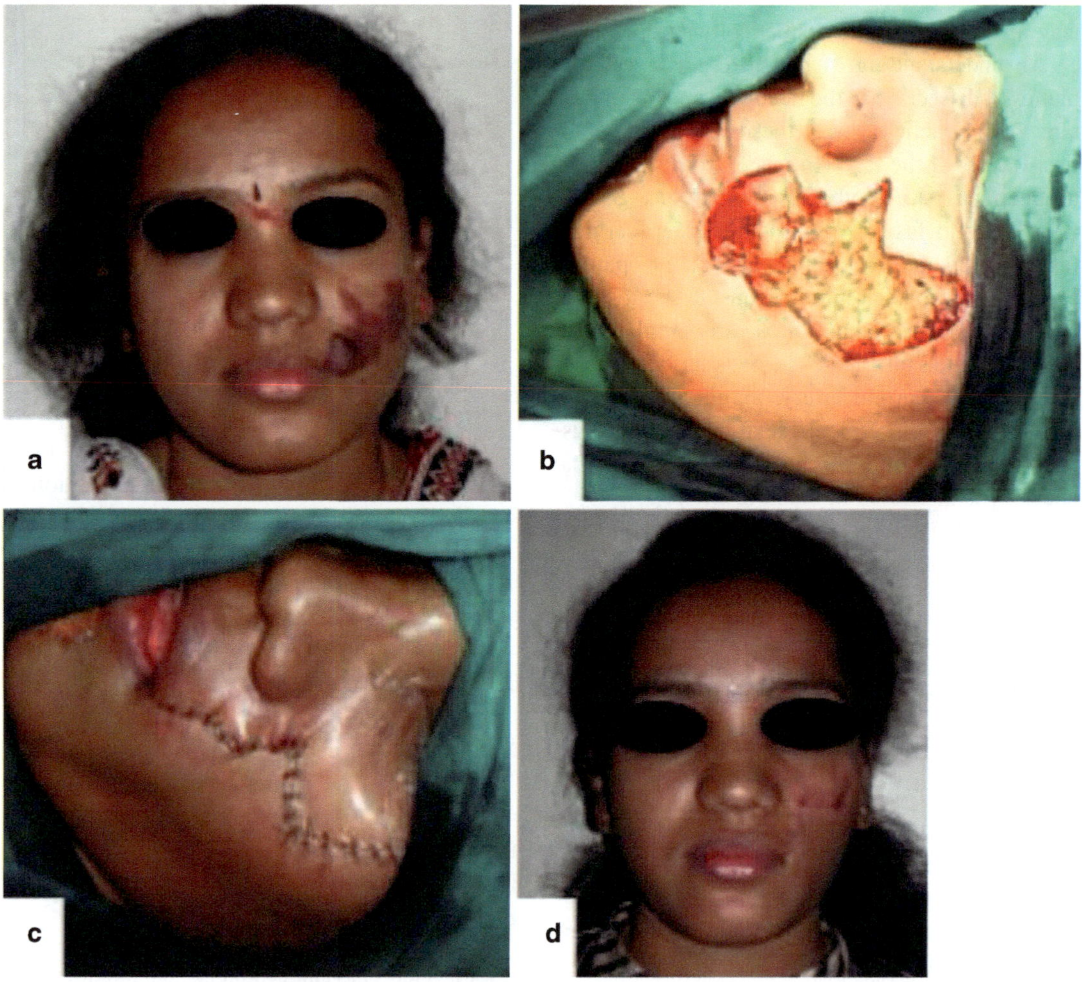

Fig. 8.3 (Case-1): Type I vascular lesion (**a**) Preoperative Left cheek involuted lesion (**b**) Excision with W-plasty (**c**) Closure (**d**) Post-operative

Functionally asymptomatic but presenting with the cosmetic problem. The lesion was excised using a w-plasty with primary closure.

Case 2 (Fig. 8.4): Sixty-eight-year-old lady with a 3 × 4 cm residual Hemangioma on the right infraorbital region. Caused superficial crusting with ulceration. Images showed the depth of lesion restricted to the skin. Primary excision with cervicofacial flap used for advancement and closure of the defect.

Case 3 (Fig. 8.5): Thirty-eight-year-old male with involuted Hemangioma of the right infraorbital region extending to the upper lip. Cosmetically unacceptable requiring excision. The lesion was excised with reconstruction using a Delto Pectoral flap. Tubed pedicle divided after 3 weeks.

Case 4 (Fig. 8.6): Fifty-nine-year-old male with a low flow Venous malformation involving the entire tongue. Macroglossia with difficulty in

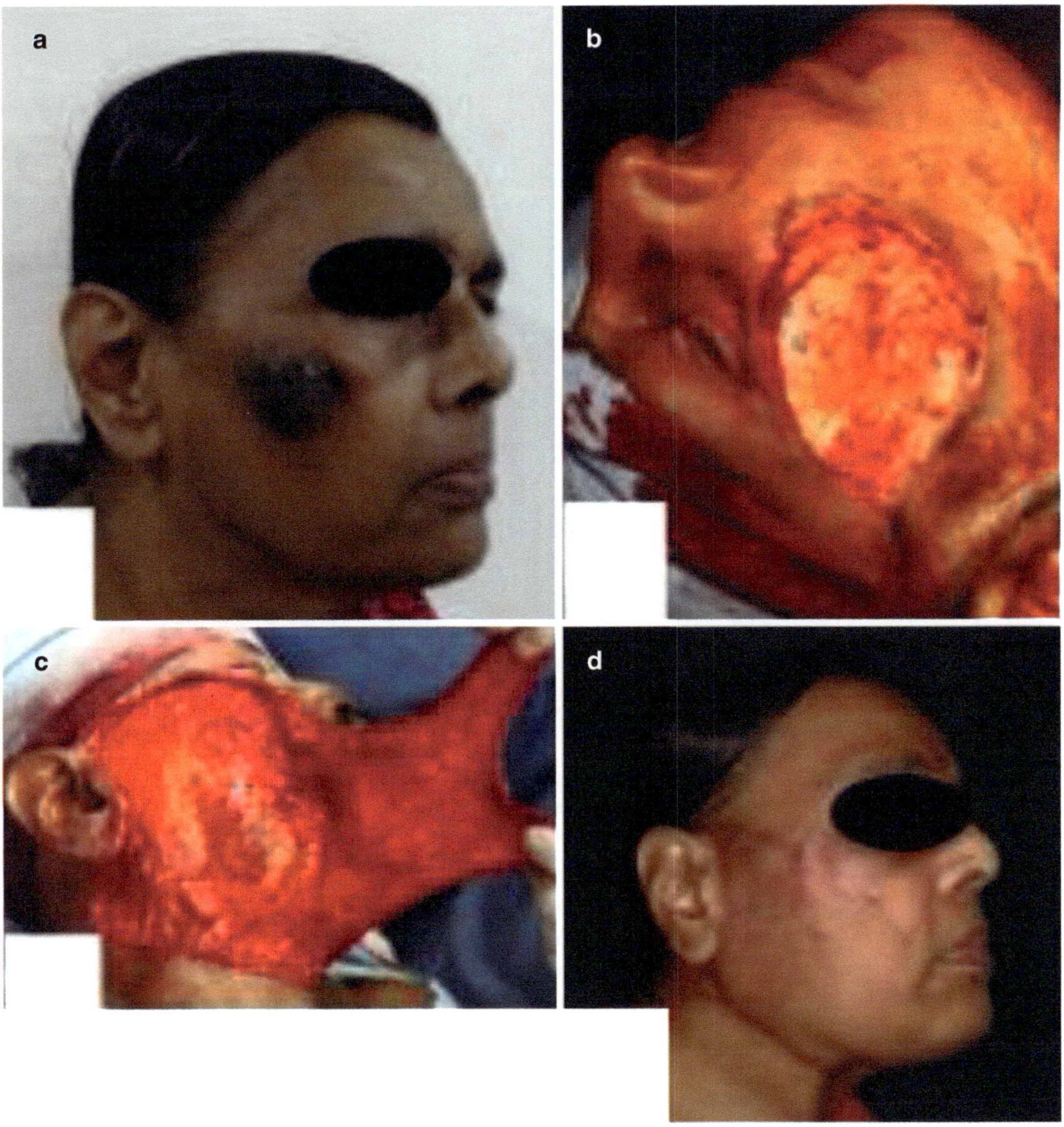

Fig. 8.4 (Case-2): Type I vascular lesion (**a**) Preoperative Residual hemangioma of right infraorbital (**b**) Excision (**c**) Cervicofascial advancement flap (**d**) Post-operative)

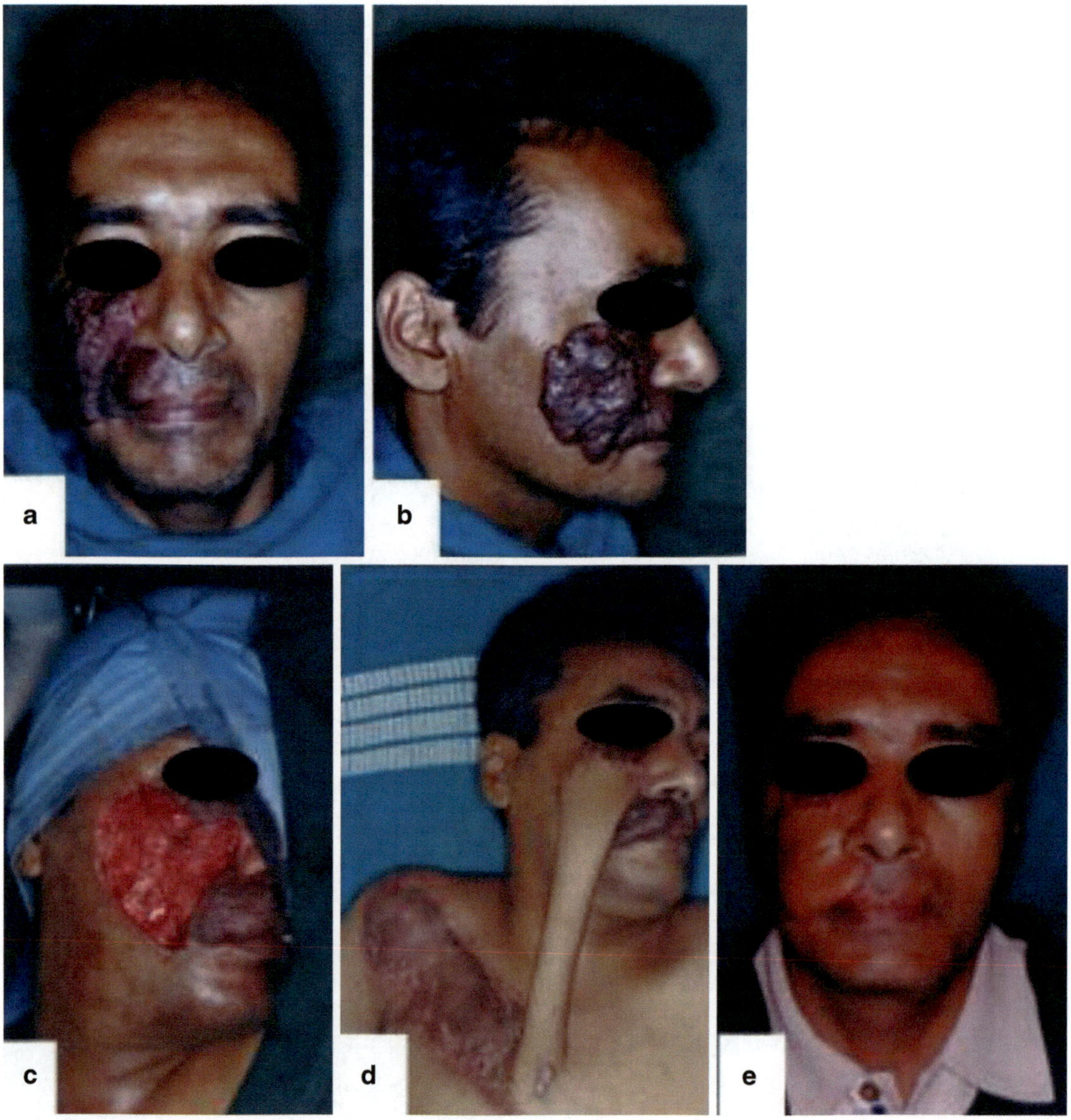

Fig. 8.5 (Case-3): Type I vascular lesion (**a**, **b**) Preoperative involuted hemangioma right infraorbital (**c**) Excision of lesion (**d**) Deltopectoral flap reconstruction (1st stage) (**e**) Post-operative following flap division

speech and swallowing. Underwent MR scan to determine the posterior extent of the lesion. Patient underwent Anterior glossectomy (V-Y excision) with primary closure. Total excision these cases would leave morbid functional defects requiring extensive reconstruction.

Type II Lesions involve the submucosal or subcutaneous tissues, which can sometimes be challenging to identify unless palpated and with the help of a Doppler or MRI scan. They present with a diffuse swelling over the face or oral cavity. These can again be low flow or high-flow lesions, with or without bruit. Small calcifications in low flow malformations can be palpated, and these are called phleboliths. These phleboliths can be a cause of pain and discomfort in many patients. Low flow venous and lymphatic lesions respond well to sclerotherapy. Bleomycin was found to be effective in the author's practice. Resistant and

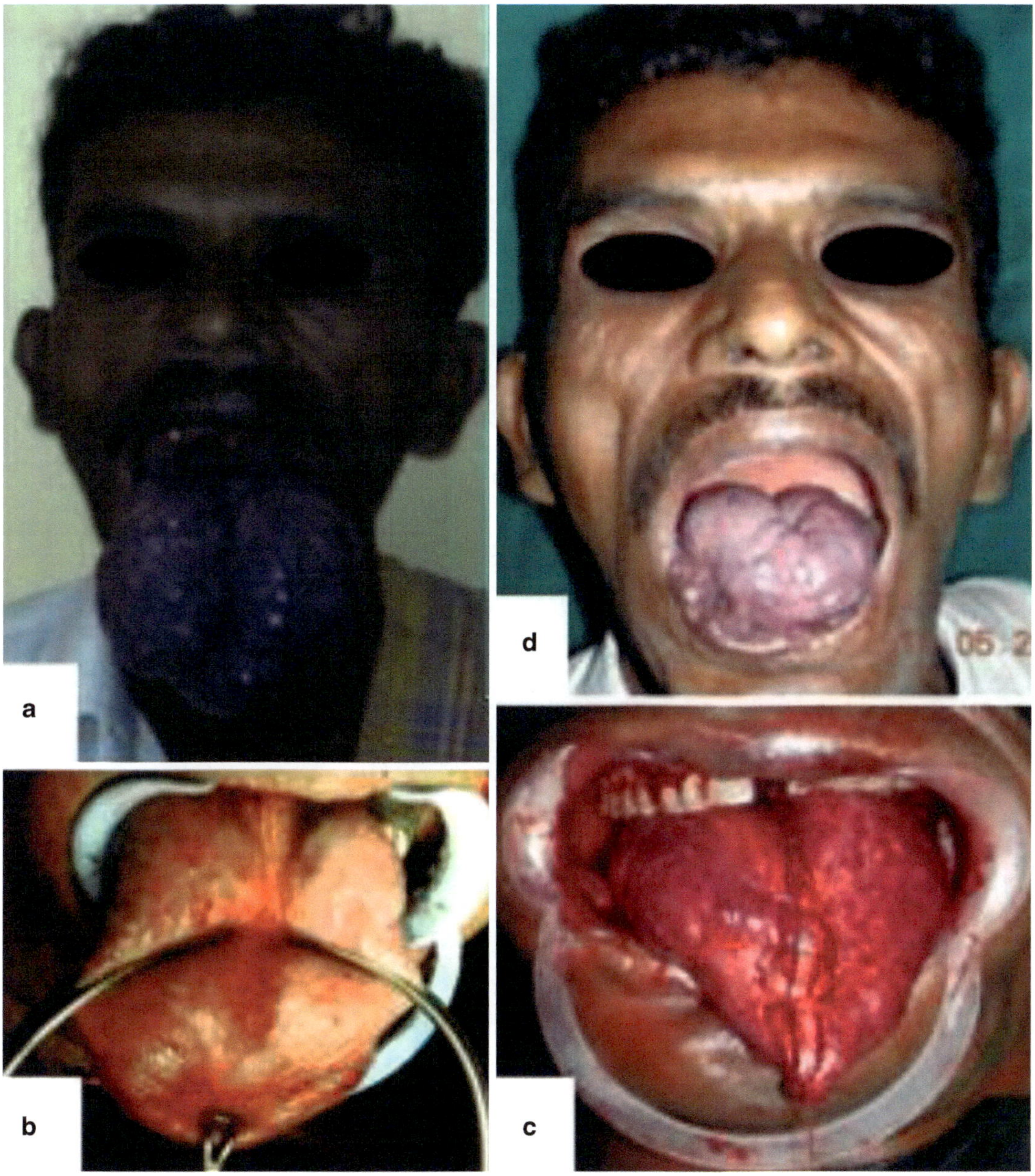

Fig. 8.6 (Case-4): Type I vascular lesion (**a**) Preoperative venous malformation of tongue (**b**) Debulking (V-Y excision using satinsky clamps) (**c**) Closure (**d**) Post-operative

untreated lesions can be operated on with complete excision and primary closure or defect reconstruction as necessary (Fig. 8.4). Any surgery should be done after raising subcutaneous flaps along skin tension lines of the face. Commonly used incisions are—preauricular with neck skin crease or temporal extension, neck crease incision alone, nasolabial approach, coronal approach, etc. Every attempt is made to maintain a sub-SMAS plane. There is always a risk of thinning the skin flap excessively, and care should be taken to avoid button-holing and avascular necrosis of the skin. The lesion is excised completely or debulked depending on the size.

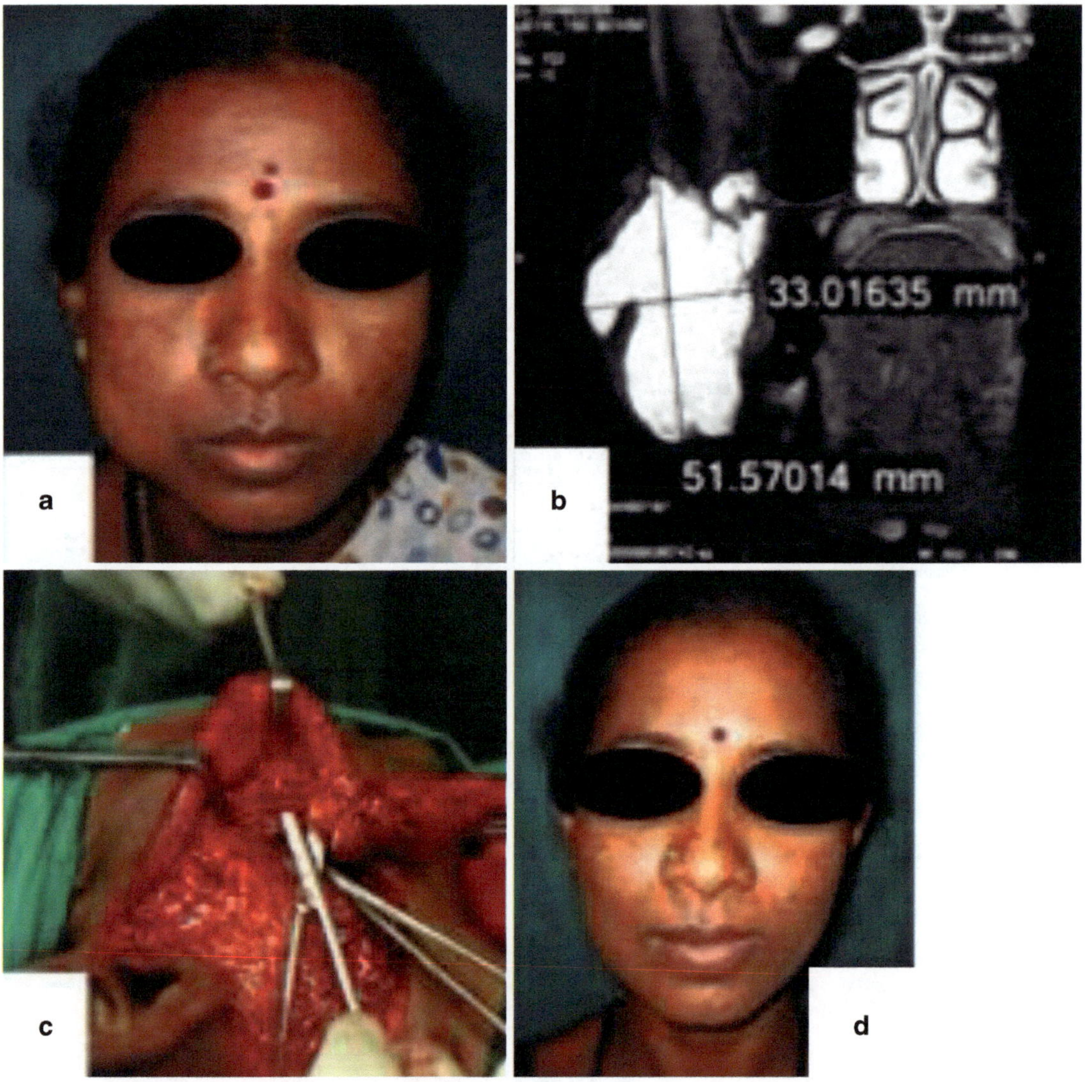

Fig. 8.7 (Case-5): Type II vascular lesion (**a**) Preoperative venous malformation of Right buccal space (**b**) Post contrast T2 weighted MRI image (**c**) Excision of lesion (**d**) Post-operative

Corseting is used for large low flow malformations, as will be described later on in this chapter.

Case 5 (Fig. 8.7): Thirty-eight-year-old female with low flow VM in the Buccal space anterior to the Parotid. Clinically swelling with occasional pain. MR scan showing the extent of the lesion in the Buccal space, superficial to Buccinator and deep to the skin. A diagnosis of low flow Venous/lymphatic malformation was made. Blairs preauricular incision with dissection along the SMAS layer. VM is totally excised. Closure with drains. Facial nerve functions are intact. Note the Phleboliths present within the lesion.

Case 6 (Fig. 8.8): Twenty-three-year-old healthy male with a swelling and sagging of his left side of the face. On palpation, there is a distinct thrill felt over the swelling in the nasolabial region. Scans detected a hi-flow arterial lesion. Feeders were seen arising from the Facial and Internal Maxillary artery.

Surgical excision was planned through an incision in the Naso Labial fold. Vascular control obtained with temporary clamping of External

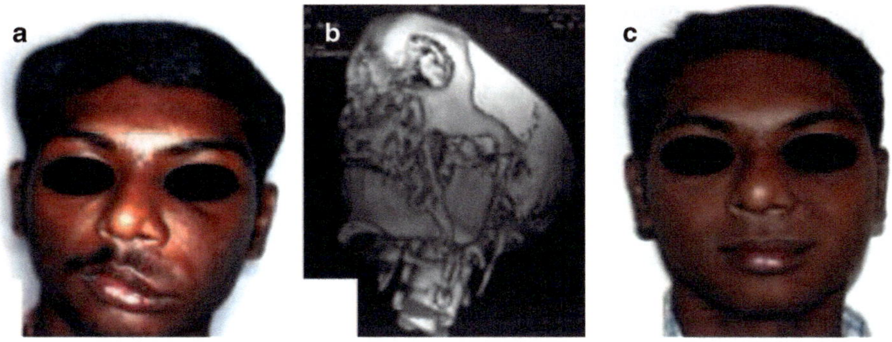

Fig. 8.8 (Case-6): Type II vascular lesion (**a**) Preoperative arterial malformation of left cheek/upper lip (**b**) 3D Reconstructed image using VRT (**c**) Post-operative showing healed left nasolabial crease incison) *VRT* Volumetric rendering technique

Carotid artery. The arterial malformation was excised along with redundant tissue. Facial skin excess was trimmed and sutured, allowing subtle facelift of the site. The incision scar was concealed in the Nasolabial skin crease.

Type III Depending on the gland involved, lesions present with diffuse swelling of the preauricular, submandibular, floor of mouth and thyroid regions. The lesion is excised completely or debulked based on the size. They are present with vascular networks within the glandular tissue. These lesions are treated either with complete excision of the involved gland or corseting, demanding multiple surgeries in the future (Fig. 8.4). Meticulous dissection with homeostasis helps in reducing morbidity consequent to nerve damage. When Corseting is used with absorbable suture material like PDS, it allows faster recovery of the involved nerve.

Case 7 (Fig. 8.9): Twenty-five-year-old female with a preauricular swelling. First seen at birth with the gradual increase in size. Irregular surface with bluish discoloured areas of overlying skin. Compressible with no palpable thrill. The outline of the swelling resembled the Parotid gland. An MRI showed presence of multicystic spaces within the Parotid gland. Aspirate drew colourless fluid, which was rich in lymphocytes. A diagnosis of Megacystic Lymphatic Malformation was made. A failed attempt at excision of the lesion was done at the age of 5. Subsequent injections of sclerosants were tried at different intervals.

Planned excision of the lesion with the superficial parotid was done. The facial nerve trunk and its branches were identified, and the lesion peeled off the nerve. Primary closure done with drains in situ postoperatively.

Case 8 (Fig. 8.10): Twenty-two-year-old female with pulsatile compressible swelling left the submandibular area. Five years history with occasional pain. Clinical examination showed thrill and scan showing arterial malformation involving the submandibular gland. Under ECA control, the lesion was excised along with the submandibular gland.

Type IV Anomalies are intraosseous lesions. They may be confined within the bone or perforate bone to involve overlying soft tissues. Clinical appearance of a bony swelling, severe pain in the jaw or bleeding from the gingiva may be seen. It is not uncommon to find these patients coming to the emergency with significant bleeding from an extraction socket on attempted extraction by a dentist. A CT with contrast/CT angiogram helps in revealing the true extent and nature of the lesion. Packing the area with gauze might be of little help in the emergency room. These patients presenting as an emergency will require endovascular embolisation followed by surgery. The lesions are treated with curettage or segmental resection of bone followed by recon-

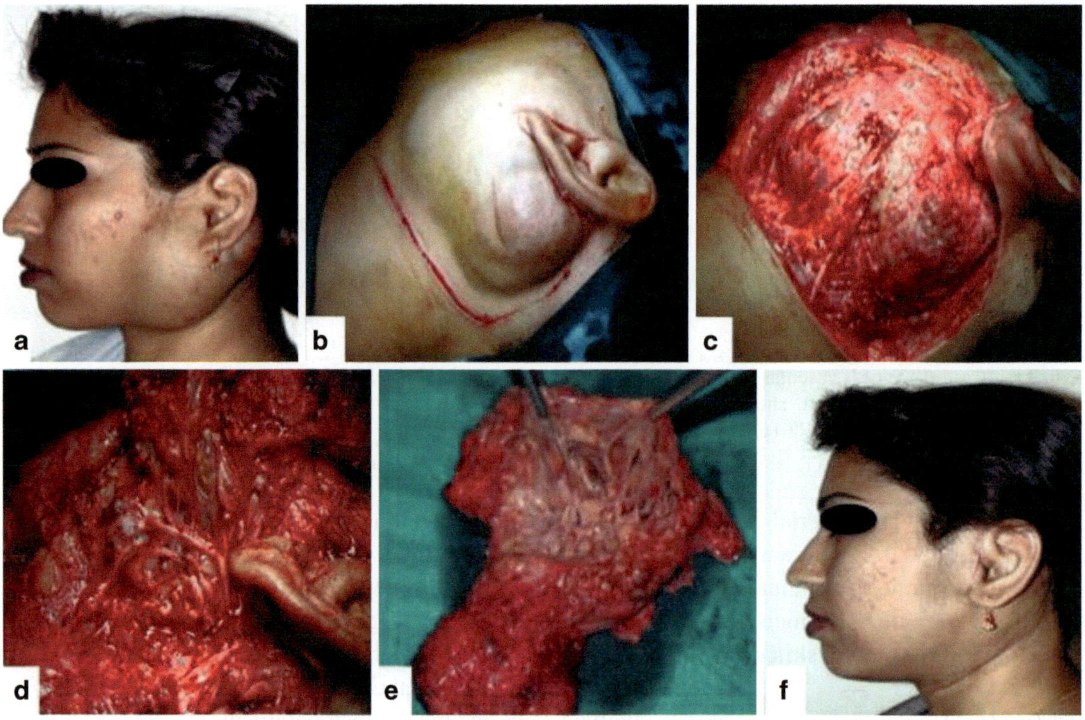

Fig. 8.9 (Case-7): Type III vascular lesion (**a**) Preoperative Left parotid lymphatic malformation (**b**) Incision (**c**) Exposure (**d**) Facial nerve dissection and excision of lesion (**e**) Excised specimen (**f**) Post-operative

struction. Curettage with intact walls encourages natural bone formation; Extracorporeal reimplantation of the curetted bone is possible in mandible or Zygoma (Fig. 8.12). Complete removal minimises the chances of recurrence. Segmental resection of mandible or maxilla warrants reconstruction. Alveolar lesions are resected with attached mucosa leading to smaller upper border defects. Local flaps can be used for soft tissue cover. In segmental defects of over 6 cm. Vascularised Fibula and iliac are the preferred donor sites of bone (Fig. 8.12).

Case 9 (Fig. 8.11): The 28-year-old patient reported complaints of mobility of teeth in her lower posterior quadrant and episodes of spontaneous bleeding from around the teeth. Panorex reveals mottled radiolucency of mandible from the midline to angle of the mandible , loss of alveolar bone with the mobile teeth splinted together with a wire. Her haemogram revealed an alarmingly low Hb of 6 gm % and correspondingly haematocrit value. Contrast-enhanced CT showed a substantial arterial malformation involving the submandibular region extending into the mandibular medullary space.

She was planned for urgent surgical intervention with vascular control using serial embolisation of all the branches of ECA sparing the Superficial temporal artery using Poly vinyl alcohol (PVA particles). Through a cervical incision, the submandibular area and the mandibular cortical bone was exposed, the submandibular malformation was excised. The Mandible was osteotimised in the midline, the teeth extracted, and the lesion was curetted through bone windows created on the buccal cortex.

Postoperative panorex, after 6 months showed the formation of good stock bone in the mandible. Further denture rehabilitation was done after 3 months.

Case 10 (Fig. 8.12): The 16-year-old-male patient was brought into the ER with profuse bleeding from the mouth. There was an attempt at the extraction of a left mandibular molar, which

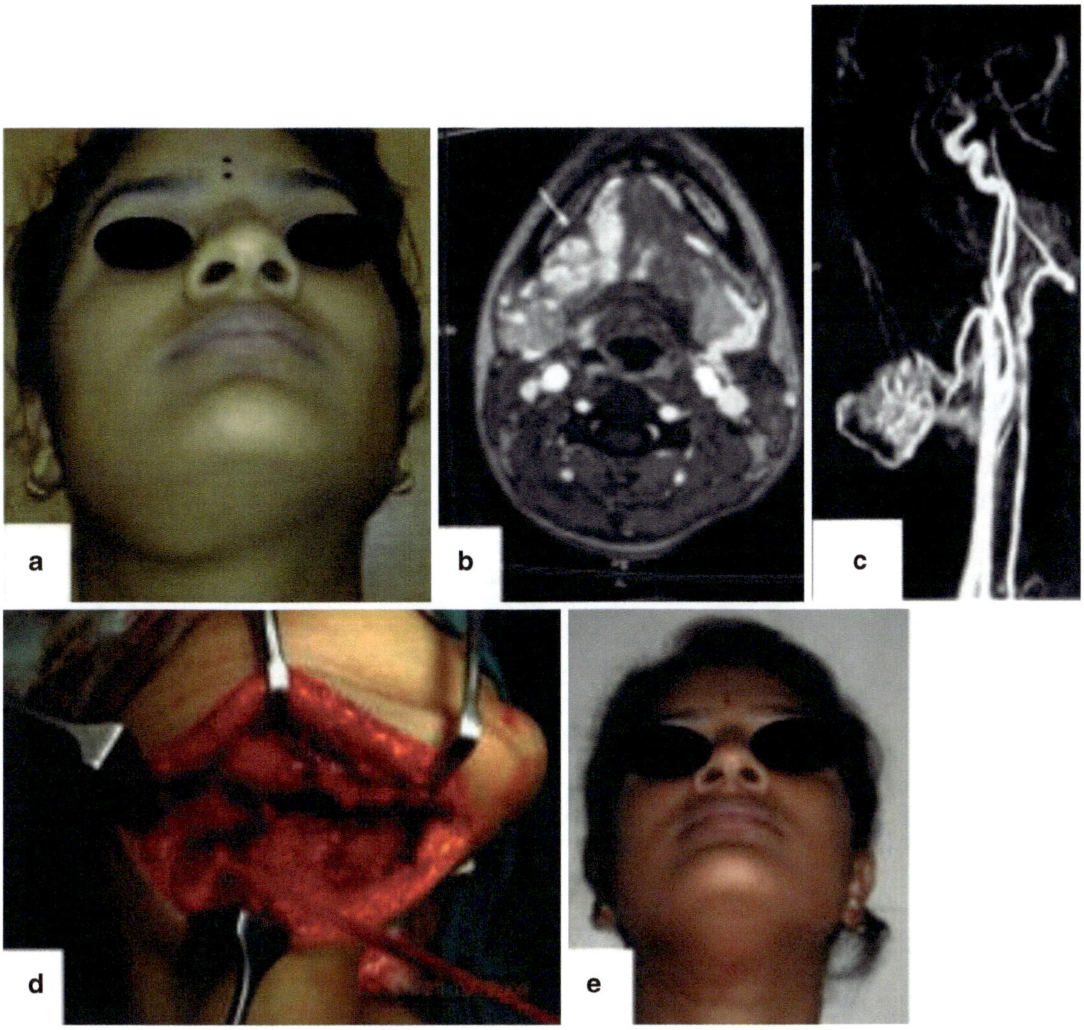

Fig. 8.10 (Case-8) Type III vascular lesion (**a**) Preoperative Right submandibular arterial malformation (**b**, **c**)-T1 weighted MRI image and DSA image (**d**) Excision of submandibular gland (**e**) Post-operative

resulted in a profuse haemorrhage. The surgeon had thoughtfully plugged the socket by replacing the tooth back in it.

The patient required a tracheostomy to secure his airway, followed by exposure and clamping of his ECA. After partial control of the haemorrhage the mandible was excised. The lesion was curetted from the medullary space, and teeth within the lesion extracted. The scaffold of the mandible was then extracorporeally re-implanted and fixed with mini plates. This helped avoid the use of a microvascular bony reconstruction.

Type V Anomalies present with difficulty in swallowing/speech/deglutition, bleeding on expectoration and symptoms depending on the site of the lesion. These lesions may involve the oropharynx, the hypopharynx, infratemporal fossa or infraorbital areas of the head and neck. Laryngo Pharyngeal lesions are visualised using direct or indirect laryngoscopy, taking care not to puncture the lesions. These can sometimes be seen extending into the trachea or oesophagus. Asymptomatic lesions should be left alone and periodically monitored, symptomatic laryngeal

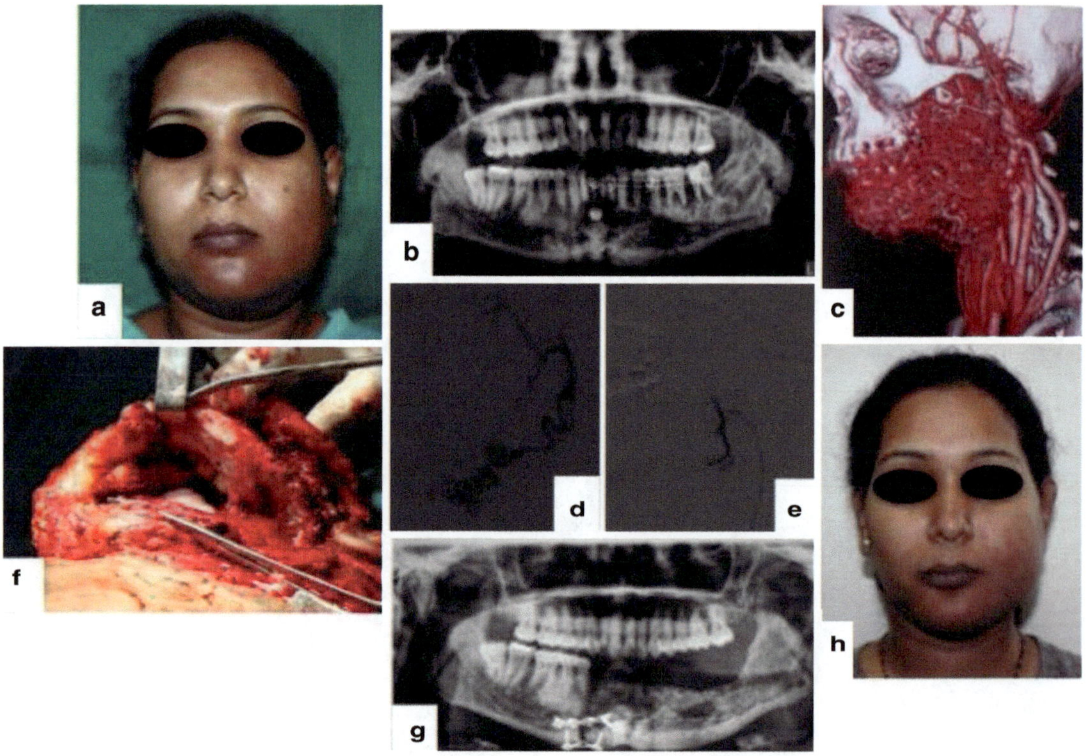

Fig. 8.11 (Case-9): Type IV vascular lesion (**a**) Preoperative Left mandible and submandibular arterial malformation (**b**) Preoperative OPG (**c**) Preoperative DSA image (**d** and **e**) pre and post embolisation (**f**) Intraoperative curettage of mandible (**g**) Postoperative OPG (**h**) Postoperative

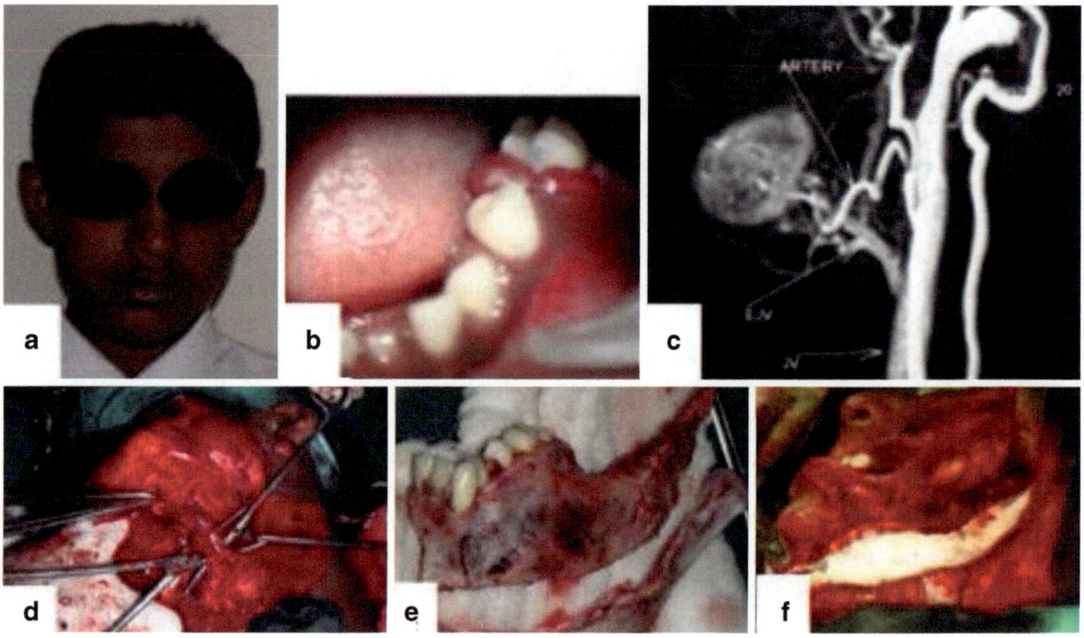

Fig. 8.12 (Case-10): Bleeding following dental extraction-Extracorporeal currettage of high flow bony vascular lesion and fixation of mandible (**a**) Preoperative (**b**) intraoral (**c**) Post contrast MR angiogram of lesion (**d**) Ligation of main feeder (**e**) extracorporcal currettage and excision of diseased bone (**f**) Fixation of mandible as free graft

or oesophageal varies are dealt with using lasers or banding. Any surgery on these lesions has a risk of life-threatening bleed with challenges in achieving haemostasis, especially those involving the major blood vessels in the skull base area. Access osteotomies should be used liberally in these cases, not to compromise on the visibility and to aid in adequate haemostasis followed with excision of the lesion.

Access is obtained through:

1. Mandibulotomy [3].
2. Maxillary Le Fort Osteotomy [4]
3. Orbital Osteotomy
4. Zygomatic Osteotomy

Case 11 (Fig. 8.13): Thirty-four-year-old male presented with throbbing headaches and intact vision. Clinical appearance showed orbital dystopia, reducible swelling in front orbital area with exophthalmos. No transmitted pulsations were elicited. CT Angiogram showed vascular dilated sacs in the supra orbital tissue with dilated superior ophthalmic vein.

The vascular sacs were injected with Cyanoacrylate glue under CT guidance. Subsequent angiograms failed to show any additional flow into the lesion. Through a coronal flap frontal craniotomy followed by superior orbitotomy was done to access and excise the coagulated vascular sacs. Postoperative appearance after 6 months showed almost 90% correction of his dystopia and exophthalmos. Vision continued to be normal.

Case 12 (Fig. 8.14): Twenty-one-year-old-male patient had swelling left preauricular (Parotid) area with difficulty in swallowing and OSA. The symptoms worsened in the last few years. A 5 × 7 cm reducible swelling outlining the Parotid gland was seen. Intraoral inspection showed bluish areas over a medially displaced left pharynx reducing the oropharyngeal space. CT with contrast revealed enhancing areas in the lateral and post pharyngeal space with the considerable displacement of the medial pharyngeal

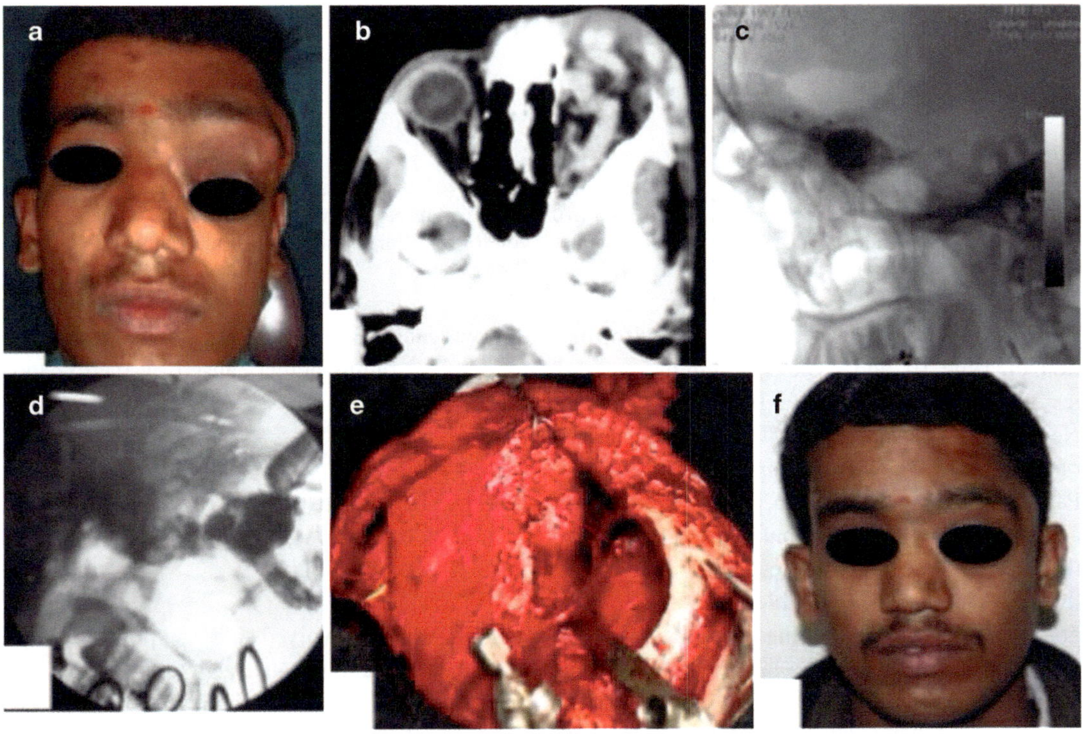

Fig. 8.13 (Case-11): Type-V vascular lesion (**a**) Preoperative left orbital vascular malformation (**b**) CT angiogram (**c**) Injection of cyanoacrylate glue (**d**) DSA image of lesion (**e**) Superior orbitotomy and excision of lesion (**f**) Postoperative

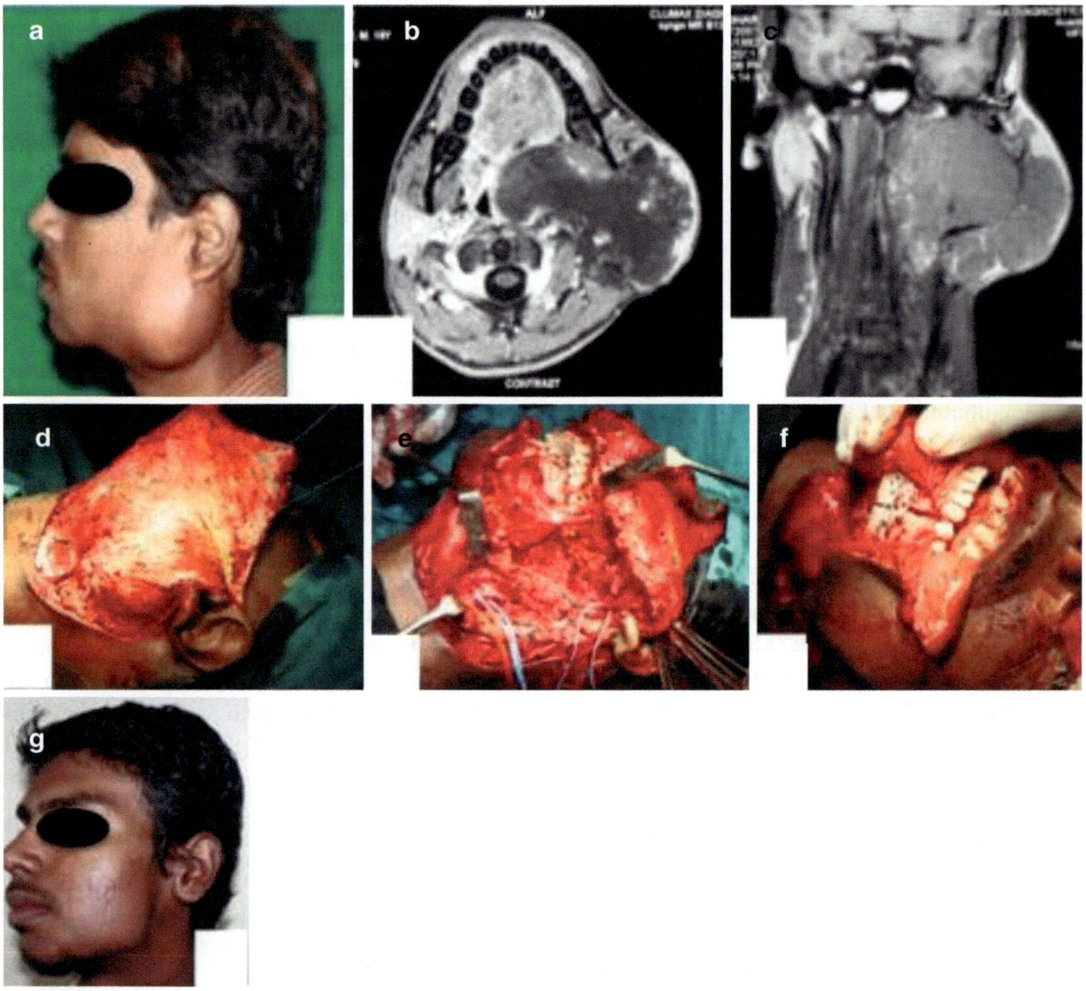

Fig. 8.14 (Case-12): Type V vascular lesion (**a**) Preoperative Left lateral pharyngeal venous malformation (**b** and **c**) Post contrast T1 weighted image (**d**) Exposure of lesion (**e**) Excision via access mandibulotomy and ECA control (**f**) Miniplate fixation of mandibulotomy site (**g**) Postoperative

wall. Diagnosed as low flow Venous malformation of Type III and Type V combination, the lesion was exposed with a Blair incision, VII Nerve and its branches identified superficial part of the lesion along with the superficial lobe of the Parotid was dissected, the deep part of the lesion accessed through a mandibular osteotomy with the lateral swing. The muscles are stripped along the medial part of the mandible. The lateral pterygoid and temporalis stripping provides adequate access and exposure to the lateral and posterior pharyngeal space. Total excision of the venous malformation was achieved. Mandible refixed using miniplates and drains placed in the lateral pharyngeal space. Postoperative images show the mandibular ramus defect caused by the expanding VM.

8.4 Technique of External Carotid Artery (ECA) Control [1]

The ECA of the involved side is exposed through a cervical incision, usually in the visible skin crease of the neck. This incision may form part of the access for exposure of the lesion. The sternocleidomastoid muscle is retracted posteriorly at the level of greater cornu of the hyoid bone, exposing the carotid sheath. The external carotid closer to the carotid bifurcation is identified at this level. The vessel is snared with a vascular sling passed through a rubber catheter. Gentle strangulation of the vessel can be accomplished by advancing the catheter. Even in situations where presurgical embolisation has been done, this additional compression of the vessel serves to reduce blood flow to the lesion. Ligation of the ECA must be avoided as far as possible. Aggressive local control of bleeding may require control of the contralateral ECA, which happens when there is the extensive collateral blood supply to the lesion.

Case 13 (Fig. 8.15): Eighteen-year-old male patient with swelling of the angle of the jaw, mobility and bleeding from the gums surrounding his second molar. Panorex showed a radiolucent area extending from the molar to the angle. CT Angio revealed hi-flow arterial lesion with feeders from the facial and lingual branches of ECA.

A planned exposure of the mandible (notice bicortical swelling) along with exposure of ECA was done. ECA was cannulated and injected with a dye to reveal the extent of vascular blush using a C-arm. Further feeders, facial and lingual were clamped using a vascular 3v clamp and reimaged with reinfection of the dye. There was considerable reduction in the vascular blush indicating a reduction in blood flow to the anomaly. The mandible was decorticated and the vascular pathology curetted along with the extraction of the mobile second molar. Post-operative panorex after 6 months showed the satisfactory bone formation of the previous pathologic site.

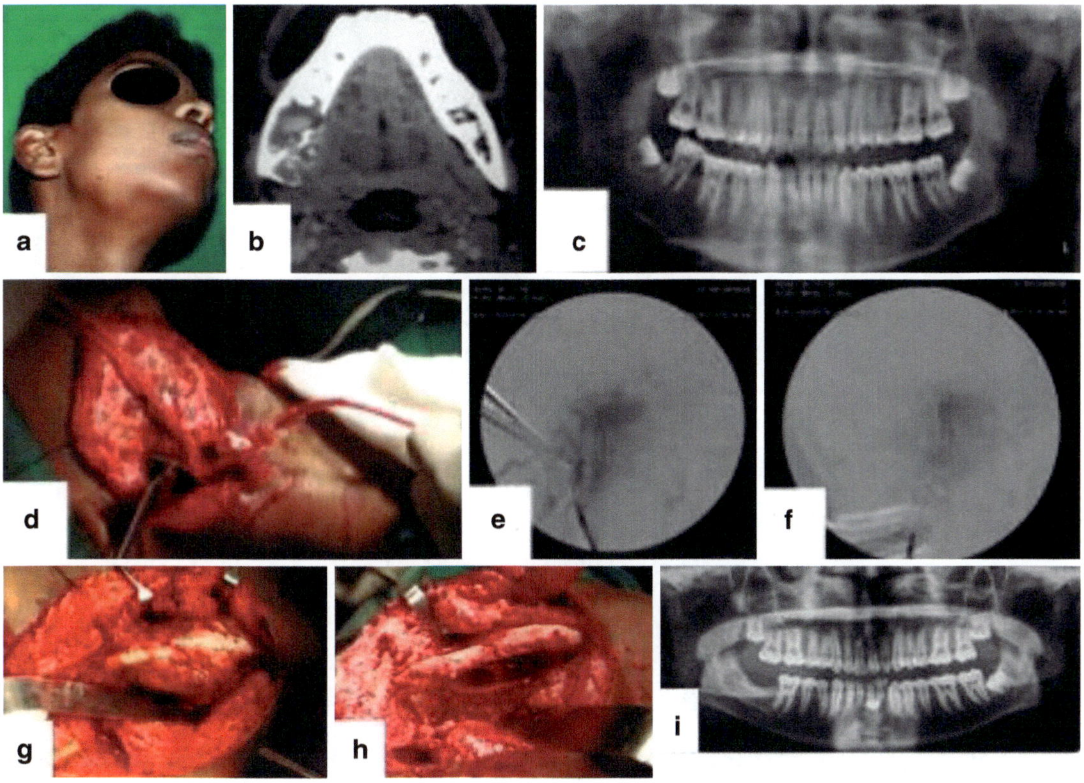

Fig. 8.15 (Case 13): Type IV vascular lesion showing ECA control (**a**) Preoperative AVM right mandible (**b**) Axial post contrast CT image (**c**) Pre operative OPG (**d**) ECA control and injection of radiopaque dye (**e**) intraoperative C-arm picture following dye injection before occluding of ECA (**f**) intraoperative C-arm picture following dye injection and occlusion of ECA (**g**) Lesion exposure (**h**) Currettage of lesion (**i**) Post operative OPG

8.5 Combination of ECA Control with Intralesional Embolisation

Using Nectacryl for a AVM of the buccal space (Type II) lesion (Fig. 8.16): 38 year Male with pulsatile expansile swelling of the Buccal space of 10 year duration. The MRA demonstrates an AVM with a large venous pool. The feeders were Facial and Temporal branches of the ECA. Decision to control the ECA followed by intra lesions injection of the venous sac with Cyanoacrylate (Nectacryl) glue was done. The thrombosed Venous sac was successfully enucleated from the Bucco temporal space. The postoperative results are demonstrative of the functional and cosmetic outcome.

8.6 Corset Suturing Technique [2]

Corset suturing is a proven technique in the management of large low flow venous malformations of the head and neck, especially in lesions where complete excision is not practically possible due to their size and approximation with important structures like internal carotid artery (ICA), common carotid artery (CCA), trachea, oesophagus,

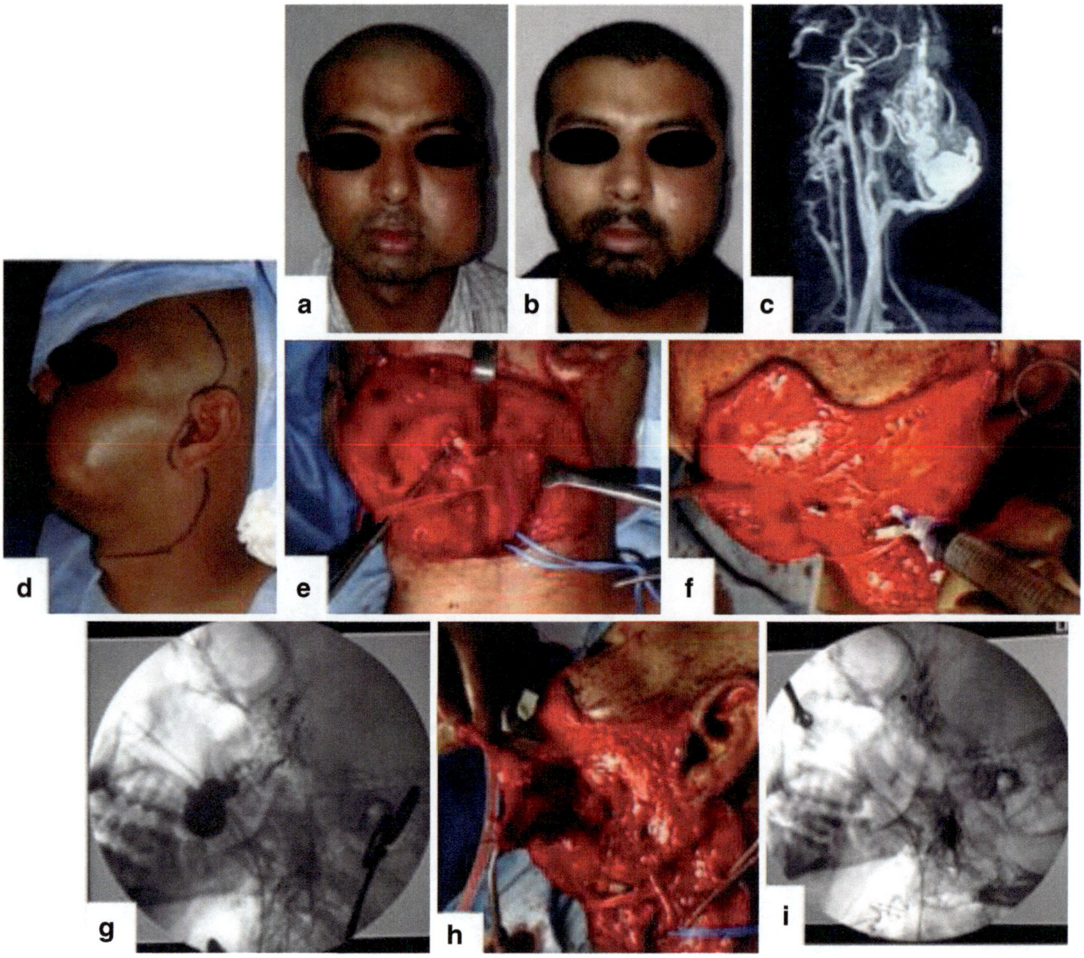

Fig. 8.16 Combination of ECA control and intralesional embolisation using Nectacryl for AVM of left buccal space-Type II (**a**) Preoperative (**b**) Postoperative (**c**) Preoperative post-contrast MR angiogram (**d**) Flap marking (**e**) Exposure with ECA control (**f**) Intralesional injection of Nectacryl (**g**) Intraoperative radiograph post injection of sclerosant (**h**) Excision of sclerosed lesion (**i**) Intraoperative radiograph post-excision of lesion

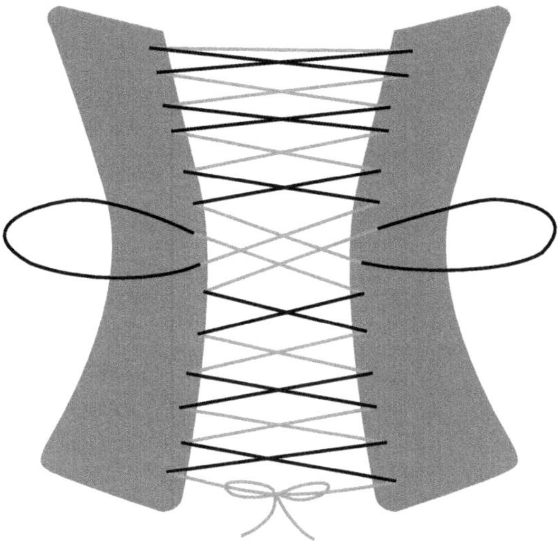

Fig. 8.17 Corset (schematic)

cervical spine, facial nerve, spinal accessory nerve, internal jugular vein and patients with significant medical issues where reduced intra-operative time is paramount.

'Corset', is a garment worn to hold and train the torso into a desired shape for aesthetic or orthopaedic purposes (Fig. 8.17).

The procedure employed is raising a flap in the sub-SMAS or subcutaneous plane depending upon the type of lesion, followed by placement of a bioresorbable suture (polydioxanone) that runs in a continuous vertical looping fashion from subcutaneous to deep layer and from one end to another, incorporating the bulk of lesion within the sutures. The suturing is advanced at regular and equidistant intervals resulting in compression of the vascular spaces and obstruction of afferent and efferent vessels. In large lesions, care is taken to make the loops of suturing parallel to each other, covering the whole lesion from superior to inferior and medial to lateral, obliterating the blood circulation within the tumour. The procedure decompresses the lesion completely and reduces the risk of postoperative haemorrhage. Excess of skin flap is then excised and closure done primarily with a drain secured in the most dependent position, and skin sucked down to the underlying tissues. The final scar is fairly acceptable due to its initial design and position in adequate access. These lesions have been uncapsulated are rarely excised completely but improve the quality of life and reduce risk of mortality due to pressure symptoms on the airway and haemorrhage. In the authors's experience, the use of corseting has proven to be beneficial, and life saving in these cases.

The excess skin flap is always excised to give a near-normal appearance. As emphasised previously, the use of adequate number of drains and meticulous hemostatic closure is imperative to achieve acceptable and aesthetic results.

Most large lesions require further excision and repeated debulking procedures as age advances until growth is complete. Large low flow lesions have a potential to be excised completely at a second stage once shrinkage is achieved using the corset suturing technique.

Case 14 (Fig. 8.18): Male patient aged 34 with a diffuse swelling right cheek. Mild facial asymmetry was seen at birth. Progressively increased in size. He had multiple therapeutic interventions, including sclerosant injections and one attempt at the surgery which was abandoned due to profuse bleeding. MRI showed a diffuse lesion from his preauricular area extending unto the zygomatic arch superiorly and unto the nasolabial fold anteriorly.

Surgical approach through a preauricular incision with cervical extension was done with the elevation of a skin flap at the level of the superficial fascia. Considering the diffuse nature and extent of the lesion into the sub zygomatic area interlocking mattress sutures were played using Polydioxanone (PDS). Similar to the ties on a corset hence named corset suturing.

The objective being compression of the large vascular sacs into smaller ones. The redundant margin of the facial flap was excised and sutured. Post-operative result at the end of 6 months showed a considerable but not total reduction of facial swelling.

8.7 Complications

Usually related to the therapeutic technique used. Pain and short-term swelling is common and can occur with sclerosing agents. Life-threatening

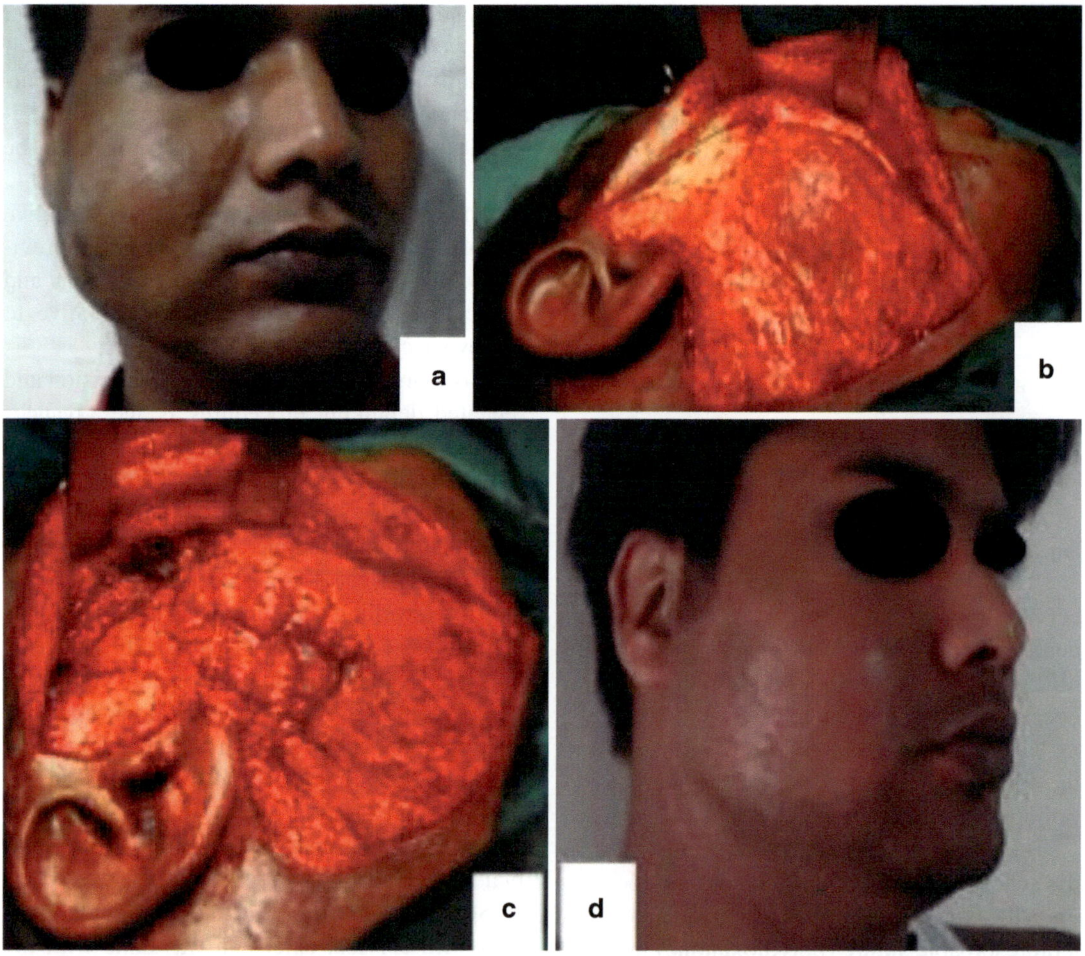

Fig. 8.18 (Case-14): Corset Suturing technique (**a**) Preoperative Venous malformation right check (**b**) Lesion exposure (**c**) CORSET SUTURING of lesion (**d**) Post operative

complications may occur in lesions of the oropharynx post-injection, causing airway distress.

Ulceration of overlying skin is also possible, especially in lesions that are close to the epidermis (Fig. 8.19). Anomalies on units such as lip, Pinna of the ear Fig. 8.20), Nasal tip are susceptible to vascular ischemia and occasionally necrosis.

Pre-operative embolisation has a risk of patients developing thromboembolism due to uncontrolled passage of embolic material into the ICA. Blindness due to retinal artery spasm or thrombosis. Therapeutic radiologic intervention must therefore be performed with utmost care and skill.

Apart from life-threatening haemorrhage and other complications such as haematoma , overlying flap necrosis, there is a possibility of damage to branches of the Facial Nerve (Fig. 8.20). Facial Nerve identification and dissection, therefore, is mandatory.

Case 15 (Fig. 8.21): Thirty-two-year-old female 7 months into her gestation reported with postauricular bleeding. She was treated elsewhere for a hi-flow arterial lesion of the right Pinna. She underwent pre-operative embolisation of her occipital and Superficial temporal arteries followed by injection of sclerosants into the anomalous Pinna. She also had circumferential transcutaneous sutures placed to control the

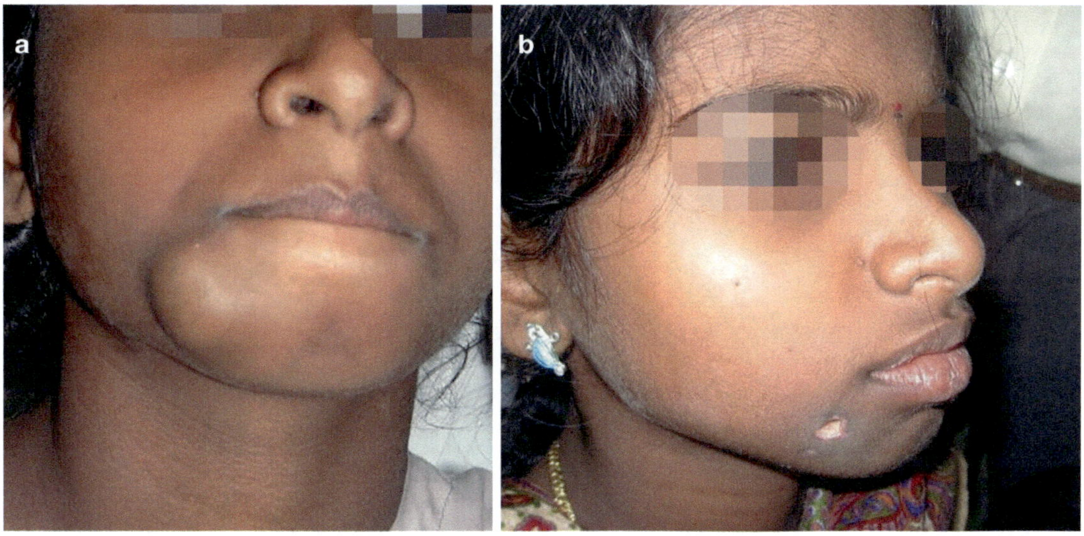

Fig. 8.19 Ulceration of overlying skin, following injection of intralesional sclerosant (**a**) Pre opertaive VM of right mentolabial region (**b**) 3 weeks post intralesional propanolol injection

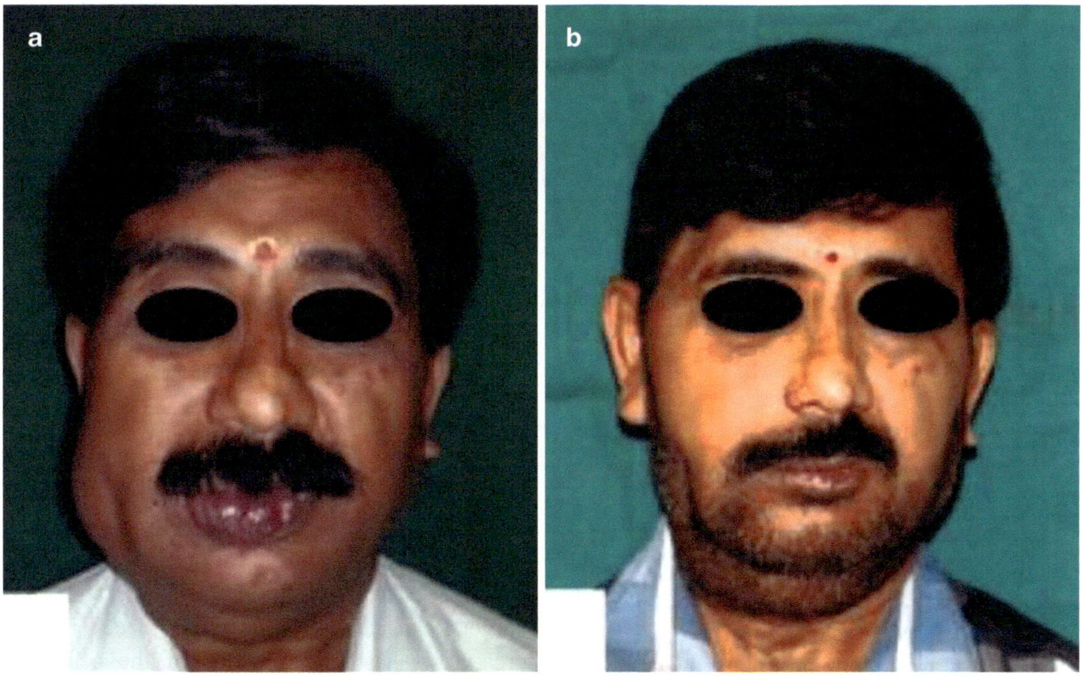

Fig. 8.20 Transient Right facial nerve palsy (**a**) Pre opertaive VM of right check (**b**) Post operative Corset suturing

bleed.This resulted in gradual ischemia with necrosis of the pinna.

The surgical decision was made to excise the ischemic Pinna with the surrounding flap leaving a raw surgical bed. Split skin graft was used to cover the surgical defect. She would require a prosthetic Ear rehabilitation in the future.

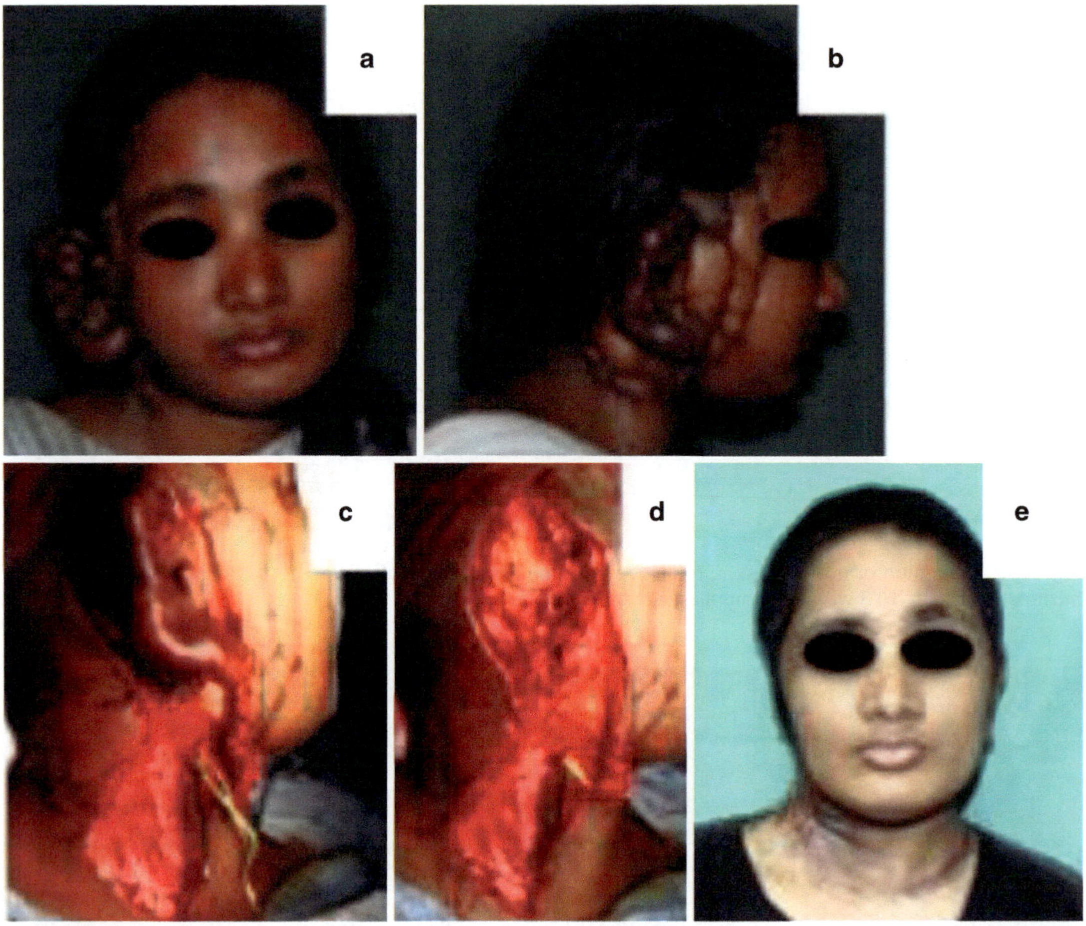

Fig. 8.21 (Case-15): Multiple interventions—Embolisation, sclerosants, surgery (**a**) and (**b**) Preoperative AVM of Right ear (**c**) Excision of lesion (**d**) Post excision defect (**e**) Post operative following advancement flap closure

8.8 Conclusion

Decision-making regarding surgical ablation of vascular lesions depends on symptomatic correlation. In the presence of functional or cosmetic problems and if non-surgical techniques like pharmacotherapy or sclerosants have been tried and exhausted with little or no improvement, surgery may be the only solution.

The diagnosis of hemangioma from a vascular malformation allows planning of the treatment. Most hemangiomas respond favourably to medical management [5], e.g Propranolol or other Beta-blockers. Partially involuted, residual lesions require surgical excision. VM, on the other hand, can be treated using intralesional sclerosants [5]. Bleomycin is the author's favourite. Non-responsive lesions would require adequate vascular control followed by surgical excision. Considering the cosmetic challenge surgery can cause, incisions are placed in skin creases or aesthetic subunits of the head and neck, which conceal postoperative scars effectively. A table showing the surgical solution depending on the type of lesion according to the authors' classification. The algorithm also guides the clinician in the steps involved in the management of the vascular anomalies.

References

1. Nair SC, Spencer NJ, Nayak KP, Balasubramaniam K. Surgical management of vascular lesions of the head and neck: a review of 115 cases. Int. J. Oral Maxillofac. Surg. 2011;40:577–83.
2. Nair SC, Chawla JP, Shroff SS, Kumar B, Shah A. Corseting: a new technique for the management of diffuse venous malformations in the head and neck region. Int. J. Oral Maxillofac. Surg. 2018;47:1534–40.
3. Johnson AB, Richter GT. Vascular anomalies. Clin Perinatol. 2018;45:737–49.
4. Vaidya S, Tozer KR, Chen J. An overview of Embolic agents. Semin Intervent Radiol. 2008;25:204–15.
5. Nair SC, Sridhar KR, Shah A, Kumar B, Shetty P. Maxillectomy through mandibulotomy—a retrospective clinical review. J Oral Maxillofac Surg. 2011;69:2040–7.

Reconstruction

9

Janarthanan Ramu, Madangopalan Ethunandan, and Subramania Iyer

9.1 Introduction

Head and neck vascular malformations are complex. Surgical resection and reconstruction are extremely challenging in these areas. The management depends upon the type of the lesion, flow in the lesion, and size of the lesion. Anatomically, the presence of major vessels, nerves, laryngeal and tracheal airway, oral cavity and esophagus makes the head and neck region a complex one for resection and reconstruction of vascular malformations. However, resection often proceeded by embolization of the lesion and its feeding vessels remain a mainstay of the treatment of these malformations.

Reconstruction of the defect after excision is essential to restore the form and function to provide cover for the major nerves and vessels, to restore the functions of the maxilla and mandible and, to avoid cosmetic disfigurement. Apart from these reasons, placement of normal healthy tissues in the diseased area has a role in the prevention of recurrences by changing the local hemodynamics.

Magnetic Resonance Imaging with MR angiogram is the best investigation to assess the extent of the lesion, the underlying neurovascular structures involvement and, to delineate the feeding vessels. High-resolution CT will be beneficial for the assessment of bony involvement. Digital subtraction Angiography (DSA) is particularly useful for preoperative embolization of the lesion, and it also shows the vascular tree, which is helpful in selecting the vessels for anastomosis away from the diseased if free tissue transfer is considered. All these investigations will be helpful in identifying the patients who need reconstruction and counsel them preoperatively.

9.2 Indications for Reconstruction and Tissue Requirements

Small vascular malformations, especially of the neck, cheek or scalp will not need reconstruction. But when the lesion is large or affecting multiple regions of the head and neck in different planes reconstruction becomes mandatory after their excision. The surgical morbidity associated with the resection in the head and neck area varies from anatomical disintegration to vital functional disturbances like speech, mastication,

J. Ramu
Department of Plastic and Reconstructive Surgery, Amrita School of Medicine, Kochi, India

M. Ethunandan
Department of Oral and Maxillofacial Surgery, University Hospital Southampton, Southampton, UK

S. Iyer (✉)
Department of Plastic and Reconstructive Surgery, Head and Neck Surgery, Amrita School of Medicine, Kochi, India

S. C. Nair, S. R. Chandra (eds.), *Management of Head and Neck Vascular Lesions*,
https://doi.org/10.1007/978-981-15-2321-2_9

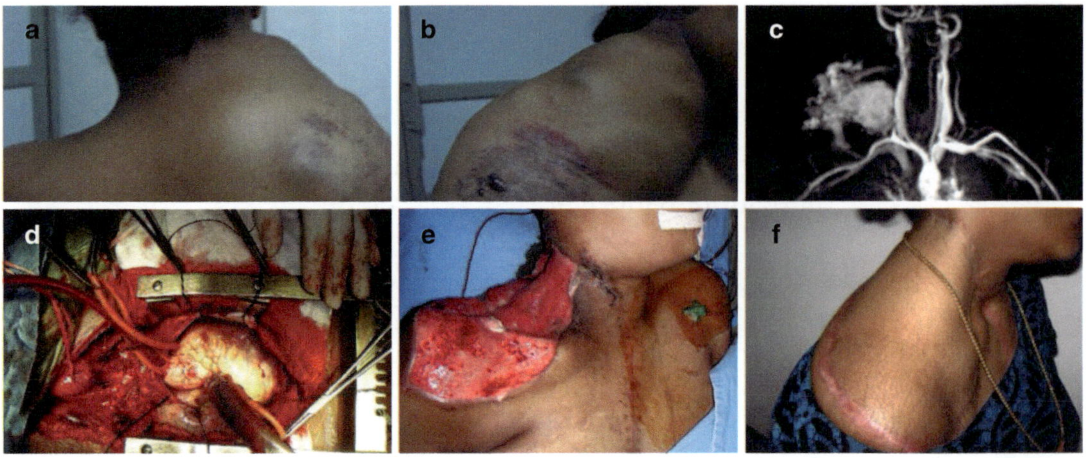

Fig. 9.1 (**a**, **b**) Large vascular malformation involving neck and shoulder (**c**) MRI angiogram showing the feeders and extensive lesion (**d**) Cardiopulmonary bypass (CPB) assisted resection (**e**) Defect at 7 days post-excision and wound packing (**f**) Free anterolateral thigh flap for soft tissue cover at 6 months follow-up

swallowing, speech, and facial expression. Provision of skin cover and providing the integrity of mucosal lining becomes the priority goals.

When mandible or maxilla is involved, they will need radical resections. Reconstruction of these structures becomes mandatory to provide skeletal support as well as the best possible dental and functional rehabilitation. Reanimating the facial units for the defects caused by accidental or purposeful damage to the facial nerve will have to be included in the goals of reconstruction in some lesions involving the parotid. Achieving aesthetically pleasing reconstruction by using the appropriate method and tissue is important, especially when a large amount of the skin and soft tissue is lost or the defects involve structures like nose or pinna.

Special points of consideration in the reconstruction of defects following excision of vascular malformations include preparing the area for reconstruction as follows:

- Achieving secure hemostasis is mandatory to a successful reconstruction. Use of tools like harmonic scalpel, liberal use of ties, clips, and electrocautery may help in getting a bloodless bed for reconstruction. The author's group has resorted to Cardio Pulmonary Bypass (CPB) to have bleeding control and to achieve bloodless field for complete excision of complex malformations where resection could not be possible without its assistance (Fig. 9.1). Wound packing is one of the effective ways of controlling bleeding. Wound packing for at least 24–48 h after the excision may be the best option for securing a bloodless field for reconstruction.

9.3 Methods of Reconstruction

The options for reconstruction range from direct closure, skin grafting, locoregional flaps, free tissue transfers and use of tissue expanders. The selection of these options varies depending upon the type of the defects, patient factors and surgeon factors.

9.3.1 Type of Lesion

Vascular malformations vary according to the type of vascular components capillary, arterial, venous, lymphatic or variable different combinations of the above components. The presence of large arterial component or arteriovenous connetion makes the physiology of the lesion high-flow, which makes the resection and reconstruction difficult. The pathological nature and fast-flow in these malformations may lead to a high chance of flap failure, and the recurrence rate makes the management complicated. In hemangioma, the role of surgery is mostly limited to removal of the residual deformed skin and subcutaneous tissue, and the objective is mostly aesthetic enhancement.

9.3.2 Type of the Defects

The defect components could be skin, mucosal lining, intervening soft tissue, as well as the bone.

9.3.2.1 Bony Defects

The goals of reconstruction are to maintain the continuity of bony defect, arch form, and alveolar height to achieve anatomical integrity and functional restoration. The optimal reconstruction of the mandible and alveolar part of the maxilla requires vascularized bone grafts and osseointegrated implants. Apart from these, the management of the orbital floor is a concern in the maxillary defect. The options for orbital floor reconstruction are placement of titanium mesh, non-vascularized bone graft, pedicled bone grafts like coronoid bone with temporalis and calvarial bone, and a free vascularized bone graft. In bony reconstruction, vascularized bone flaps are ideal as most of these patients are young helping to achieve good long-term results. Free fibula flaps are considered the gold standard in these reconstructions. Pre-plating of the mandible may not be possible in all cases as these lesions can present as expansile growth in the mandible. In such cases, virtual planning using CT images will guide us to get better outcomes in terms of osteotomy and plating.

9.3.2.2 Soft Tissue Defects

In major vascular malformations, the skin and entire subcutaneous tissue are involved. In the oral cavity, the lesion affects mucosa as well. Hence the soft tissue defect encountered usually will be large and may be through and through. Although preservation of facial muscles and facial nerves is important for functional significance, it may need resection and plan of reconstruction of the facial nerve should be considered (Fig. 9.2).

9.3.3 Timing of Reconstruction

The reconstruction can be carried out primary (immediately), delayed primary (within 7 days) or secondary (after 7 days). The key to successful reconstruction is perfect hemostasis. Any bleeding beneath the reconstructed tissue is a risk for failure of the flaps. Up to 20% flap failure has been reported in patients undergoing immediate free tissue reconstruction following resection of head and neck arteriovenous malformations. The risk of bleeding is more with fast-flow malformations like arteriovenous malformations. It may be prudent to do wound packing immediately after resection to control hemostasis. This is followed

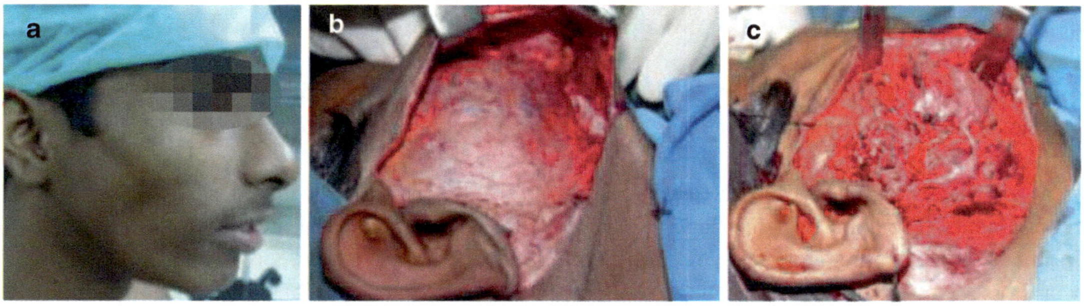

Fig. 9.2 (**a**) Vascular malformation involving right parotid region (**b**) Intraoperative image showing the malformation (**c**) Intraoperative image showing preserved facial nerve post-excision

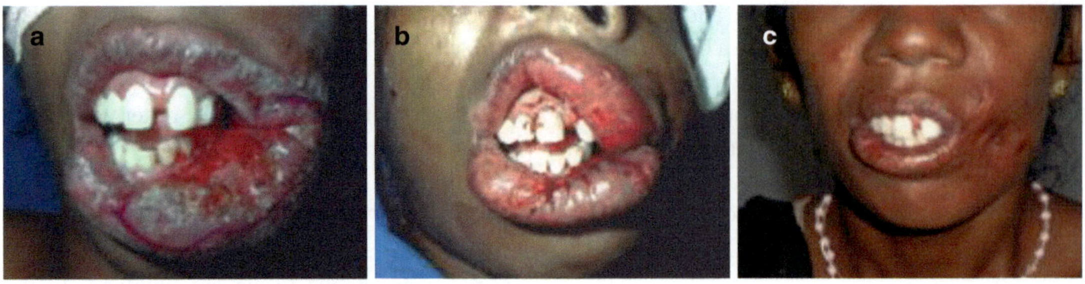

Fig. 9.3 (**a**) Preoperative image of vascular malformation with partial involvement of lower lip (**b**) Immediate postoperative image after excision and primary closure (**c**) At 1 year follow-up

by reconstruction as a delayed primary or secondary manner, being ideal in reconstructing these malformations. The primary reconstruction may be carried out only if complete hemostasis is possible.

9.3.4 Options of Reconstruction

Similar to any oncologic reconstructions, the options vary from locoregional flaps to free tissue transfer. The methods chosen will depend on the size, site as well as age of the patient. Local tissue is preferable to achieve the best cosmesis in some parts of the face. Methods of using local tissue include direct closure and the use of local flaps. Regional flaps like deltopectoral, forehead, pectoralis major flaps may be used in larger defects. But their usefulness is quite limited in the reconstruction of these defects because the aesthetic and functional issues involved with these flaps are unacceptable in a benign condition like this. In certain scenarios like nasal defects where forehead flap gives better outcomes, similarly lip defects the better cosmesis will be by replacing like with like using the adjacent lip or opposite lip. Free tissue transfers may be needed in many head and neck vascular malformations as majority of these patients belong to young age group and only free tissue transfers often satisfy the tissue requirements. The choice of free flaps also helps to mitigate the donor site-related problems. The workhorse flaps were anterolateral thigh flaps and radial forearm flaps in soft tissue defects.

Direct closure is useful and possible in many situations where tissue laxity is not a concern. Lip defects upto one-third of the original lip size can be closed directly (Fig. 9.3). In tongue lesions, the expanded tongue can be excised in such a way, that allow us to directly close the defect, retaining the mobility and shape of the tongue.

9.4 Use of Tissue Expanders

The tissue expansion plays a vital role in the reconstruction of scalp, nasal defects and soft tissue defects of the face. The problem with tissue expansion is the necessity of multiple stages. It may not be feasible to use the expander at the time of primary resection and may need to be expanded and reconstructed at a later stage. In these cases, the defect is allowed to be repaired suboptimally by direct closure or with skin graft initially. When the wound is well settled the reconstruction starts. In case of nasal defects, a medially based forehead flap is the best using the supratrochlear/supraorbital vessels in the pedicle. In large nasal defects, the tissue expander is placed under the proposed flap area in order to achieve the primary closure of the donor defect. Usually, for the forehead, a rectangular tissue expander is better suited for expansion. The incision for placement of the expander is chosen in such a way that it will be included in the incision for flap rising later on. The injection port is placed at an adjacent area, preferably on a bony surface aiding its detection and easy injection of saline later on. Expansion is usually started 2 weeks later and continued till desired expansion of the flap area has been achieved. This may necessitate weekly or twice weekly injections for

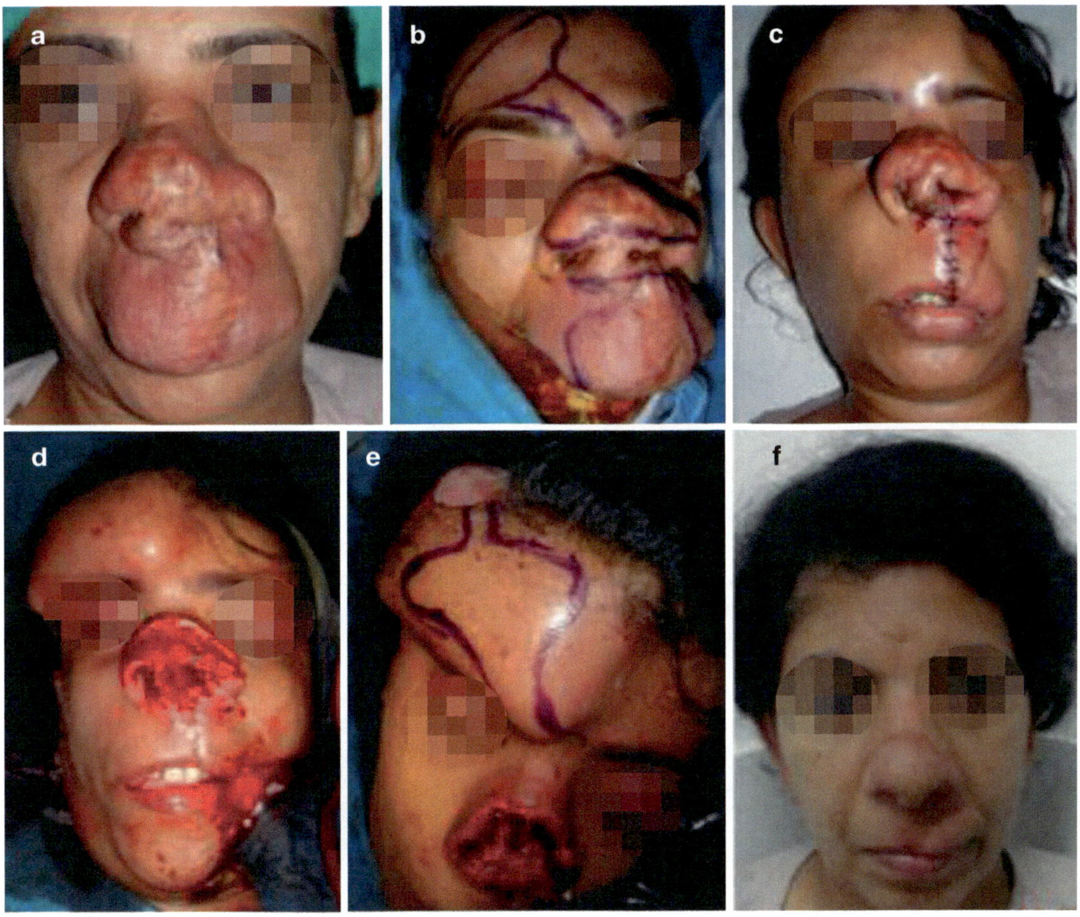

Fig. 9.4 (**a**) Vascular malformation involving the nose and upper lip (**b**) Preoperative planning for excision (**c**) Postoperative image after stage 1 excision and closure of upper lip, partial excision of nasal malformation and placement of tissue expander (**d, e**) Stage 2 excision of nasal malformation and planning of expanded oblique forehead flap for nasal defect (**f**) post-operative image at 10 months

4–6 weeks. After this, the expander is removed and the flap transferred to the nose to resurface it. The donor area is primarily closed. Allowing another 3–4 weeks for the transferred flap to settle down and the third step of surgery, i.e. The division of the pedicle and inset, is completed (Fig. 9.4).

9.5 Free Tissue Transfer in Reconstruction of These Defects

In larger defects with the requirement of composite tissues, free flaps are the choice for reconstruction (Figs. 9.5 and 9.6). The advantages of these flaps include the transfer of suitable tissue in large volumes in a single stage. The selection of the flap will depend on the tissue requirement and the safety of its transfer. Usual choices are radial forearm or anterolateral thigh flaps for soft tissue alone defects and fibula free flap for bony reconstruction. Radial forearm flap is a suitable choice for total lip reconstruction or facial resurfacing. In total lip reconstruction, the flap can be combined with reconstruction of the oral sphincter using fascia. Advantage of the radial forearm flap is the long pedicle which allows us to use the opposite side as the source vessel. Anterolateral thigh flaps are useful wherever a larger defect of soft tissue resurfacing is needed.

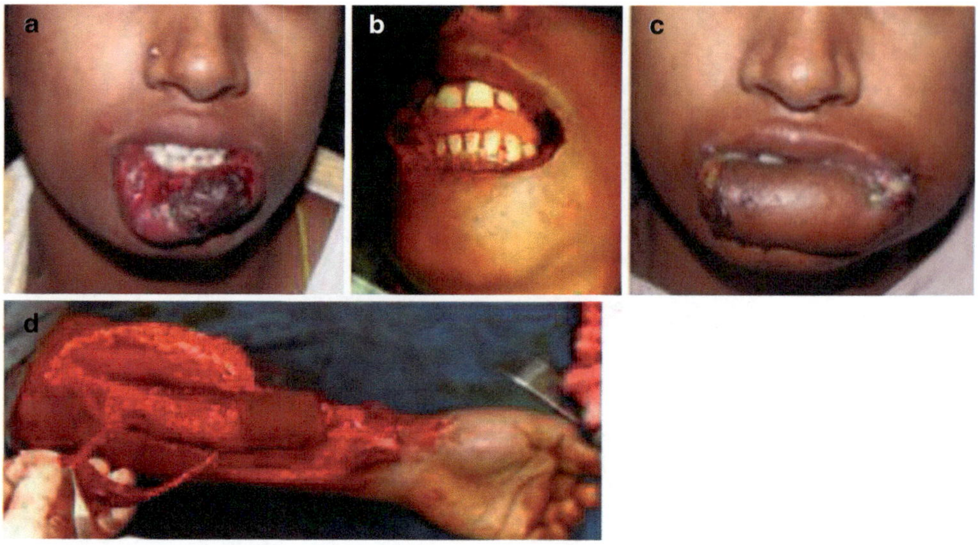

Fig. 9.5 (**a**) Preoperative image of vascular malformation involving the lower lip (**b**) Immediate postoperative image after near-total excision (**c**) 2 weeks postoperative image after reconstruction with radial forearm free flap (**d**) Harvested radial forearm free flap

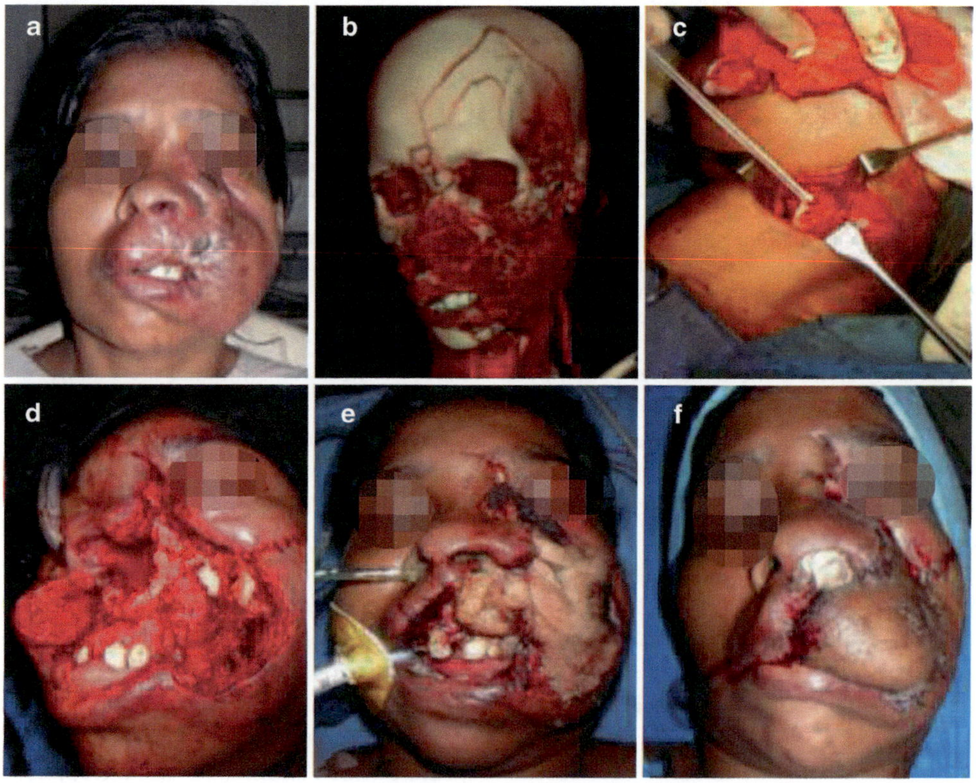

Fig. 9.6 (**a**) Recurrent vascular malformation involving cheek, upper lip (**b**) CT angiogram showing the Abnormal vasculature (**c**) Intraoperative control of facial artery prior to excision (**d**) Defect post-excision (**e**) wound packing post-excision (**f**) Delayed primary free radial forearm flap cover

Bony reconstruction can and should be attempted when the defect involves the mandible or the maxilla. Fibula becomes an obvious choice due to its excellent bone stock as well as pedicle length.

9.5.1 Pedicle Selection in Free Tissue Transfer

The selection of normal vessels for anastomosis is crucial for the success of the free faps in these cases. The vessels on the same side may be unsuitable as the arteries are hypertrophied and the veins huge. The chance of anastomotic complications was high in the diseased vessels. Hence they have to be chosen outside the area of the pathology, which may necessitate to go close to the origin of the vessel on the same side or even to use the opposite side vessels.

9.5.2 Prevention of Flap Failures

As discussed previously selection of a safe flap as well as the normal vessels as the recipients is most important in prevention of failure of free flaps in these defects. The chance of flap failure is still high mostly due to bleeding issues related to these malformations. Delaying the reconstruction by days or weeks after the excision prevents this.

9.5.3 Advantages of Free Tissue Transfer apart from its Reconstructive Benefits

Frequently post-excision, the microscopic lesions exist, which results in recurrence. There has been a report on the suppression of these malformations by placing a new vascularized tissue on the wound bed of the resected malformation. This concept of "regulatory flap" by use of free tissue changing the local hemodynamics and suppressing the collaterals or microfistula formation which results in decrease in recurrences. The free tissue transfer also reduces the postoperative complications like seroma, pain, deformity, and functional problems.

9.6 Computersied Planning, Surgical Guides and Patient-Specific Implants

Technological advances have provided the clinician with opportunities to meticulously plan the surgical resection and reconstruction in advance with the help of dedicated computer software. Intraoperative navigation and imaging provide an additional layer of control to determine if the preplanned objectives have been achieved during the operation. Though these methods can be utilised for many surgical interventions, they are most useful for operations involving bony resections and complex three-dimensional reconstruction (Fig. 9.7a, b).

A dedicated CT scan with a minimum slice thickness of 1 mm and "zero" degree gantry tilt is obtained of the area of interest. The scans are uploaded to the local laboratory or commercial organisation, which has access to the relevant software. These same scans can also be used for intraoperative navigation, if so desired.

The clinician is able to plan the surgical resection on the computer with the knowledge of the clinical and imaging parameters (Fig. 9.7c). Once the clinician is happy with the resection, the planned segment is "removed" on the computer, and the ensuing defect "reconstructed by mirroring" from the opposite (uninvolved) side (Fig. 9.7d). Modifications to the "mirrored" reconstruction can be incorporated to account for any residual lesion or other eventualities (e.g. muscle atrophy, enophthalmos, exophthalmos, etc.). A stereolithographic model can be manufactured from the final plan and utilised to construct a local or outsourced patient-specific implant using titanium mesh or sheet (Fig. 9.7e). Accurate restoration of premorbid anatomy and excellent aesthetic outcomes can be obtained by utilising patient-specific implants (Fig. 9.7f–h).

The same process can also be utilised for the creation of a "surgical guide", once the surgical resection has been finalised (Fig. 9.8a). This guide can be used once the lesion is exposed and allows quick and accurate resection of the lesion with predetermined margins (Fig. 9.8b). The guide also allows the clinician to avoid critical structures determined in the planning process and can minimise the exposure required.

Various alloplastic materials are available through commercial organisations and can be utilised for the reconstruction of complex three-dimensional defects. Each material has its merits and shortcomings, and the clinician will have to choose the most appropriate one based on the individual patient characteristics, need for cross-sectional imaging surveillance, radiotherapy, cost, etc. The illustrated case was reconstructed with PEEK (poly ether ketone) patient-specific implant (Fig. 9.8c).

The use of patient-specific alloplastic implants allows accurate and predictable reconstruction of complex three-dimensional defects, especially in the upper facial skeleton/peri-orbital region, which cannot be easily achieved with the use of autologous reconstruction. Mirroring allows the achievement of excellent symmetry, and the lack of an additional donor site helps reduce patient discomfort and surgical time. There is, however, a financial cost associated with the planning, creation of the surgical guide and patient-specific implant, which will principally be determined by the type and size of the implant and the complexity of the planning process. Care should be exercised with its use in patients with compromised soft tissue cover, potential risk of infection, especially when exposed to the sino-nasal or oral environment and those who have had or likely to have radiotherapy.

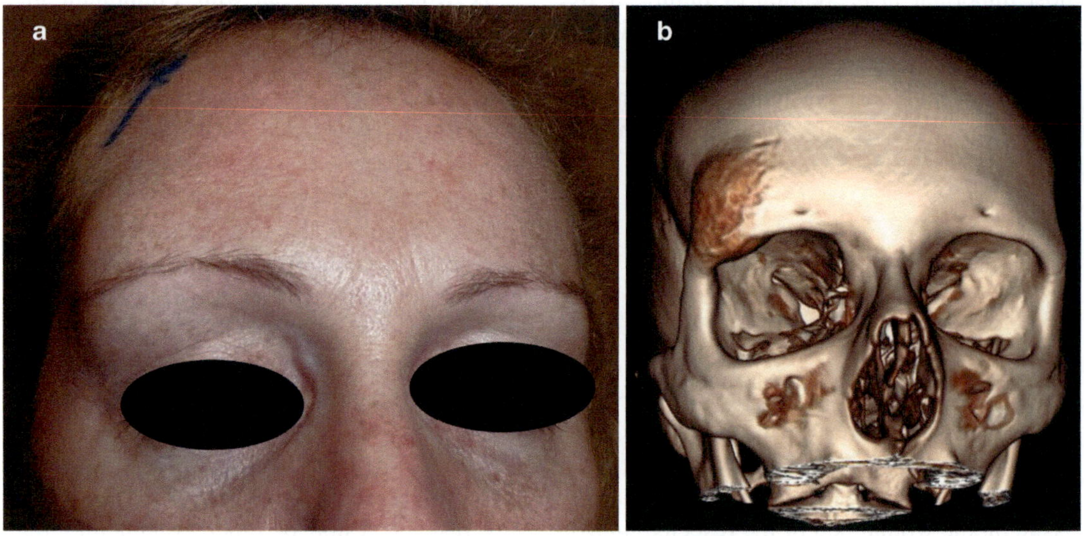

Fig. 9.7 (**a**) Right Supraorbital intra-osseous VM of the frontal bone. (**b**) 3-D reformatted CT scan demonstrating location and extent of the lesion. (**c**) Virtual surgical planning with the 3D modeling of the "excision" of the lesion. (**d**) Virtual surgical 'mirror modeling' of the contralateral side for planning following "mirroring reconstruction" of defect. (**e**) Stereolithographic model with adapted titanium mesh patient-specific implant. (**f**) Patient-specific implant in situ following resection

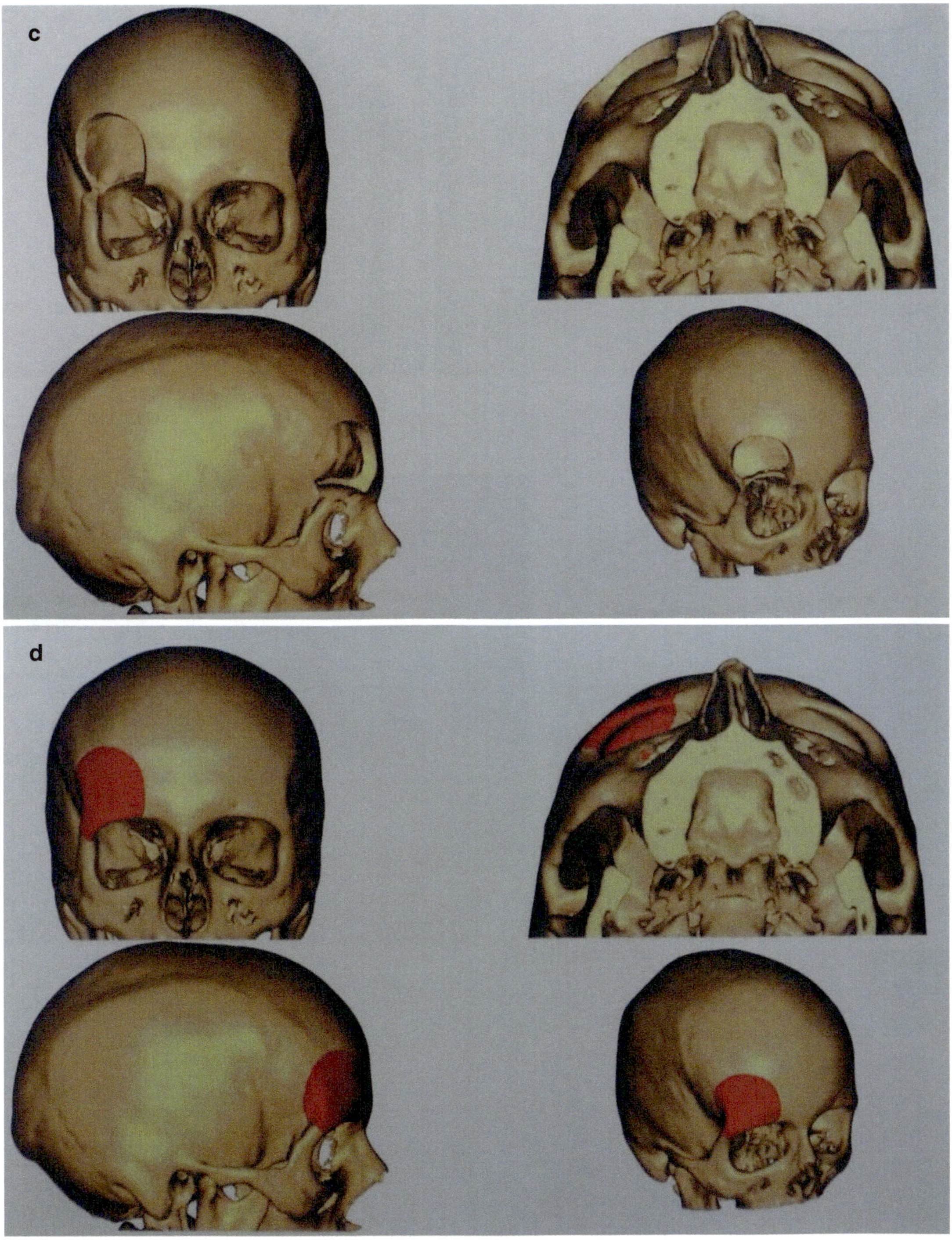

Fig. 9.7 (continued)

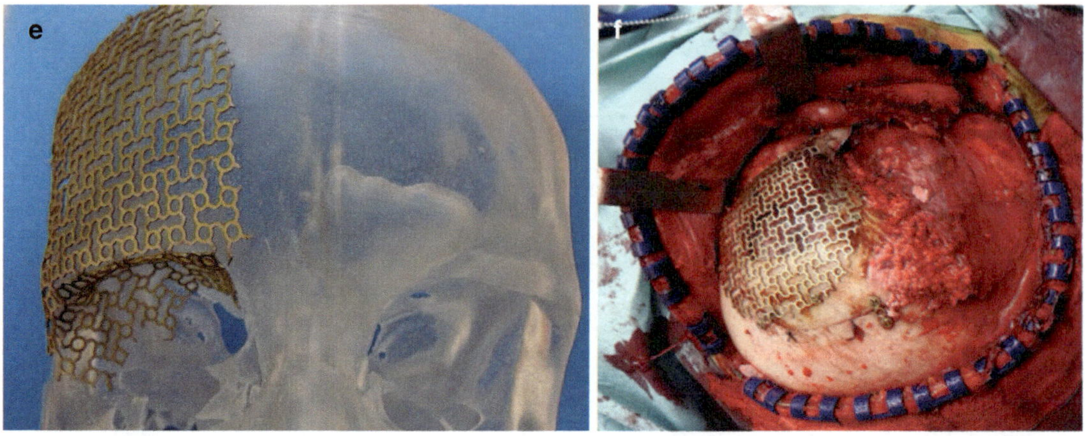

Fig. 9.7 (continued)

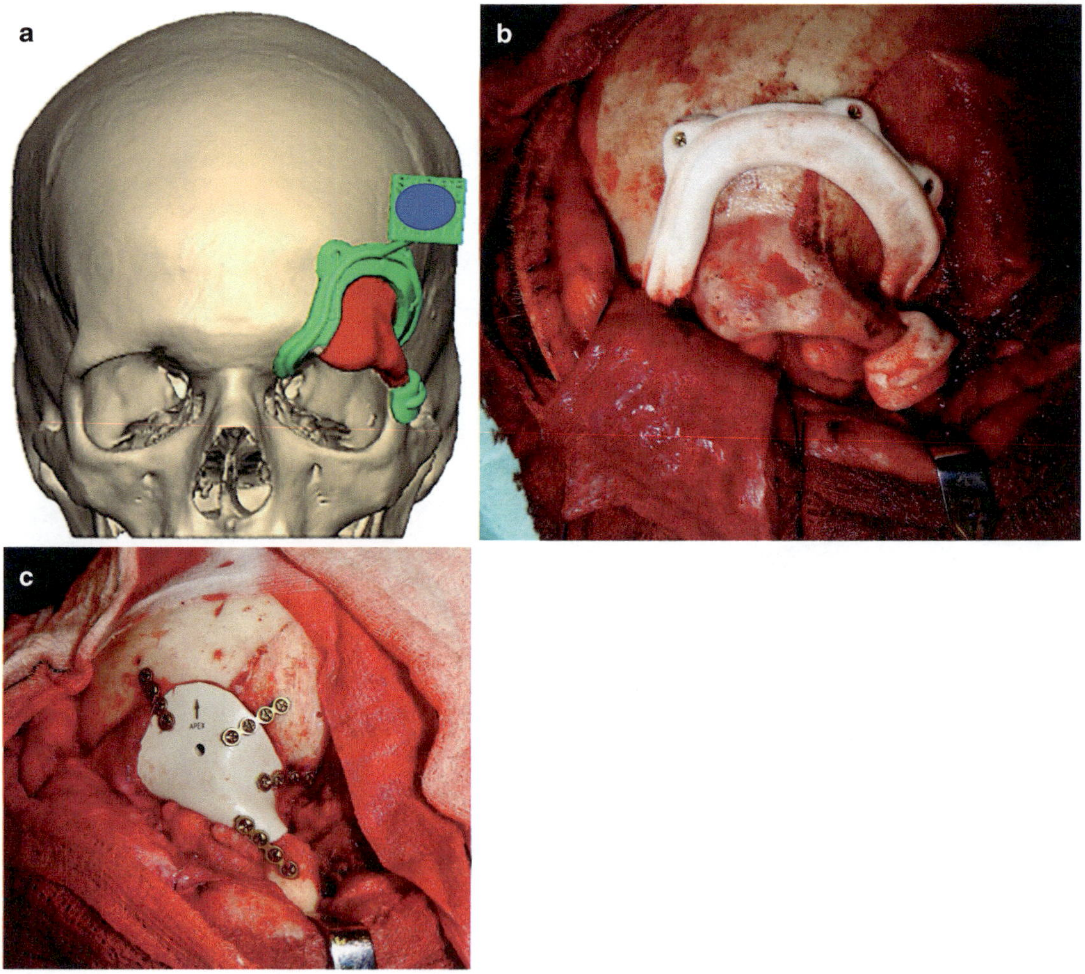

Fig. 9.8 (**a**) Computer planned surgical guide left supraorbital lesion. (**b**) Surgical guide in situ with predetermined resection margins. (**c**) Reconstruction with patient-specific PEEK implant in situ

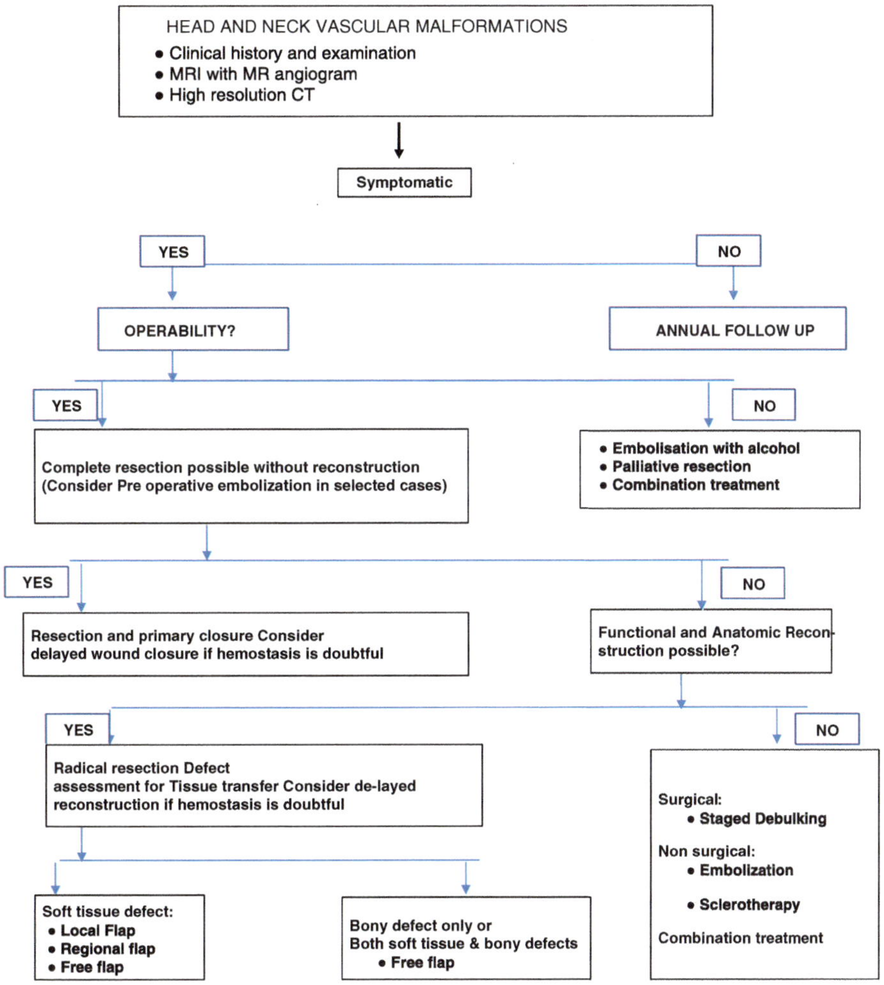

Flow chart for reconstruction of defects after resection of vascular malformations

9.7 Points to remember while undertaking reconstruction of defects after resection of major vascular malformations

- Assess the patient clinically, radiologically by MRI with MR angiogram.
- High-resolution CT will be helpful in suspected bony lesions
- Pre operative embolization should be considered in selected cases like High-flow vascular malformations where temporary surgical occlusion of the feeding vessel is not possible during surgery
- Temporary clamping of the source vessel prior to the resection in will help in controlling the blood loss and also a clear surgical field for preservation of vitals structures like facial nerve
- Complete excision in the form of radical resection in all possible cases will drastically reduce the recurrence rate
- Compression wound packing and delayed wound closure or reconstruction to be considered in cases of incomplete hemostasis
- Delayed primary reconstruction would be an ideal time for tissue transfers
- Primary closure can be done ideally after 48 h of wound packing

- Locoregional flaps gives better results in specific defects of small to moderate size (rotation flap for scalp defects, lip switching/ estlander flap for lip defects, forehead flap for nasal defects)
- Free tissue transfers are ideal for moderate to large size defects and in bony defects

Palliative resection can be considered in patients at risk for impending life threatening bleeding

Lasers and Nonsurgical Modalities 10

Huy Q. Tran, Victoria A. Manon, Simon Young, and James C. Melville

10.1 Introduction

Vascular anomalies in the head and neck regions are among the common pathologies that maxillofacial surgeons encounter in their clinical practice. While surgical excision is historically the mainstay treatment for most large, complex vascular anomalies, nonsurgical therapies have developed as excellent alternatives for the treatment of certain pathologic types (telangiectasia, capillary malformations) and as adjunctive tools for others (Figs. 10.1, 10.2, and 10.3). This group of treatments consists of medicinal use, laser therapy, radiographic-guided embolization, and sclerotherapy. More often than not, treatments involve a combination of the aforementioned techniques in order to achieve clinical response. Laser therapy in particular has emerged as one of the most promising fields behind its ability to selectively destroy the aberration while sparing

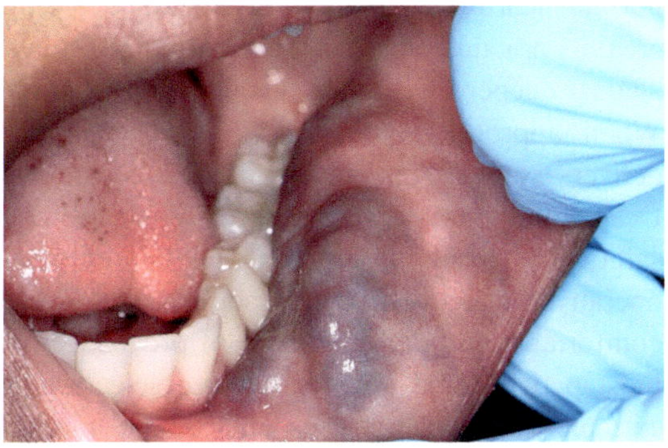

Fig. 10.1 Hemangioma of the lower lip

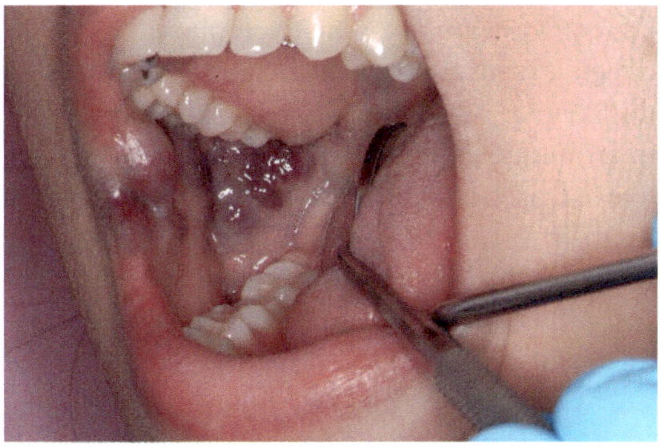

Fig. 10.2 Vascular malformation of the buccal mucosa

Figures and Art by Dr. Victoria A. Manon DDS MD

H. Q. Tran · V. A. Manon · S. Young
Katz Department of Oral & Maxillofacial Surgery, The University of Texas at Houston, University of Texas Health Science Center at Houston, Houston, TX, USA

J. C. Melville (✉)
Katz Department of Oral & Maxillofacial Surgery, The University of Texas at Houston, University of Texas Health Science Center at Houston, Houston, TX, USA

Oral, Head, and Neck Oncologic and Microvascular Reconstructive Surgery, Katz Department of Oral & Maxillofacial Surgery, The University of Texas at Houston, University of Texas Health Science Center at Houston, Houston, TX, USA
e-mail: James.C.Melville@uth.tmc.edu

S. C. Nair, S. R. Chandra (eds.), *Management of Head and Neck Vascular Lesions*,
https://doi.org/10.1007/978-981-15-2321-2_10

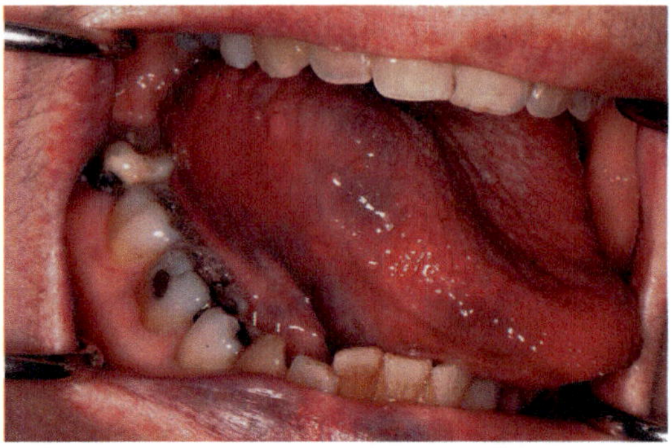

Fig. 10.3 Cavernous hemangioma of the tongue

normal nearby tissues. While still an evolving area, its practical application is currently limited against deeper and larger subcutaneous vessels. When appropriately selected and used, laser delivers excellent operative and cosmetic results. Despite the initial learning curve associated with safety, its ease of use and relatively benign post-operative period make laser therapy a relatively comfortable and preferred type of procedure for most patients and clinicians. Case selection is extremely important, as not all vascular anomalies are amenable to laser therapy, and not all types of laser are effective for one particular lesion. As laser technology continues to develop, current systems are quickly replaced by more effective and convenient models. The focus of this chapter will be the discussion of many common laser types, although by no means an exhaustive list, used to treat vascular pathology in regard to their biophysics, clinical applications, and limitations. In addition, other therapeutic modalities will be discussed as alternative or adjunctive treatment options to laser therapy.

10.2 History of Laser and Current Modalities

In 1916, Albert Einstein published the doctrine "*Zur Quantum Theorie der Strahlen*" (The Quantum Theory of Radiation) which provided the theoretical foundation for laser generation through the idea of *stimulated emission*. It was not until 1960 that the American physicist Theodore Maiman constructed and introduced to the public the first ruby diode laser. Just 1 year later, laser application gained a significant foothold in the medical community when a dermatologist, Leon Goldman, began his research at the first biomedical laser laboratory at the University of Cincinnati. The development of laser continued steadily over the next decade with the introduction of many types of laser in dermatologic surgery, such as the CO_2, argon, and Nd:YAG. These lasers emitted a continuous beam of energy capable of destroying target tissues while simultaneously maintain hemostasis through its thermal power. As such, they were used as adjuncts in surgical treatment of highly vasculated organs. The practicality of these lasers was however limited due to the destructive nature of a high-powered, continuous wave of energy to both target pathologic and nearby healthy tissues, resulting in lacerated wounds and hypertrophic scarring. The search was then underway for a type of laser that would only target the desired structures. In 1981, Anderson and Parrish came forth with the theory of selective thermolysis. This groundbreaking theory centered around the potential of laser beam to selectively cause destruction to target tissue (chromophores) while sparing others by taking advantage of the variation in light absorption spectra [1].

To achieve this feat, laser was made to be discontinuous or pulsatile. Laser wavelength can be attuned to maximize absorption by the target tissue and minimize absorption by competing constituents. Hemoglobin absorbs light at wavelength peaks of 418, 542, and 577-nm, which makes the 585- or 595-nm pulse dyed laser an extremely effective treatment for most superficial vascular malformations. Another important principle of selective thermolysis is the phenomenon of thermal relaxation, which is defined as the time required for tissue to lose 50% of its heat via diffusion. The duration of the beam, or pulse duration, must be shorter than the thermal relaxation time of the target tissue. This confines the heat emitted by the laser within the target and prevents dissipation to adjacent structures. On the other hand, the pulse duration must also be long enough for sufficient buildup of thermal energy within the target vessel lumen to be clinically effective.

While selective thermolysis works well for superficial and small types of vessels in the head and neck area, it has limited use in larger and deeper vessels. In these situations, laser wavelength must be modified to increase depth penetration, and pulse duration must be increased to allow enough time for temperature rise in larger vessels.

10.2.1 Flash Lamp Pumped Pulsed Dye Laser (585-nm, 595-nm)

Using a rhodamine dye dissolved in a solvent, the flash lamp pumps energy to produce yellow light at a distinct wavelength. The pulsed dye laser (PDL) is primarily used in the treatment of small, superficial vascular anomalies such as capillary malformations, superficial infantile hemangiomas, and telangiectasia. First-generation PDL (wavelength at 577-nm) was introduced in the 1980s and replaced argon laser as a safer and more effective treatment for capillary malformations. Current PDL today produces light at 585- or 595-nm with an increased depth of penetration, and most systems are equipped with a cooling device for added protection of nearby tissues. Delivered by fiberoptic technology, the energy generated is preferentially absorbed by hemoglobin and oxyhemoglobin, creating a thermal-induced damage and coagulative phenomenon within the blood vessel. Thermal relaxation time for small cutaneous vessels (diameter of <100-um) is approximated to be 1- to 5-ms [2]. For this reason, the pulse duration of PDL is routinely kept at 0.45-ms. PDL is traditionally reserved for only superficial vascular lesions due to its maximum depth of only 1.2-mm [3]. Its limited depth can be partly due to the presence of melanin, a skin constituent that also absorbs light produced at this wavelength. Due to an increased concentration of competing melanin, the laser has even poorer depth penetration in dark-skinned individuals or those with Fitzpatrick skin type IV and V.

Common side effects of PDL are erythema, edema, and purpura which can last up to 2 weeks. Purpura is caused by leakage of erythrocytes due to the rapid heat buildup and resulting photoacoustic damage to the vessel walls. Patients and parents must be forewarned and be prepared of this unappealing side effect, which is a common reason for discontinuation of therapy. With current models of PDL permitting variable pulse duration, the longer pulse duration can generate a lower peak energy, and thus a slower and gentler thermal effect that does not cause vessel rupture. No purpura is noted with the use of long-pulsed PDL [4].

10.2.2 Frequency-Doubled Q-Switched Nd:YAG/KTP Laser (532 nm)

The frequency-doubled, Q-switched Nd:YAG laser, as described by its name and also known as KTP laser, utilizes a frequency doubling technique (second harmonic generation) to generate green light at 532-nm. This wavelength is well-absorbed by oxyhemoglobin and is taken advantage of in application of selective thermolysis. Initially, a diode laser pumps the Nd:YAG crystal to produce a 1064-nm laser energy that is then made to focus onto a potassium titanyl phosphate crystal. This technique ultimately produces a second light energy that is doubled in frequency and consequently halves the wavelength to 532-nm ($\lambda = v/f$; λ = wavelength, f = frequency, v = velocity of light).

Common parameter for the 532-nm laser is a pulse duration ranging from 1- to 50-ms and fluence up to 40-J/cm^2. The advantage of the frequency-doubled Nd:YAG laser lies in its longer pulse duration that allows for accumulation of sufficient thermal energy in large vessels. In comparison to flash-lamped pulse dye which is routinely set at 0.45-ms, the 532-nm laser is more effective at treating vessels that are >200-nm in diameter. The effectiveness of the 532-nm laser is conjected to be due to the reported thermal relaxation time of 1- to 10-ms in the 200-nm vessel size, which requires a longer pulse duration [5]. Additionally, when it was first introduced, the laser allowed for flexibility to adjust pulse duration and/or fluence as needed in order to achieve clinical response. In lesions refractory to PDL treatment, the frequency-doubled Nd:YAG laser is a good alternative and should be offered to the patient. Another advantage of this type of laser is the absence of purpura, a bothersome side effect that frequently occurs in PDL treatment. The longer pulse duration applies a lower peak energy to the target, which eliminates the vicious thermal buildup that is responsible for vessel rupture.

Melanin in the skin absorbs the 532-nm light slightly better than at 585-nm. The frequency-doubled Nd:YAG laser is less effective in Fitzpatrick skin type IV and V due to the higher concentration of competing melanin, which may cause skin dyschromia and blistering after treatment session. The vulnerability of melanin, coupled with a longer pulse duration, necessitates the use of a cooling device perioperatively when using the 532-nm laser in order to protect the overlying tissue. Nevertheless, the laser still carries a risk of damage to healthy tissues, in particularly a higher risk of scarring (18%) compared to the PDL-treated lesion (3%) [6].

10.2.3 Long-Pulsed Nd:YAG Laser (1064-nm)

Since it was first introduced in 1964, the 1064-nm Nd:YAG laser has remained a versatile tool for the cosmetic clinician and is originally developed for procedures such as hair removal and ablation of atrophic scar. The laser secured a position in the 1990s as a valuable alternative for the treatment of certain types of vascular anomalies, which up until that point were only treated by shorter wavelength lasers. Utilizing a medium of impure yttrium-aluminum-garnet crystal that is doped by 1% neodymium ions, the laser emits light at a near-infrared wavelength of 1064-nm. With a much lower level of absorption from melanin, the laser is able to extend the depth of penetration to 5- to 6-mm, targeting deeper vessels that are unreachable by other lasers. The lack of absorption by competing melanin also allows for the use of the laser in patients with Fitzpatrick skin type IV and V. On the other hand, hemoglobin and oxyhemoglobin have lower level of light absorption at 1064-nm. To compensate, energy fluence is increased up to 300 J/cm^2 in order to generate a sufficient amount of thermal energy within the vessel lumen for the coagulation of blood. The pulse duration is routinely kept at 0.1–300-ms at this high level of energy to avoid inadvertent thermal damage to the overlying tissue. This also allowed for gentler heating of the vessel which prevents postoperative purpura.

Traditionally, the laser is applied by direct cutaneous contact with a fiberoptic cable. One to two passes are made over the lesion until blanching and/or shrinkage of the lesion is noted. Unsafe level of exposure to the skin or mucosa must be avoided by continuously moving the laser tip and avoid excessive overlapping passes. If the lesion is nodular, a glass slide can be used in an attempt to flatten the lesion to enhance the depth of laser penetration. In an inaccessible location such as the palate or floor of the mouth, a test tube with side window is an effective adjunctive tool. The fiberoptic is inserted through the window while the test tube compresses the lesion. In deeper and thicker vascular lesions, the interstitial technique is useful in order to protect the overlying mucosa or skin. The fiberoptic cable can be inserted into the lesion focus through a 14-gauge angiocatheter [7, 8]. The delivery of the laser energy is more selective with this technique that would have otherwise cause extensive damage before reaching its target, decreasing the risk of tissue sloughing and duration of postoperative pain.

Success for the long-pulsed Nd:YAG laser in treating hemangiomas and vascular malformations is generally good, with reported rate of at least 50% improvement in 71.5–80% of all treated vascular lesions [9, 10]. Another study demonstrated a complete clearance rate of 77% intraoral lesions after a single session, and the persistent lesions cleared after an additional one to two sessions [11]. While an effective therapy, the window of safety in long-pulsed Nd:YAG laser is extremely narrow. Incidence of skin damage is high with its application, including scarring and blistering. A concomitant dynamic cooling device should always be used for additional epidermal and dermal protection. Conservative approach should be taken with multiple treatment sessions as opposed to an aggressive single session to avoid risk of collateral damage.

10.2.4 CO_2 Laser (10,600-nm)

Prior to the advent of pulsatile, selective-targeted laser, the CO_2 laser is considered a constant workhorse for the surgeons in treatment of maxillofacial pathologies. At an infrared wavelength of 10,600-nm, the laser produces continuous light energy that is highly absorbed by water molecule. Considering that the human body approximates 85% of water (mucosal tissue carriers an even higher proportion), it is an effective ablative tool capable of performing surgery in a bloodless manner. The thermal energy generated upon tissue contact instantly cauterizes and seals off small blood vessels with a diameter up to 0.5-mm [12, 13]. The laser can be carried out in either excisional or vaporizing style by using it in a focused or defocused mode, respectively. The vaporizing mode, like the name suggests, instantly burns off the superficial layer of the target tissue, and multiple passes are required to remove the whole lesion. Careful pre-operative clinical and radiographic evaluation must also be made to assess for the breadth of the lesion. CO_2 laser in the vaporizing mode is frequently used in treating biopsy-proven precancerous lesions due to the ease of use and benign postoperative healing period. A major drawback of the layer-by-layer technique is the uneven and unpredictable depth penetration (possibly due to variation in water concentration within the laser field) and thus a greater degree of control is needed by the surgeon to avoid any iatrogenic damage to important underlying anatomic structures. This mode should only be used if the target is known pathologically or biopsy-proven prior to the treatment session. If a concurrent biopsy is required, the focused mode should be used as a scalpel to excise the lesion with an understanding that the tissues near the laser margins are generally altered histologically and will not be of use to the pathologist. A morphological, histochemical, and immunocytochemical study demonstrated blisters, erosions, clefts of the epithelium, as well as nuclei changes in specimens excised by CO_2 laser [14]. It is recommended that the surgeon should account for this issue by further extent the margins of laser excision to ensure that unaltered normal tissue is included in the submitted specimen.

Advantages of the CO_2 laser includes decreased operative blood loss, shorter surgical time, and a relatively benign postoperative healing period. In regard to the latter, the CO_2 laser creates an immediate wound site filled with charred flesh, which is later replaced by fibrinous tissue. One characteristic of the laser wound is the delayed and reduced inflammatory response that attribute to minimal postoperative swelling. Pain is subjectively reported to be minimal after laser therapy, possibly due to the lack of intense inflammatory response and the incineration of nerve endings. There is also a decreased amount of myofibroblasts, which are cells responsible for wound contracture and healing. Thus, CO_2 laser causes significantly less scarring compared to conventional surgical treatment. This is extremely advantageous when treating pathology in certain anatomical regions such as the floor of the mouth. On the other hand, the healing process after laser treatment is also delayed due to the lack of contracture as well as a lack of blood flow from laser cauterization. In spite of this, no suturing or dressing is necessary, and wound site is left to heal by secondary intention. The effects of CO_2 laser on tissues is dependent on duration of application and selected energy power, which should be adjusted accordingly to the individual skin or mucosal integrity to avoid excessive damage.

10.2.5 Diode Laser (532-, 800-, 810-, 940-, and 980-nm)

Perhaps one of the most widely used laser technology in modern maxillofacial surgery, the diode laser works via a solid-state semiconductor to emit light at varying intensity and wavelengths. The laser is conveniently housed in a portable, cost-effective unit system and is powered by standard wall electricity. In accordance to the principle of selective thermolysis, the pulsed mode at 532-nm works similarly to PDL and allows for treatment of superficial vascular anomalies while sparing healthy nearby tissues. Unlike the PDL, the diode laser can deliver energy at a longer pulse duration (1–100-ms) and does not induce purpura due to the lack of rapid vaporization and vessel rupture [15]. At a wavelength of 800–900-nm and approximately 3–5-W, the diode laser can penetrate the skin more deeply than PDL while maintaining selectivity for hemoglobin chromophores. This near-infrared setting is generally used to approach deep vascular lesions that are refractory to standalone PDL or KTP laser. The flexibility to adjust wavelength, power, and pulse duration allows the diode laser to be commonly used in an office environment for a diverse array of maxillofacial procedures, including treatments for superficial capillary malformations, telangiectasia, and deep venous malformations. The diode laser can closely emulate a number of aforementioned laser technology by simply modifying its settings. When used in continuous mode, the laser can also be used effectively as a scalpel in excising highly vasculated lesions such as fibrous hyperplasia while maintaining excellent hemostasis and avoiding the need for sutures [16].

10.3 Laser Application in Vascular Anomalies

10.3.1 Capillary Malformations

Capillary malformations (CM), frequently referred to as port wine stains, are observed in 0.3–0.5% of infants as a pink macular or patch stain and tend to increase in size as the child grows [17]. A high suspicion for syndromic involvement and subsequent workup is necessary if CM occurs in the V1 dermatome (Sturge–Weber), is associated with asymmetrical limb hypertrophy (Klippel–Trenaunay), or with acute onset sensory and motor disturbances (Cobb). CM occurs due to the absence of neural innervation to the aberrant vessels within the superficial papillary nexus, leading to a lack of sympathetic drive, blood-pooling, and resulting vessel dilation. This pathologic behavior is hypothesized to be the reason for the high recurrence rate post-treatments. Most clinicians advocate for CM to be treated as early as possible to avoid increased growth and thickness of the lesion, which necessitate the use of higher intensity laser and increased number of treatments. Additionally, early treatment of CM precludes the psychogenic burden placed on the young patients (Table 10.1).

Prior to the introduction of pulse dye laser (PDL), CM was frequently treated with argon laser with 60% success rate in adults. Argon laser was unsuitable in children due to severe pain experienced during treatment and the resulting high level of scarring in this age group. In adults, the high-intensity energy of argon laser is also associated with unacceptable side effects including a significant rate of hypertrophic and atrophic scarring, hyper- and hypo-pigmentation [18]. When first introduced, first-generation PDL (577-nm) was effective for CM and permitted use in the infancy period. Second-generation PDL (585-nm, 595-nm) was even better and includes a dynamic cooling device (DCD) that cools the skin surface and reduces pain perioperatively.

Table 10.1 Type of laser and its application in head and neck vascular pathology

Type of laser	Wavelength	Color	Application in head and neck vascular pathology
Flash-lamped pumped pulsed dye laser (PDL)	585-nm, 595-nm	Yellow	Capillary malformations; superficial infantile hemangiomas; telangiectasia
Frequency-doubled Q-switched Nd:YAG (KTP) laser	532-nm	Green	Capillary malformations that are resistant to PDL, such as syndromic CMs that are larger and thicker; telangiectasia; venous malformations
Long-pulsed Nd:YAG laser	1064-nm	Invisible	Capillary malformations that are resistant to PDL, such as syndromic CMs that are deeper, larger, and thicker; telangiectasia; venous malformations
Diode laser	532-, 800-, 810-, 940-, and 980-nm	Various	Telangiectasia; venous malformations; excision of highly vascularized lesions such as fibrous hyperplasia

Treatments are routinely set with spot size of 5–10-mm, energy fluence between 5 and 8 J/cm^2, and pulse duration of 0.45-ms. Clinical end goal of each treatment session is the cessation of blanching in the aberrant region, or when the dark-purple coloration of purpura is noted. Slight overlap of laser field is attempted to avoid a reticulated pattern of pigmentation. However, overlapping should be minimized to decrease inadvertent thermal damage to the healthy tissues. Parents must also be informed that multiple treatments of PDL are frequently required to promote clearance. Multiple studies have shown that patients with CM require an average of 10 or more treatments to achieve clearance, with one treatment occurring every 2–4 weeks [19, 20]. The success rate is especially enhanced in patients with Fitzpatrick skin type I-III due to decreased concentration of competing melanin. Darker-skinned individuals may need to wait a longer period between treatments to allow resolution of post-inflammatory pigmentation.

Partial or complete recurrence of CM is high, with study indicating recurrence rate of 3% within a 1-year period and 40% within a 3-year period [21]. Touch-up laser procedures can be offered to the patient when early signs of recurrence are noticed. CM that are large and thick, such as those associated with Klippel–Trenaunay syndrome, is generally refractory to traditional PDL treatment and necessitates the use of other lasers. For these types of CM (estimated 20–30% of total cases), the frequency-doubled and long-pulsed 1064-nm Nd:YAG are the better alternatives [22]. The longer pulse duration in these types of laser also allows for a slower and gentler buildup of thermal energy, preventing vicious rupture of the involved vessels and the resulting, unsightly purpura.

10.3.2 Infantile Hemangiomas (IHs)

While laser is an effective treatment for capillary malformations, its application in infantile hemangiomas is debatable among clinicians. Hemangiomas, as a group, affect approximately 2.6% of newborns, particularly in 10% of Caucasians [23]. They are usually absent at birth but tend to appear shortly after and exponentially grow within the first year (proliferative phase). The majority of IHs begin the involution phase by 12 months of life, with 50% of these lesions involute by the age of 5, 70% by the age of 7, and 90% by the age of 9 [24]. However, involuted IH can still leave heavy scars, persistent fibrofatty protuberance, and telangiectasia. Up to 80% of lesions that had not involuted by 6 years of age will leave behind some level of disfiguring remnants [25]. It is also somewhat difficult to predict which lesion will have a benign clinical course, and which can negatively affect the patient's quality of life. While the decision to treat for IH remains controversial, the conservative "watch and wait" approach is losing ground due to the associated complications observed in the past decades. Ulceration is the most frequent complication with growing IHs, and lesions occurring in esthetic zones create various social issues for the growing patients. It is not the authors' intention in this chapter to support one particular approach, and it must be emphasized that at the moment there is no one-treatment-fits-all therapy for IH. In other word, treatment must be individualized, and more often than not, a combination of therapies is necessary to achieve clinical response. Regardless, the goals in treating hemangiomas remain absolute, that is, to promote an uncomplicated clinical course and optimize resolution of the disease.

In recent years, new advocates have come forth, albeit with skepticisms, with the idea that the most ideal period for IH to be treated is when the lesion has yet to begin its proliferative phase. This period is referred to as the precursor phase and is best treated with pulsed dye laser (PDL). At a setting of 595-nm, 7 J/cm^2, 0.150–0.300-ms, PDL has been shown to induce an earlier involution course and prevent development of deeper lesions when used in this precursor period [23]. Outside of this window period, the application of laser in uncomplicated IH is uncertain. On the one hand, early signs of ulceration or potential functional impairment (airway and visual obstruction) are strong indications for the initiation of treatment. If the hemangioma is in its proliferative stage, medical intervention with propranolol or oral corticosteroid is first-line therapy. PDL (595-nm, 7 J/cm^2, 0.45 ms) should be initiated when the ulcerated lesion is nonresponsive to medical treatment, as laser can induce healing, alleviate pain, decrease infection and bleeding [26]. In vitro study has positively demonstrated the significance of PDL treatment in decreasing vascular endothelial growth factor (VEGF) expression, which is believed to be one of the key signals behind aberrant tumor growth [27]. Ablative laser (CO_2, continuous Nd:YAG) is used in adjunct with surgical and medical therapies when life-threatening situations arise such as obstructing subglottic hemangioma with potential for massive intraoperative hemorrhage. In the involuting period, PDL is an effective tool in treating unappealing remnants such as telangiectasia and erythematous skin. The laser, however, cannot treat disfiguring lesions. While PDL does not offer contouring capability, it can help in decreasing the extent of wound size created by surgical therapy.

The most important factor in laser success lies in the location of the hemangioma within the skin layers (superficial, deep, or mixed). It is important to emphasize that PDL is only effective in superficial lesions due to their maximal depth penetration of only 1.2-mm. Vessels that lie in the deeper level of dermis must be treated with the longer-wavelength Nd:YAG. Tolerance to this alternative laser is significantly reduced, and the clinician must be mindful about overzealous treatments in deep or mixed lesion to avoid significant scarring, atrophy, and dyschromia. Compared to CM, PDL therapy in hemangiomas has yet to achieve the same success as a monotherapeutic modality due to its pathologic nature. The laser still has a therapeutic role in ulcerative IH and has been documented to be an excellent adjunct to other types of treatments (timolol maleate 0.5% gel, oral propranolol, and surgical excision) [28–30].

10.3.3 Telangiectasia

PDL and diode lasers are effective therapy for the treatment of facial telangiectasia because the involved vessels are generally small (0.1–1-mm) and lie in the superficial layer of the skin. In deeper and larger vessels, longer-wavelength lasers such as the Nd:YAG are the more preferred modes of therapy. Telangiectasia is a condition in which a small vessel (capillary, arteriole, or venule) is persistently dilated and visually appreciated in the skin or mucosa. While a benign condition, the lesion can be esthetically unpleasant when located in the head and neck areas such as nasal tip, cheeks, and chin. Associated symptoms such as burning pain and itching may accompany the lesion.

Common PDL setting used in the treatment of isolated telangiectasia is 585-nm, 5–7 J/cm^2, and pulse duration of 0.45-ms. Concomitant use of cooling device or cryogen spray is recommended for analgesic and epidermal protection. The laser targets the telangiectasia with overlapping spots of 1-mm. Extensive spot overlap at this laser setting runs the risk of damaging the overlying skin, including ulceration, blisters, and hyperpigmentation. When there is a cluster of capillaries feeding into a central arteriole in an arborizing pattern (spider angioma), all aberrant vessels must be completely eradicated by the laser to prevent recurrences. Clinical endpoint of PDL treatment is the disappearance of the involved vessels or when a light-colored purpura is noticed. Immediate dark gray coloration indicates damage to normal tissues and so a lower fluency should be adjusted. Generally, one to two treatments are needed for focal type of telangiectasia [31]. While PDL is effective in treating telangiectasia and erythema associated with rosacea, recurrence is observed to be high due to a chronic inflammatory nature of the disease. In this case, laser therapy is approached as a symptomatic rather than curative treatment. Oral pharmacologic agents (tetracyclines, macrolides, metronidazole, and isotretinoin) and topical gels (brimonidine tartrate, metronidazole, and azelaic acid) are also used for symptoms relief and to decrease chance of disease relapse. Telangiectasia associated with rosacea is commonly refractory to laser treatment. Although its mechanism in treating rosacea is unclear, a daily 40-mg dose of modified-release doxycycline is an effective course of therapy with proven anti-inflammatory action [32]. Nevertheless, the most effective treatment of the disease is still by avoidance of trigger agents and other lifestyle modifications [33].

The most significant side effects of traditional PDL treatment in telangiectasia are the postoperative period of purpura that may last up to 2 weeks. As this side effect may understandably be unacceptable for certain patient, longer-pulsed dye laser (595 nm, 6–40-ms, 7 J/cm^2) or KTP laser may be used albeit with a diminished rate of clearance and need for multiple laser passes and treatment sessions [4, 34, 35]. The longer pulse duration also allows for increase in laser fluency up until the purpuric threshold. Telangiectasia treated with frequency-doubled Nd:YAG laser is reported to achieve a moderate success with clearance rate of 66% in isolated telangiectasia and 93.5% in spider angioma. The number of treatment to achieve clearance ranges from 1 to 3 sessions [36]. The rate of success in treating facial telangiectasia is even higher, most likely related to the thin layer of head and neck skin compared to that of the extremities. One study shows that 93.9% of facial lesions achieved at least 75% clearance, and the remaining lesions requiring one more treatment to achieve clearance [37]. When this laser is used, clinical endpoint is set arbitrarily with blanching of vessel or when mild erythema is noted. No purpura should be seen when longer-pulsed PDL is used. However, thicker telangiectasia still requires the use of purpura-induced setting in order to achieve clinical response [38].

10.3.4 Venous Malformations

Venous malformations (VM) are a collection of thin-walled, slow-flowing anomalous vessels and have an estimate incidence of 1 in 10,000 [39]. Approximately 40% of VM occur in the head and neck area [40]. Like other types of vascular malformations, they exist at birth but may not be clinically diagnosable and instead grow proportionally with the rest of the body. Puberty, trauma, and pregnancy can dramatically trigger the increase in size of the lesion. VM are clinically soft, blue-purple lesions that are compressible and can change in size depending on body position and/or Valsalva maneuver. The low flow of the lesion increases risk of thrombus formation and subsequent calcium deposition, which frequently lead to phleboliths capable of causing pain and swelling [41]. Phleboliths can be visualized radiographically as radiopaque or radiolucent lesions and can be confused with salivary calculi if occurred near major or minor salivary glands.

Treatment of VM is dependent on the size and location of the lesion. Conservative approaches such as compression and positional elevation is generally used for lesions in the extremity but may not be appropriate for those in the head and neck. Sclerotherapy is historically the treatment of choice for head and neck VM. Ethanol in absolute concentration (100%) and in mixture (Ethibloc), bleomycin, and OK-432 are sclerosant agents that have yielded good results but carry high risk of damage and fibrosis to local structures. Additionally, systemic complications exist with the use of sclerosants such as renal and cardiac toxicity. Care must be taken when treating patients with medical history of end-stage renal disease or arrhythmia. Alternatively, laser therapy has a valuable role in the treatment of VM, especially in locations where injection of sclerosants is deemed unsafe or when immediate ablative surgery may sacrifice a large amount of tissues requiring reconstruction. Long wavelength lasers such as the Nd:YAG and diode lasers (810-nm) are generally used in VM of the head and neck because they have adequate skin/mucosal penetration and good light absorption by deoxyhemoglobin and oxyhemoglobin. Serial treatments of laryngeal VM by Nd:YAG laser have yielded significant shrinkage and improvement in symptoms [42]. While recurrence of VM is high, because any remnant of abnormal vessel can grow and recanalize, the application of laser is still effective when being considered as a symptomatic type of treatment. Furthermore, laser therapy can be used as an adjunct to sclerosing or surgical therapy by debulking and reducing the size of the lesion, thus limiting the extent of surgical wound.

10.4 Conclusion

Laser therapy has proven to be a valuable instrument in treating vascular anomalies when used with safety and precautions. The most advantageous feature of laser is the ability to selectively target the aberrant vessels while sparing normal, healthy tissues. While the principle of selective thermolysis lends the technology a way to maintain acceptable cosmetic and functional outcomes, the same idea also limits it to a level of energy that may not be effective in more resilient pathologies. In an attempt to strike the right balance, laser technology has significantly progressed since its first introduction to the medical community. New systems and models are continuously presented, and an increasing number of clinicians are opting to receive training in laser treatments. As interest in the technology continues to grow, the future of laser therapy is undeniably promising due to current research and developments being done in the field (Figs. 10.4 and 10.5).

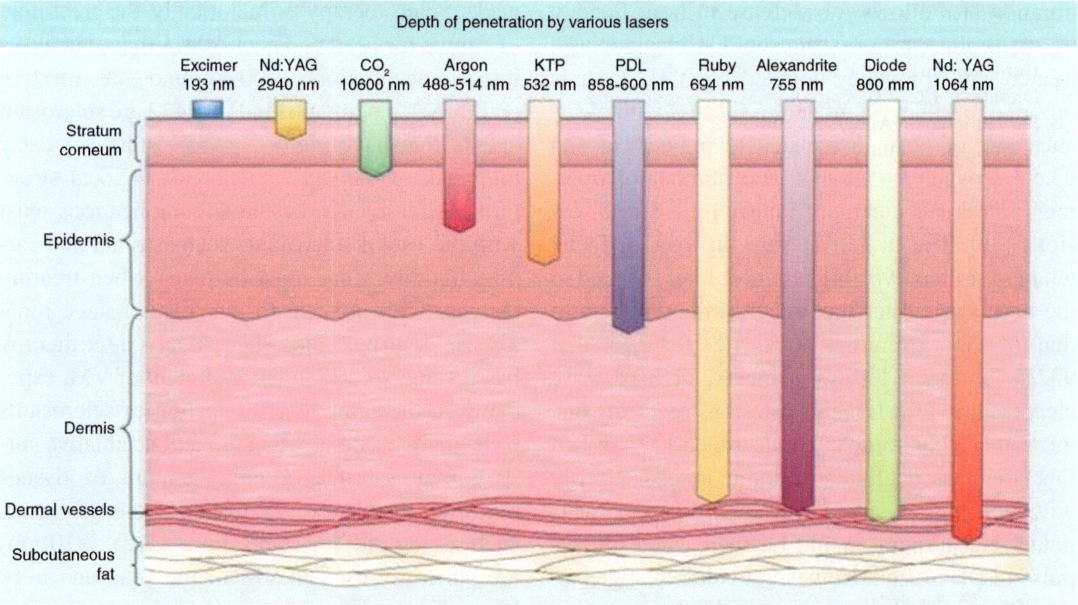

Fig. 10.4 Depth of penetration by different types of lasers

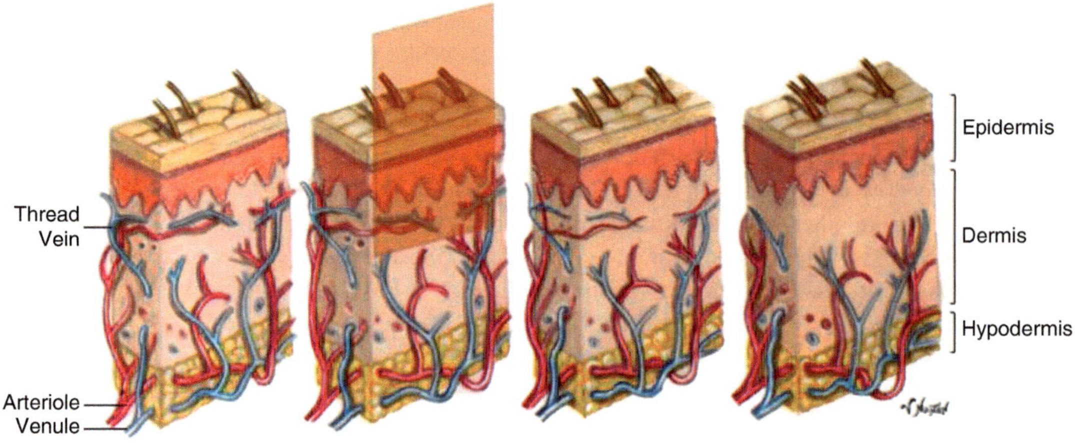

Fig 10.5 Laser therapy and effects on superficial vascular lesions. (1) Vascular abnormalities visibly seen on the skin. (2)The laser safely passes through the skin and the heat energy is absorbed by the blood vessels making up the thread vein, breaking down the vessels and causing it to coagulate. (3) Effective treatment allows the thread vein to collapse. (4) The collapsed vessels gradually breaks down and replaced by scar tissue. Drawings by Dr. Victoria A. Manon

References

1. Geiges ML. History of lasers in dermatology. In: Basics in dermatological laser applications, vol. 42. Basel: Karger Publishers; 2011. p. 1–6.
2. Waldorf HA, Lask GP, Geronemus RG. Laser treatment of telangiectasias. In: Cosmetic laser surgery. New York, NY: Wiley; 1996. p. 71–107.
3. Ng MSY, Tay YK. Laser treatment of infantile hemangiomas. Indian J Paediatr Dermatol. 2017;18(3):160.
4. Jasim ZF, Woo WK, Handley JM. Long-pulsed (6-ms) pulsed dye laser treatment of rosacea-associated telangiectasia using subpurpuric clinical threshold. Dermatol Surg. 2004;30(1):37–40.
5. Dierickx CC, Casparian JM, Venugopalan V, Farinelli WA, Anderson RR. Thermal relaxation of port-wine stain vessels probed in vivo: the need for 1-10-millisecond laser pulse treatment. J Invest Dermatol. 1995;105(5):709–14.
6. Lorenz S, Scherer K, Beatrix Wimmershoff M, Landthaler M, Hohenleutner U. Variable pulse frequency-doubled Nd: YAG laser versus flashlamp-pumped pulsed dye laser in the treatment of port wine stains. Acta Derm Venereol. 2003;83(3):210.
7. Clymer MA, Fortune DS, Reinisch L, Toriumi DM, Werkhaven JA, Ries WR. Interstitial Nd: YAG photocoagulation for vascular malformations and hemangiomas in childhood. Arch Otolaryngol Head Neck Surg. 1998;124(4):431–6.
8. Vesnaver A, Dovšak DA. Treatment of large vascular lesions in the orofacial region with the Nd: YAG laser. J Craniomaxillofac Surg. 2009;37(4):191–5.
9. Civas E, Koc E, Aksoy B, Aksoy HM. Clinical experience in the treatment of different vascular lesions using a neodymium-doped yttrium aluminum garnet laser. Dermatol Surg. 2009;35(12):1933–41.
10. Groot D, Rao J, Johnston P, Nakatsui T. Algorithm for using a long-pulsed Nd: YAG laser in the treatment of deep cutaneous vascular lesions. Dermatol Surg. 2003;29(1):35–42.
11. Yang HY, Zheng LW, Yang HJ, Luo J, Li SC, Zwahlen RA. Long-pulsed Nd: YAG laser treatment in vascular lesions of the oral cavity. J Craniofac Surg. 2009;20(4):1214–7.
12. Frame JW. Removal of oral soft tissue pathology with the CO2 laser. J Oral Maxillofac Surg. 1985;43(11):850–5.
13. Strauss RA, Fallon SD. Lasers in contemporary oral and maxillofacial surgery. Dent Clin North Am. 2004;48(4):861–88.
14. Zaffe D, Vitale MC, Martignone A, Scarpelli F, Botticelli AR. Morphological, histochemical, and immunocytochemical study of CO2 and Er: YAG laser effect on oral soft tissues. Photomed Laser Surg. 2004;22(3):185–9.
15. Niamtu J III. The treatment of vascular and pigmented lesions in oral and maxillofacial surgery. Oral Maxillofac Surg Clin North Am. 2004;16(2): 239–54.
16. Amaral MBF, De Ávila JMS, Abreu MHG, Mesquita RA. Diode laser surgery versus scalpel surgery in the treatment of fibrous hyperplasia: a randomized clinical trial. Int J Oral Maxillofac Surg. 2015;44(11):1383–9.
17. Stratigos AJ, Dover JS, Arndt KA. Laser therapy. Dermatology. 2003;2:2153–75.
18. Landthaler M, Hohenleutner U. Laser therapy of vascular lesions. Photodermatol Photoimmunol Photomed. 2006;22(6):324–32.
19. Tomson N, Lim SPR, Abdullah A, Lanigan SW. The treatment of port-wine stains with the pulsed-dye laser at 2-week and 6-week intervals: a comparative study. Br J Dermatol. 2006;154(4):676–9.
20. Anolik R, Newlove T, Weiss ET, Brightman L, Hale EK, Karen JK, et al. Investigation into optimal treatment intervals of facial port-wine stains using the pulsed dye laser. J Am Acad Dermatol. 2012;67(5):985–90.
21. Orten SS, Waner M, Flock S, Roberson PK, Kincannon J. Port-wine stains: an assessment of 5 years of treatment. Arch Otolaryngol Head Neck Surg. 1996;122(11):1174–9.
22. Savas JA, Ledon JA, Franca K, Chacon A, Nouri K. Pulsed dye laser-resistant port-wine stains: mechanisms of resistance and implications for treatment. Br J Dermatol. 2013;168(5):941–53.
23. Stier MF, Glick SA, Hirsch RJ. Laser treatment of pediatric vascular lesions: port wine stains and hemangiomas. J Am Acad Dermatol. 2008;58(2):261–85.
24. Ronchese F. The spontaneous involution of cutaneous vascular tumors. Am J Surg. 1953;86(4):376–86.
25. Finn MC, Glowacki J, Mulliken JB. Congenital vascular lesions: clinical application of a new classification. J Pediatr Surg. 1983;18(6):894–900.
26. David LR, Malek MM, Argenta LC. Efficacy of pulse dye laser therapy for the treatment of ulcerated haemangiomas: a review of 78 patients. Br J Plast Surg. 2003;56(4):317–27.
27. Cao Y, Wang F, Jia Q, Xu R, Dang W, Chen Q, Wang Y. One possible mechanism of pulsed dye laser treatment on infantile hemangioma: induction of endothelial apoptosis and serum vascular endothelial growth factor (VEGF) level changes. J Lasers Med Sci. 2014;5(2):75.
28. Reddy KK, Blei F, Brauer JA, Waner M, Anolik R, Bernstein L, Geronemus RG. Retrospective study of the treatment of infantile hemangiomas using a combination of propranolol and pulsed dye laser. Dermatol Surg. 2013;39(6):923–33.
29. Asilian A, Mokhtari F, Kamali AS, Abtahi-Naeini B, Nilforoushzadeh MA, Mostafaie S. Pulsed dye laser and topical timolol gel versus pulse dye laser in treatment of infantile hemangioma: a double-blind randomized controlled trial. Adv Biomed Res. 2015;4:257.
30. Park KH, Jang YH, Chung HY, Lee WJ, Kim DW, Lee SJ. Topical timolol maleate 0.5% for infantile hemangioma; it's effectiveness and/or adjunctive pulsed dye laser–single center experience of 102 cases in Korea. J Dermatol Treat. 2015;26(4):389–91.

31. Wall TL. Current concepts: laser treatment of adult vascular lesions. Semin Plast Surg. 2007;21(3):147.
32. Feldman SR, Huang WW, Huynh TT. Current drug therapies for rosacea: a chronic vascular and inflammatory skin disease. J Manag Care Pharm. 2014;20(6):623–9.
33. Weinkle AP, Doktor V, Emer J. Update on the management of rosacea. Clin Cosmet Investig Dermatol. 2015;8:159.
34. Tanghetti E, Sherr E. Treatment of telangiectasia using the multi-pass technique with the extended pulse width, pulsed dye laser (Cynosure V-Star). J Cosmet Laser Ther. 2003;5(2):71–5.
35. Iyer S, Fitzpatrick RE. Long-pulsed dye laser treatment for facial telangiectasias and erythema: evaluation of a single purpuric pass versus multiple subpurpuric passes. Dermatol Surg. 2005;31(8):898–903.
36. Solak B, Sevimli Dikicier B, Oztas Kara R, Erdem T. Single-center experience with potassium titanyl phosphate (KTP) laser for superficial cutaneous vascular lesions in face. J Cosmet Laser Ther. 2016;18(8):428–31.
37. Cassuto DA, Ancona DM, Emanuelli G. Treatment of facial telangiectasias with a diode-pumped Nd: YAG Laser at 532nm. J Cutan Laser Ther. 2000;2(3):141–6.
38. Alam M, Dover JS, Arndt KA. Treatment of facial telangiectasia with variable-pulse high-fluence pulsed-dye laser: comparison of efficacy with fluences immediately above and below the purpura threshold. Dermatol Surg. 2003;29(7):681–5.
39. Boon LM, Mulliken JB, Enjolras O, Vikkula M. Glomuvenous malformation (glomangioma) and venous malformation: distinct clinicopathologic and genetic entities. Arch Dermatol. 2004;140(8):971–6.
40. Mulliken JB, Fishman SJ, Burrows PE. Vascular anomalies. Curr Prob Surg. 2000;37(8):517–84.
41. Scolozzi P, Laurent F, Lombardi T, Richter M. Intraoral venous malformation presenting with multiple phleboliths. Oral Surg Oral Med Oral Pathol Oral Radiol Endod. 2003;96(2):197–200.
42. Glade R, Vinson K, Richter G, Suen JY, Buckmiller LM. Endoscopic management of airway venous malformations with Nd: YAG laser. Ann Otol Rhinol Laryngol. 2010;119(5):289–93.

Correction to: General, Surgical, and Functional Anatomy for Vascular Lesions of Head and Neck

Srinivasa R. Chandra, Sunil Shroff, Steven Curry,
Amelia Christabel Rajasekaran, and Sanjiv C. Nair

Correction to:
Chapter 7 in: S. C. Nair, S. R. Chandra (eds.), *Management of Head and Neck Vascular Lesions*, https://doi.org/10.1007/978-981-15-2321-2_7

The original version of this book was inadvertently published with incorrect name of the chapter author.

Author name corrections have been updated in this revised version.

The updated version of this chapter can be found at https://doi.org/10.1007/978-981-15-2321-2_7

S. C. Nair, S. R. Chandra (eds.), *Management of Head and Neck Vascular Lesions*,
https://doi.org/10.1007/978-981-15-2321-2_11